The Shoulder

OPERATIVE TECHNIQUE

The Shoulder

OPERATIVE TECHNIQUE

Melvin Post, MD

Professor, Department of Orthopaedic Surgery
Rush Medical College
Chicago, Illinois
Senior Attending,
Department of Orthopaedic Surgery
Rush-Presbyterian-St. Luke's Medical Center
Chicago, Illinois

Evan L. Flatow, MD

Professor of Orthopaedic Surgery
College of Physicians and Surgeons,
Columbia University
Associate Chief, The Shoulder Service
New York Orthopaedic Hospital,
Columbia-Presbyterian Medical Center
New York, New York

Louis U. Bigliani, MD

Professor of Orthopaedic Surgery
College of Physicians and Surgeons,
Columbia University
Chief, The Shoulder Service and Vice Chairman,
Department of Orthopaedic Surgery
New York Orthopaedic Hospital,
Columbia-Presbyterian Medical Center
New York, New York

Roger G. Pollock, MD

Assistant Professor of Orthopaedic Surgery
College of Physicians and Surgeons,
Columbia University
Assistant Attending, The Shoulder Service
New York Orthopaedic Hospital,
Columbia-Presbyterian Medical Center
New York, New York

Illustrations by Vaune J. Hatch, MEd, MA

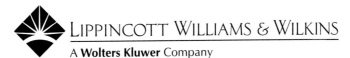

LIPPINCOTT WILLIAMS & WILKINS
A **Wolters Kluwer** Company
Philadelphia • Baltimore • New York • London
Buenos Aires • Hong Kong • Sydney • Tokyo

Editor: Darlene Cooke
Managing Editor: Fran Klass
Marketing Manager: Diane Harnish
Production Coordinator: Danielle Hagan
Project Editor: Lisa J. Franko
Design Coordinator: Mario Fernandez
Typesetter: Graphic World, Inc.
Printer/Binder: RR Donnelley & Sons Company

Copyright © 1998 Lippincott Williams & Wilkins
351 West Camden Street
Baltimore, Maryland 21201-2436 USA

Rose Tree Corporate Center
1400 North Providence Road
Building II, Suite 5025
Media, Pennsylvania 19063-2043 USA

Accurate indications, adverse reactions, and dosage schedules for drugs are provided in this book, but it is possible that they may change. The reader is urged to review the package information data of the manufacturers of the medications mentioned.

Printed in the United States of America

First Edition,

Library of Congress Cataloging-in-Publication Data

The shoulder : operative technique / authors, Melvin Post ... [et al.].
    p. cm.
    Includes bibliographical references and index.
    ISBN 0–683–06947–0
    1. Shoulder—Surgery. I. Post, Melvin, 1928–   .
    [DNLM: 1. Shoulder—surgery. 2. Shoulder Fractures—surgery.
    3. Musculoskeletal Diseases—surgery. 4. Orthopedics—methods.   WE
    810 S55865 1998]
    RD557.5.S547 1998
    617.5′72059—dc21
    DNLM/DLC
    for Library of Congress   97–42619
                                           CIP

The publishers have made every effort to trace the copyright holders for borrowed material. If they have inadvertently overlooked any, they will be pleased to make the necessary arrangements at the first opportunity.

To purchase additional copies of this book, call our customer service department at **(800) 638-0672** or fax orders to **(800) 447-8438.** For other book services, including chapter reprints and large quantity sales, ask for the Special Sales department.

Canadian customers should call **(800) 665-1148,** or fax **(800) 665-0103.** For all other calls originating outside of the United States, please call **(410) 528-4223** or fax us at **(410) 528-8550.**

99 00
2 3 4 5 6 7 8 9 10

To our wives and families, for their love and support.

Preface

The shoulder is an extremely interesting and complex area of the body. Over the last decade, interest in shoulder surgery has increased. This has resulted in the development of new operative techniques offering surgeons more options in the surgical treatment of patients with shoulder problems. The success of shoulder surgery starts with a thorough knowledge of the anatomy and pathophysiology and depends on an accurate diagnosis as the foundation on which to apply sound, practical surgical techniques.

In this volume, we will share with you many of the surgical approaches and techniques that have had a high percentage of successful outcomes. We have outlined many of the common surgical procedures that you will encounter in your practice. Included are many tips that will facilitate your procedures and improve your outcomes.

Acknowledgment

We would like to thank all of those who helped make this volume possible, especially Vaune Hatch, our illustrator, who has thoughtfully and clearly depicted our surgical approaches and techniques. We also thank Caroline Reidy, our academic coordinator, who was responsible for helping to collate all of the material. Dr. Patrick Conner and Dr. William Levine were instrumental in assisting in the collection of needed information for this volume. Finally, we would like to thank the editors and staff at Williams & Wilkins for their patience and persistence in the completion of this volume.

Contents

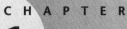

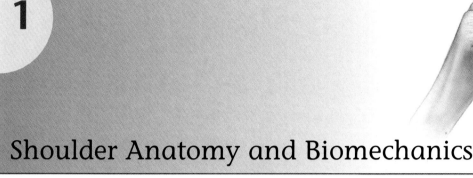

Shoulder Anatomy and Biomechanics

EVAN L. FLATOW

Introduction

Although a thorough understanding of anatomy is at the heart of all orthopaedics, it is especially vital in shoulder surgery. The skeletal anatomy, easily seen on radiographs, is of less relative importance, compared with the soft tissues, than in other joints. Furthermore, it is difficult to carry out an operative intervention without fully understanding the complex relationship among the many muscles, ligaments, and five articulations (glenohumeral, acromioclavicular, sternoclavicular, subacromial, and scapulothoracic) that make up the shoulder girdle. Finally, the proximity of so many major nerves, arteries, and veins to the operative field in the shoulder presents special risks to the surgeon not fully prepared for their usual and unusual locations.

Biomechanics is also of great importance in shoulder surgery. Although most orthopaedic procedures aim either explicitly or implicitly to restore normal mechanics in joints damaged by disease or injury, shoulder operations must correct a joint that is prone to both instability and stiffness and for which a complex interplay of muscles, ligaments, and articular surfaces is required for normal functioning.

This chapter reviews the anatomy and biomechanics of the shoulder in the context of operative reconstruction.

Anatomy

BONES

Proximal Humerus

The shaft of the humerus connects with the proximal portion at the surgical neck, just below the lesser and greater tuberosities at the metaphyseal flare (Fig. 1.1). This is a common site of fractures due to relative osteoporosis in this area, especially in older patients (49, 106). It has also been suggested that this region may abut on the acromion in extreme positions, either leveraging the head out in dislocations or initiating a surgical neck

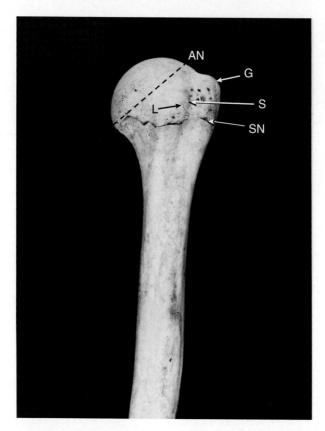

Figure 1.1.   Proximal humerus of a cadaver specimen. The greater (G) and lesser (L) tuberosities as well as the anatomical (AN) and surgical neck (SN) of the humerus are shown. The bicipital sulcus (S) is located between the tuberosities.

fracture (22). The anatomic neck is above the tuberosities, between the articular margin of the head and the attachment of the articular capsule. The head is inclined relative to the shaft at an angle of 130 to 150°, and its center is offset approximately 6 mm medially and 3 mm posteriorly from the axis of the shaft (14).

Humeral retroversion has been extensively studied (Fig. 1.2). Because the proximal humerus lacks a structure analogous to the femoral neck (whose axis is reliably measured to assess hip version), the determination of humeral version requires defining the edges of the proximal humeral articular surface. However, the articular margin is irregular and varies from the top of the head to the bottom. Because of this and the varying radiographic techniques and choices for the distal axis (especially a 6° difference between the transepicondylar axis and the distal humeral articular surface), estimates of "normal" humeral retroversion have varied. Although most studies have reported average humeral retroversion to be from 26 to 31° (31, 53, 64, 66, 99, 111), average values of 18 to 20° (13, 83) and of 40° (97) have also been found. However, the finding that there is a wide range of retroversion in shoulders of patients free of known shoulder disorders, even varying between the two shoulders of one individual, is perhaps more important (13, 31). This has led to a shift in emphasis in shoulder replacement surgery from putting the humeral component in the "correct" amount of retroversion to adjusting the version to that particular shoulder, being guided more by the local anatomy such as the cuff insertion and biceps groove than by an exact predetermined number (120).

The greater tuberosity has three facets into which insert the tendons of the supraspinatus, the infraspinatus, and the teres minor. Recognizing these facets on radiographs can be helpful in localizing calcium deposits and in determining the extent of involvement of a greater tuberosity fracture. The tendon of the subscapularis muscle inserts on the anterior surface of the lesser tuberosity. The bicipital groove, bridged by the transverse humeral ligament, separates the two tuberosities. The tendon of the long head of the biceps and the arcuate artery, a branch of the anterior humeral circumflex artery, lie in this sulcus (20, 55).

Scapula

The scapula is a thin, triangular bone that glides on the muscles of the posterolateral thoracic cage, extending from the second to the seventh ribs (Fig. 1.3). The scapular spine separates the infraspinatus and supraspinatus fossas, extending superiorly and laterally to form the base of the acromion (20).

Coracoid

The coracoid process projects anteriorly and laterally from the neck of the scapula at the level of the superior glenoid. Coracoid impingement syndromes have been described and have been related to the length of the coracoid, which should normally not project laterally more than 2 cm beyond a line drawn tangentially to the glenoid face (37, 38). The coracoid is an important and easily palpated landmark defining the rotator interval between

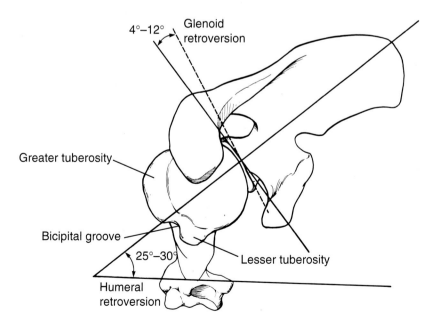

Figure 1.2 The humeral head is retroverted 25–30° relative to the distal humerus. The glenoid is retroverted 4–12°. (Redrawn from Neer CS II. Shoulder reconstruction. Philadelphia: WB Saunders, 1990:1–39).

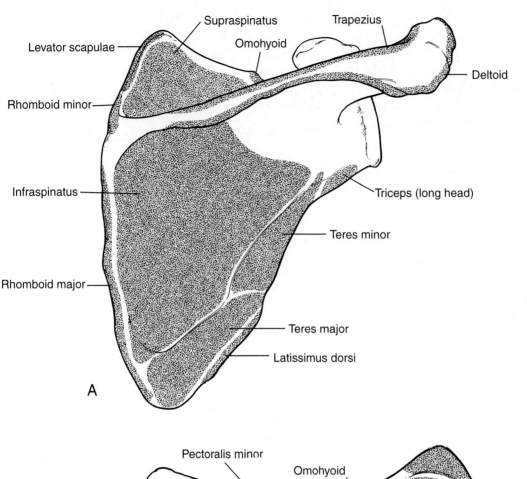

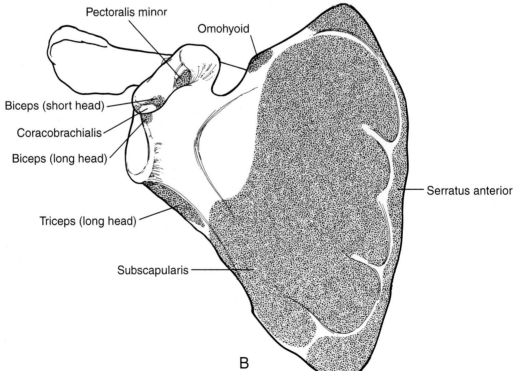

Figure 1.3. Posterior **(A)** and anterior **(B)** views of the scapula showing the muscles that attach to or take origin from it. (Redrawn from Gray's anatomy. 30th ed. Clemente CD, ed. Philadelphia: Lea & Febiger, 1984:233–235, 370, 375, 512–528).

the supraspinatus and infraspinatus muscles, locating the joint line anteriorly (e.g., as a guide for the introduction of an arthroscope posteriorly), and
marking the medial extent of the surgical field, beyond which lie the major
neurovascular structures. There is occasionally a true joint between the coracoid and the overlying clavicle (72, 90).

The scapular notch for the suprascapular nerve lies just medial to the
base of the coracoid and is spanned by the transverse scapular ligament.
Variations in the shape of the notch and in the arrangement of the ligament
(119) may be important in suprascapular nerve entrapment.

Glenoid

The glenoid cavity, or fossa, is bordered superiorly and inferiorly by the
supraglenoid and infraglenoid tuberosities, which serve as attachment sites
for the long head of the biceps and the long head of the triceps, respectively.
The glenoid is shaped like an inverted comma, with the superior aspect being
narrower than the inferior aspect. The glenoid is divided into two unequal
portions by an epiphyseal line that is located at the junction of the upper and
middle third of the glenoid fossa. The epiphyseal line probably represents the
old epiphyseal scar of the glenoid cavity (36).

The articular surface is concave and is covered with hyaline cartilage,
which is typically thinner in the center (Fig. 1.4). The articular surface of the
glenoid is only approximately one-third to one-fourth that of the humeral

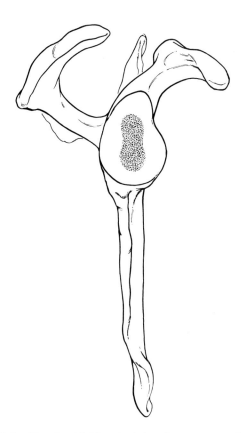

Figure 1.4.   The glenoid. The stippled region represents the center
of the glenoid cavity where the articular cartilage is thinner.

head (112). Because of the position of the scapula on the kyphotic thorax, the glenoid faces anteriorly. The superior-inferior line of the glenoid is angled at an average of 15° medially, with the scapular plane as the reference point (94). There is an average retroversion of 4 to 12° of the glenoid articular surface (30, 99, 104). This can be difficult to quantify because the version tends to change depending on the level (upper, middle, or lower) examined (53, 99).

Acromion

The acromion extends from the spine of the scapula anteriorly and laterally to articulate with the distal end of the clavicle. It is a part of the roof of the space for the rotator cuff, and variations in its shape may affect contact and wear on the cuff (impingement) (10, 85). Failure of fusion of the acromial epiphysis to the scapula occurs in approximately 1.4% of cases and has been classified into the following four types: preacromial, mesacromial, metacromial, and basiacromial centers (73). The relationship of the unfused acromial epiphysis to subacromial impingement is controversial (88).

Clavicle

The clavicle connects the scapula to the thoracic cage through its articulations at the acromioclavicular joint and the sternoclavicular joint. The bone has a double curvature and is shaped like an "S" when viewed in the transverse plane (Fig. 1.5). The medial curve is convex anteriorly, whereas the lateral curve is convex posteriorly. The bone tends to be thicker and more cylindrical at the medial end and broad and flat at the lateral end (35). The clavicle serves as a frame for muscle attachments, a strut (to the midline) to

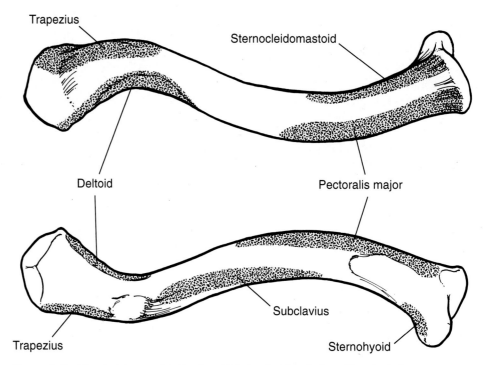

Figure 1.5. The clavicle, superior **(top)** and inferior **(bottom)** views. The stippled areas represent the origin and insertion of muscles from the clavicle. (Redrawn from Gray's anatomy. 30th ed. Clemente CD, ed. Philadelphia: Lea & Febiger, 1984:233–235, 370, 375, 512–528).

guide scapulothoracic motion, and a barrier to protect underlying neurovascular structures.

By spacing the shoulder complex from the midline, the clavicle acts as a lateral fulcrum so that the axiohumeral muscles, especially the pectoralis major, do not expend their effort pulling the shoulders medially, but rather rotate and adduct the humerus. The result is that tremendous forces are generated along the clavicle. When internal fixation is (rarely) required, strong devices must be used.

Joints

GLENOHUMERAL JOINT

Articular Surfaces

The humeral head and glenoid articular surfaces are spherical, and the radii of curvature of matched glenoid and humeral surfaces are surprisingly conforming (108, 112). Cartilage thickness measurements partially explain prior misperceptions of a less curved glenoid. The glenoid articular cartilage is thicker peripherally; thus, measurements taken from radiographs will indeed yield a more shallow (i.e., larger radius) glenoid bone surface (112). Therefore, the lack of bony stability of this joint in comparison with the hip, for example, is not due to a relatively flat glenoid as has often been stated, but rather to the small surface area of the glenoid which does not enclose the humeral head. The stabilizing effect of the articular surfaces is magnified by muscle pull, which produces a concavity-compression effect (75).

Joint Capsule

The glenohumeral articulation relies heavily on the soft tissues for stability. The musculotendinous units of the rotator cuff provide dynamic stability, whereas static stability comes from the joint capsule, the glenohumeral ligaments, and the labrum. The surface area of the capsule is approximately two times that of the humeral head. The capsule is watertight, and negative intraarticular pressure can help stabilize the glenohumeral joint (20). The capsule encloses the shoulder joint in a "cylindrical fashion" (really a truncated cone due to the discrepancy in the diameters of the humeral head and glenoid) that extends medially from the base of the coracoid process and the rim of the glenoid, where the labrum attaches, to insert laterally at the distal border of the anatomic neck and the proximal humeral diaphysis (19). The inferior portion of the capsule, the axillary pouch, is lax and redundant with the arm in the neutral position (91, 92). The cuff serves to reinforce the capsule through a tight adherence between the capsule and the overlying musculotendinous units. The capsule is weakest inferiorly where there are no tendinous cuff attachments (19, 20).

The inner aspect of the capsule is covered by a thin synovial membrane. As the long head of the biceps tendon penetrates the capsule, it becomes encased in this synovial membrane, which travels with the biceps down the proximal humerus (20) (Fig. 1.6). This is why any condition causing shoulder inflammation and synovitis may also produce tenderness over the proximal biceps long head tendon.

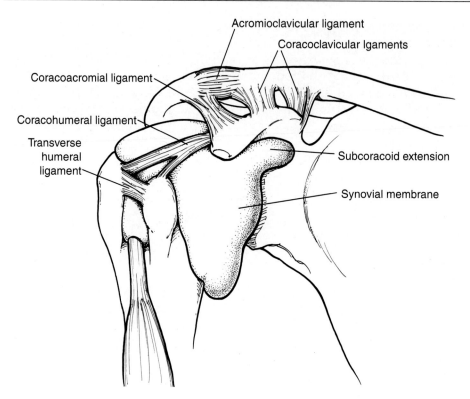

Acromioclavicular ligament

Coracoclavicular lgaments

Coracoacromial ligament

Coracohumeral ligament

Transverse
humeral
ligament

Subcoracoid extension

Synovial membrane

Figure 1.6. The synovial membrane and the coracoacromial arch. The subcoracoid extension of the joint can be appreciated. Note the ligaments that bind the coracoacromial arch. The transverse humeral ligament spans the lesser and greater tuberosities and bridges the roof of the bicipital groove. (Modified with permission Gray's anatomy. 30th ed. Clemente CD, ed. Philadelphia: Lea & Febiger, 1984:233–235, 370, 375, 512–528).

Ligaments

Coracohumeral Ligament

The coracohumeral ligament is a thick band of capsular tissue that extends from the base and lateral border of the coracoid, transversely, to its insertion into the rotator interval between the supraspinatus and subscapularis tendons (Fig. 1.7). It tethers external rotation of the adducted arm and may contribute to vertical stability of the joint (4, 20, 35, 36). This ligament must frequently be released during surgery for massive rotator cuff tears, as this allows mobilization of the retracted tendon (87).

Glenohumeral Ligaments

The glenohumeral ligaments represent thickenings of the anterior joint capsule. Three distinct glenohumeral ligaments—the superior, middle, and inferior—have been described (121) (Fig. 1.8). There can be significant variation in their presence, size, and attachments (20, 44, 109, 121). The advent of arthroscopy has allowed an additional view of the functional anatomy of these ligaments; the synovial surface of these ligaments can now be examined without otherwise opening the joint capsule. This has resulted in the re-examination of these ligaments and further documentation of their functional significance (61, 102).

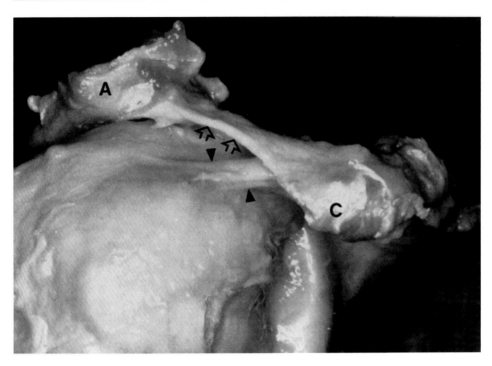

Figure 1.7. Anatomic dissection of a cadaveric specimen showing the coracohumeral ligament (closed triangle) and the coracoacromial ligament (open arrows). The acromion (A) and the coracoid (C) are labeled. (Reproduced with permission from Neer CS II, Satterlee CC, Dalsey RM, et al. The anatomy and potential effects of contracture of the coracohumeral ligament. Clin Orthop 1992;280: 13–16).

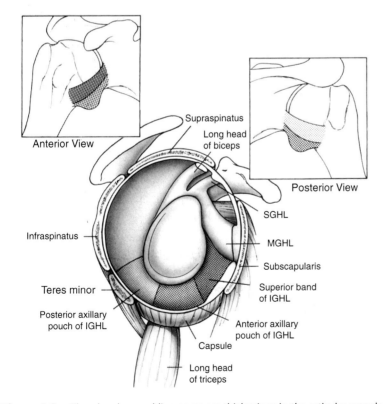

Figure 1.8. The glenohumeral ligaments are thickenings in the articular capsule and serve as passive check veins, especially at the extremes of motion.

Superior Glenohumeral Ligament

According to DePalma et al. (36), the superior glenohumeral ligament was the most constant of the three ligaments and was present as a distinct entity in more than 90% of the specimens they dissected. However, there can be great variation in its size and consistency. It originates just anterior to the origin of the long head of the biceps tendon and courses laterally along the medial head of the tendon to insert into the fovea capitis, just superior to the lesser tuberosity (36, 91, 92, 121, 123). According to DePalma (33), this ligament tends to hypertrophy with age.

Middle Glenohumeral Ligament

The middle glenohumeral ligament is the most variable of the three ligaments. It was present in approximately 80% of the specimens dissected by DePalma et al. (36), and there was considerable variability in its size and attachments. It usually originates from that region of the glenoid labrum or glenoid rim, just below the superior glenohumeral ligament, to insert on the medial aspect of the lesser tuberosity. Here it can blend with the subscapularis tendon and become part of the anterior lateral capsule. This ligament serves as restraint to anterior translation of the humeral head (36, 91, 92, 121).

Inferior Glenohumeral Ligament

The inferior glenohumeral ligament is the thickest and most consistent of the three ligaments. It is a triangular structure that originates from the anterior-posterior and inferior margins of the glenoid labrum and the glenoid rim to insert on the inferior aspect of the anatomic neck and the superior aspect of the surgical neck of the humerus (36, 121). The anterior portion of the ligament is thicker and has been named the superior band of the inferior glenohumeral ligament (11, 121). In between these two distinct bands is the so-called axillary pouch; this represents the inferior redundancy of the capsule. A posterior thickening, termed the posterior band, has been reported (91, 92). However, other studies have found this to be an inconsistent structure (118). The superior band is the thickest region, and all three regions of the inferior glenohumeral ligament are thicker near the glenoid than near the humerus (118).

Glenoid Labrum

The glenoid labrum is composed of dense fibrous tissue. It represents a thickening of the joint capsule that is continuous through a fibrocartilaginous transition zone with the glenoid cartilage, joint capsule, and periosteum of the neck of the scapula. It is triangular in cross-section, with its base at the glenoid rim. It is present in some form circumferentially around the glenoid. Suggestions that the labrum functions as a "chock block" implicitly assume a glenoid surface that is less curved than the humeral head and thus in need of a peripheral wedge to provide conformity. Because the articular surface of the glenoid and humeral head are conforming, the labrum and soft tissues adjacent to the glenoid add to stability by extending the load-bearing area of the socket. In other words, although these structures do not add to the congruence of the opposing surfaces, they do add to stability by increasing the size of the already congruent surfaces (Fig. 1.9) (112).

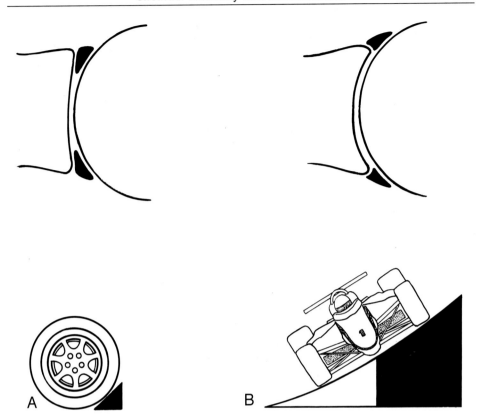

Figure 1.9. **(A)** It has been suggested that the labrum functions as a "chock block," deepening and increasing the curvature of a socket that is flatter than the head. This is not the case, however, because exact measurements have shown that the humerus and glenoid have, on average, the same curvature. **(B)** The labrum's role can be better thought of as extending the surface area of the socket, much as adding to the bank of a road deepens a curve.

Cooper et al. (28) suggested that the labrum is more firmly attached inferiorly (i.e., below the epiphyseal line) and more loosely attached superiorly. The primary attachment site superiorly appears to be either into the long head of the biceps tendon or somewhere around the supraglenoid tuberosity where the tendon attaches. The inferior glenohumeral ligament inserts into the inferior aspect of the labrum (28, 36, 82, 91, 92). The blood supply to the labrum comes from branches of the suprascapular, subscapular, and posterior humeral circumflex arteries (28).

SUBSCAPULARIS BURSA

The subscapularis bursa is located between the subscapularis tendon and the underlying joint capsule. It communicates with the joint cavity through openings in the capsule between the superior and middle glenohumeral ligament. The subscapularis bursa is a prime location for intraarticular loose bodies as well as synovial folds and fringes (1).

ACROMIOCLAVICULAR JOINT

The acromioclavicular joint is a diarthrodial joint between the lateral border of the clavicle and the medial border of the acromion. The articular surfaces are separated by a fibrocartilaginous intraarticular disc, which may be partial or complete (34, 35, 122). The joint is covered by a capsule that is relatively thicker on the superior and anterior surfaces. It is reinforced by the acromioclavicular ligaments (5) and by fascia from the trapezius and deltoid muscles, which tend to reinforce the joint's superior aspect (Fig. 1.6).

The average size of the adult acromioclavicular joint is 9 mm wide by 19 mm long (16, 109). The angle of inclination of the joint can be variable (34, 35). Higher degrees of torsion at the lateral one-third of the clavicle, as well as increasing inclination of the acromial facet of the acromioclavicular joint, may be associated with increased degenerative changes of the acromioclavicular joint (34, 35). When performing arthroscopy or arthrocentesis of the acromioclavicular joint, it is important to keep the variable inclination in mind, because it is extremely difficult to introduce instruments or needles that are not in the plane of the joint.

Because of the small area of the acromioclavicular joint and the high loads transmitted from the chest to the humerus by the muscles (e.g., pectoralis major), the stress on the distal clavicular articular surfaces may be high, and compressive failure (e.g., osteolysis of the distal clavicle in weight lifters) is not uncommon.

Ligaments

Coracoclavicular Ligaments

The coracoclavicular ligaments consist of two distinct parts—the conoid and trapezoid ligaments (Fig. 1.6). The coracoclavicular ligament helps to reinforce the acromioclavicular articulation by serving as the "primary suspensory ligament of the upper extremity" (103). An actual joint between the coracoid and the clavicle may exist (72, 90).

Trapezoid Ligament

The trapezoid ligament is anterior and lateral to the conoid ligament. It arises from the posterior half of the superior surface of the coracoid to insert on the trapezoid ridge, which is located on the inferior surface of the lateral clavicle. The ligament is trapezoidal or quadrangular and is oriented in the sagittal plane (34, 35).

Conoid Ligament

The conoid ligament is located medially and posterior to the trapezoid ligament. It originates from the superior surface of the coracoid, medially and posteriorly, to insert on the conoid tuberosity at the undersurface of the lateral clavicle (34, 35). Fukuda et al. (46) have performed biomechanical studies of the contributions of specific ligaments to acromioclavicular joint stability. They found that the coracoclavicular ligaments provide vertical stability to the acromioclavicular joint at large displacements, whereas the acromioclavicular ligaments provide vertical stability at small displacements and are the primary restraints to posterior instability at all displacements tested.

The stability of the acromioclavicular joint is such that very little relative motion occurs between the clavicle and the scapula, which rotate in a synchronous fashion (39).

STERNOCLAVICULAR JOINT

The sternoclavicular joint is the only true articulation between the upper extremity and the axial skeleton (Fig. 1.10). It is formed by the medial or sternal end of the clavicle and the upper portion of the sternum. There is a discrepancy in size between the medial end of the clavicle and the sternal portion of this articulation, so that there is relatively little bony congruity. Stability in the sternoclavicular joint is provided by the intraarticular disc and the surrounding ligamentous structures (33–35).

The capsule is reinforced anteriorly and posteriorly by the strong, anterior and posterior sternoclavicular ligaments (Fig. 1.10). The posterior sternoclavicular ligament is the stronger of the two and prevents inferior depression of the lateral end of the clavicle (6, 60). The costoclavicular ligament is extraarticular and extends from the first costal cartilage to its relatively broad insertion on the proximal end of the clavicle. The interclavicular ligament connects the proximal portion of both clavicles on either side of the sternum, usually through an attachment with the sternum. This ligament may be absent or nonpalpable in some individuals (60). The sternoclavicular ligament is thought to prevent drooping of the clavicle laterally (6). However, the precise role of the ligaments around the sternoclavicular joint is unknown and likely depends on arm position and the loading configuration (32).

Major structures of clinical importance behind the sternoclavicular joint include the trachea, the esophagus, the dome of the pleura, and the great vessels of the neck. Given this proximity to important structures and the fact that most scapulothoracic motion occurs through the sternoclavicular joint

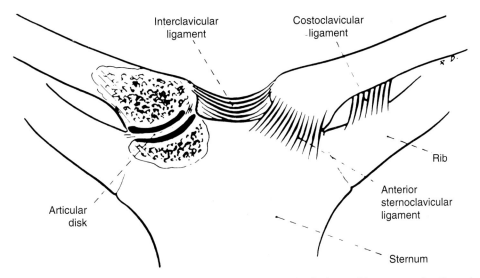

Figure 1.10. The sternoclavicular joint with the ligaments clearly shown. The cross-section through the joint shows the disc separating the joint into two compartments. (Reproduced with permission from Hollingshead WH. The shoulder. In: Anatomy for surgeons. 3rd ed. Philadelphia: Harper Row, 1952;3:300–337).

(because little occurs at the acromioclavicular joint), internal fixation of the sternoclavicular joint with metallic devices has been fraught with peril and generally abandoned.

SCAPULOTHORACIC ARTICULATION

The scapulothoracic articulation is probably the most neglected of the articulations that make up the shoulder complex. This is not a true joint, but a space between the concave surface of the anterior scapula and the convexity of the posterior chest wall. It is occupied by neurovascular, muscular, and bursal structures and allows relatively smooth motion of the scapula on the underlying thorax (35). Any scapular irregularities or growths, such as an osteochondroma, can impair this gliding.

Seventeen muscles either attach to or take origin from the scapula. It is through these muscular and ligamentous attachments that the scapula remains in position along the thorax during the scapular excursion that occurs with shoulder motion (Fig. 1.11). Among the most important of these are the serratus anterior, which holds the medial angle against the chest wall, and the trapezius, which is important in rotating and elevating the scapula in synchrony with glenohumeral motion.

Although the classic understanding had been that different portions of shoulder motion were controlled by either glenohumeral or scapulohumeral motion, it was soon appreciated that scapulohumeral rhythm is smooth, and that the muscles that rotate the scapula are active throughout the range of arm elevation. Unfortunately, this realization may have led to the opposite extreme, an expectation that there was some sort of fixed proportion to scapulothoracic rhythm, and many studies sought to find out whether it was 2:1, 1.5:1, etc. It turned out that although there is, on average, approximately 2° of glenohumeral elevation for every 1° of scapulothoracic elevation, the actual ratio during any portion of the arc of elevation is highly variable (45, 59, 126) and likely volitional and task-dependent (110). For example, it has been proposed that for heavy tasks, a person may lower his or her scapula while elevating the glenohumeral joint to tighten the ligaments for stability and power.

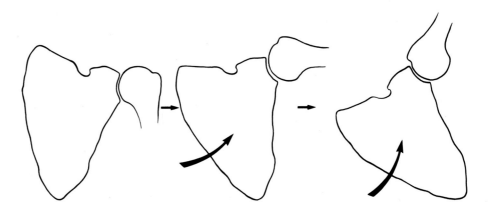

Figure 1.11.   Smooth gliding of the scapula on the chest wall is essential for arm motion.

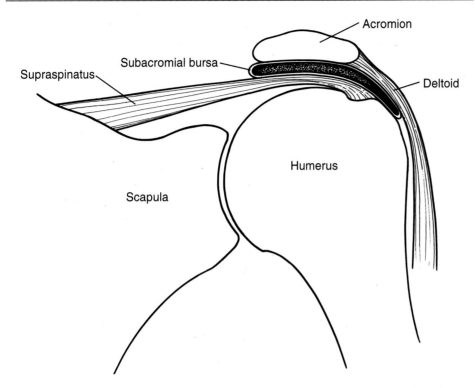

Figure 1.12. Schematic coronal section through the glenohumeral joint illustrating the subacromial bursa and its relationship to the overlying acromion and deltoid. The supraspinatus tendon separates the subacromial bursa from the glenohumeral joint.

Scapulothoracic Bursae

Three bursae around the scapulothoracic articulation have been described in association with scapulothoracic bursitis and "snapping scapula" (78). There is a bursa at the superomedial angle of the scapula between the serratus anterior and the subscapularis muscle. The second bursa exists between the serratus anterior and the lateral chest wall. The last and most inconsistent one may be located at the inferior angle of the scapula (79, 95).

CORACOACROMIAL ARCH/SUBACROMIAL SPACE

The subacromial space (96) is located between the coracoacromial arch superiorly and the rotator cuff tendons and humeral head inferiorly. The head is susceptible to impingement in the subacromial space by the undersurface of the acromion and the leading edge of the coracoacromial ligament, which may contribute to rotator cuff failure and biceps tendon ruptures (84).

Subacromial Bursa

The subacromial bursa is attached superiorly to undersurface of the acromion and the coracoacromial ligament (Fig. 1.12). Inferiorly, it is attached to the superior aspect of the greater tuberosity. It is bordered medially by the coracoid process and laterally by the deltoid muscle (116). The subacromial bursa generally does not communicate with the glenohumeral joint unless there is a tear of the rotator cuff (21, 23–25). Better appreciation of bursal anatomy has improved visualization during arthroscopic acromioplasty.

Coracoacromial Ligament

The coracoacromial ligament is triangular, and its most common configuration is two bands, anterolateral and posteromedial, arising separately from the coracoid and extending laterally to join at the insertion site of the ligament at the anterolateral aspect of the acromion (Fig. 1.7). Spurs tend to occur in the anterolateral band, suggesting that the ligament bears load. This may occur due to direct contact on the underlying head and rotator cuff and also because the ligament tethers the acromion to the coracoid, preventing deformation upward of the acromion whenever the humerus translates upward against it. The coracoacromial arch has a passive stabilizing role against superior humeral subluxation, especially important when there is a large rotator cuff tear and loss of dynamic head depression.

Muscles

SCAPULOTHORACIC MUSCLES

The scapulothoracic muscles connect the upper extremity to the axial skeleton through their attachments to the scapula, the vertebral column, and the thoracic cage.

Trapezius

The trapezius has an extensive origin from the base of the skull to lower thoracic and upper lumbar vertebrae. It is the most superficial of the scapulothoracic muscles. The muscle can be divided into three portions. A superior portion originates from the external occipital protuberance and the ligamentum nuchae to insert on the lateral one-third of the clavicle. A middle portion originates from the cervical and upper thoracic spinous processes (C6 to T3) to insert on the spine of the scapula. The inferior portion originates from the thoracic spinous processes, and as low as the second lumbar vertebrae, to insert at the base of the scapular spine (7, 20) (Fig. 1.13). The trapezius functions mainly as a scapular retractor and as an elevator of the lateral angle of the scapula. It receives innervation from the spinal accessory nerve (CN XI), (81, 107) and receives its blood supply from the transverse cervical and dorsal scapular arteries (60).

Rhomboids

The rhomboid muscles have two portions that are considered as separate muscles: the rhomboid minor and the rhomboid major. The rhomboid minor originates from the lower portion of the ligamentum nuchae and the spinal processes of C7 to T1 to insert on the vertebral border at the base of the spine of the scapula. The rhomboid major arises from the spinous processes from T2 through T5 to insert just inferior to the insertion of the rhomboid minor at the inferior angle of the scapula (Fig. 1.13). The dorsal scapular artery and the nerves provide the blood supply and innervation to the rhomboids, respectively. These muscles act to retract and elevate the scapula (20).

Levator Scapulae

The levator scapulae takes origin from the transverse processes of the cervical spine, originating at the atlas and extending to the third or fourth cervical vertebrae. It inserts on the superior angle of the scapula (Fig. 1.13). The levator scapulae elevates the superior angle of the scapula and produces upward and middle rotation of the body of the scapula. It receives innervation

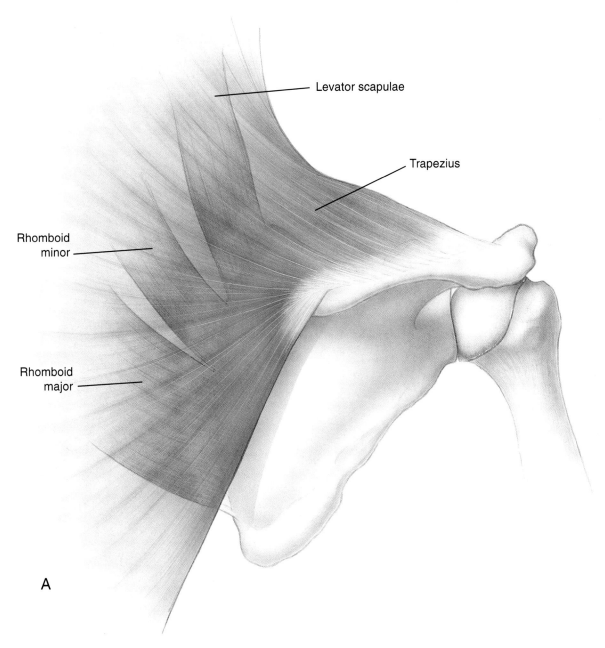

Figure 1.13. **(A)** Posterior view of the scapula with the trapezius, rhomboids and levator scapulae muscles.

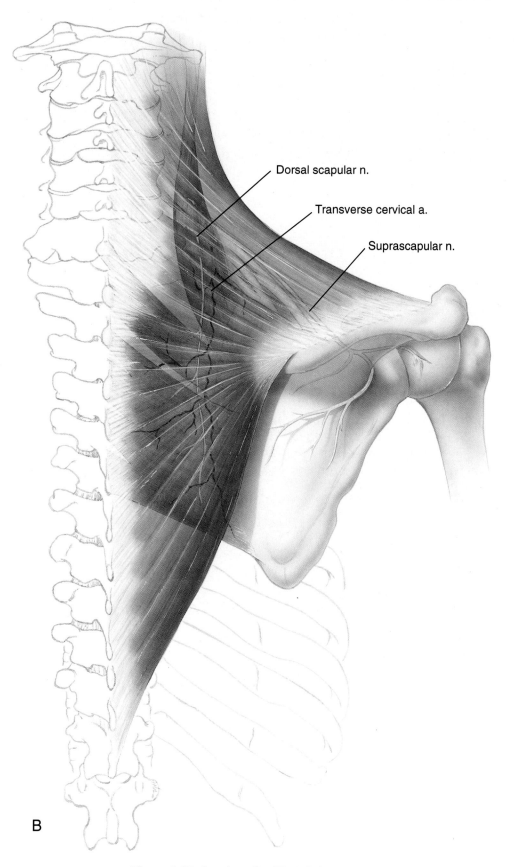

B

Figure 1.13. *(continued)*   **(B)** Underlying nerves.

from branches of the third and fourth cervical spinal nerves and receives its blood supply from the dorsal scapular artery (20).

Serratus Anterior

The serratus anterior takes origin from the body of the first nine ribs and the anterolateral aspect of the thorax. It consists of three portions that insert from the superior to the inferior angle of the scapula. The serratus anterior is responsible for scapular protraction and upward rotation of the scapula (89). It is innervated by the long thoracic nerve (56) and receives its blood supply from the lateral thoracic artery (20) (Fig. 1.14).

Pectoralis Minor

The pectoralis minor is a thin muscle located deep to the pectoralis major. It takes origin from the anterior portion of the second to fifth ribs to insert on the inner aspect of the base of the coracoid (Fig. 1.15). It protracts and rotates the scapula inferiorly (60). The medial pectoral nerve (C8, T1) provides innervation to this muscle, while its blood supply comes from the pectoral branch of the thoracoacromial artery (20).

Subclavius Muscle

The subclavius muscle has a tendinous origin from the first rib and inserts on the inferior surface of the middle third of the clavicle. The muscle acts to stabilize the sternoclavicular joint during extensive activity (101). The nerve to the subclavius, a branch from the brachial plexus, provides innervation, whereas the clavicular branches from the thoracoacromial and supraspinatus arteries provide circulation (20).

GLENOHUMERAL MUSCLES

These muscles originate from the scapula and insert on the humerus to move and stabilize the shoulder joint.

Deltoid

The deltoid is the largest of the glenohumeral muscles (Fig 1.16). It is a cone-shaped muscle that is draped over the rotator cuff and the glenohumeral joint (35). All approaches to the glenohumeral joint involve splitting or retracting the deltoid.

There are three portions of the deltoid muscle. The anterior portion is unipennate and originates from the lateral clavicle. The middle deltoid is multipennate and takes origin from the acromion. The posterior portion of the deltoid is also unipennate and comes off the spinous process of the scapula. All three portions of the muscle converge inferiorly to insert on the deltoid tuberosity of the humerus. The muscle is bordered medially by the lateral border of the pectoralis major muscle. The triangular space between them is the deltopectoral groove; it contains the cephalic vein and the acromial and deltoid branches of the thoracoacromial artery (20). The presence of these structures must be appreciated during the anterior approach to the shoulder joint via the deltopectoral interval.

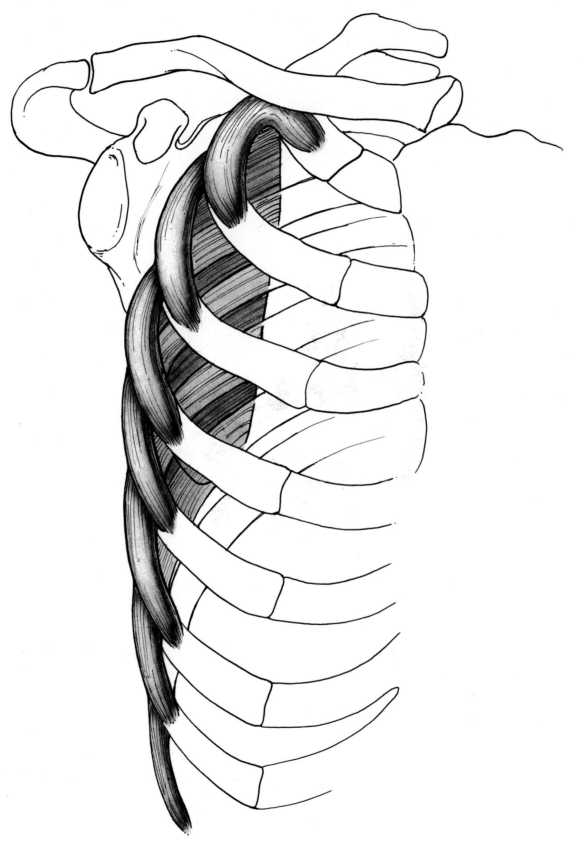

Figure 1.14.   The serratus anterior showing its origin from the ribs
to insert on the medial border of the scapula.

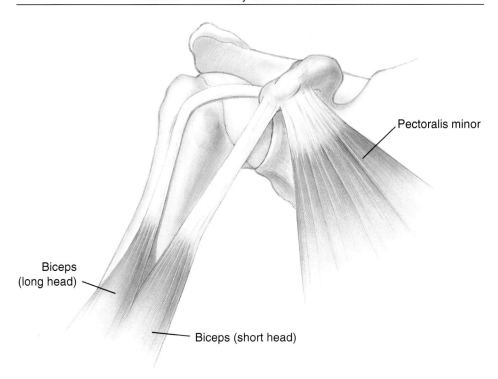

Pectoralis minor

Biceps
(long head)

Biceps (short head)

Figure 1.15. The long head of the biceps originates from the superior rim of the glenoid, whereas the short head takes origin from the coracoid along with the pectoralis minor. (Modified with permission from Gray's anatomy. 30th ed. Clemente CD, ed. Philadelphia: Lea & Febiger, 1984:233–235, 370, 375, 512–528).

The anterior and middle portions of the deltoid allow for elevation in the scapular plane. They also flex the shoulder with help from the pectoralis major and biceps tendon. However, the principle action of the deltoid is abduction in the coronal plane (60). The posterior humeral circumflex artery and the deltoid branches of the thoracoacromial artery provide circulation. Innervation is provided by the axillary nerve. The axillary nerve and the posterior humeral circumflex vessel course circumferentially along the deep surface of the muscle. The axillary nerve is usually located approximately 6 cm inferior to the lateral edge of the acromial border (108).

Rotator Cuff

The rotator cuff is made up of the supraspinatus, infraspinatus, teres minor, and subscapularis muscles. It provides dynamic stabilization of the glenohumeral joint by depressing the humeral head into the glenoid cavity and by balancing the forces of the other major muscles around the shoulder.

Supraspinatus Muscle

The thick muscular fibers of the supraspinatus arise from the supraspinatus fossa to extend forward and laterally, deep to the coracoacromial arch, to the superior aspect of the greater tuberosity (Fig. 1.17). The tendon blends into the joint capsule and the tendon of the infraspinatus muscle below (19, 20, 55).

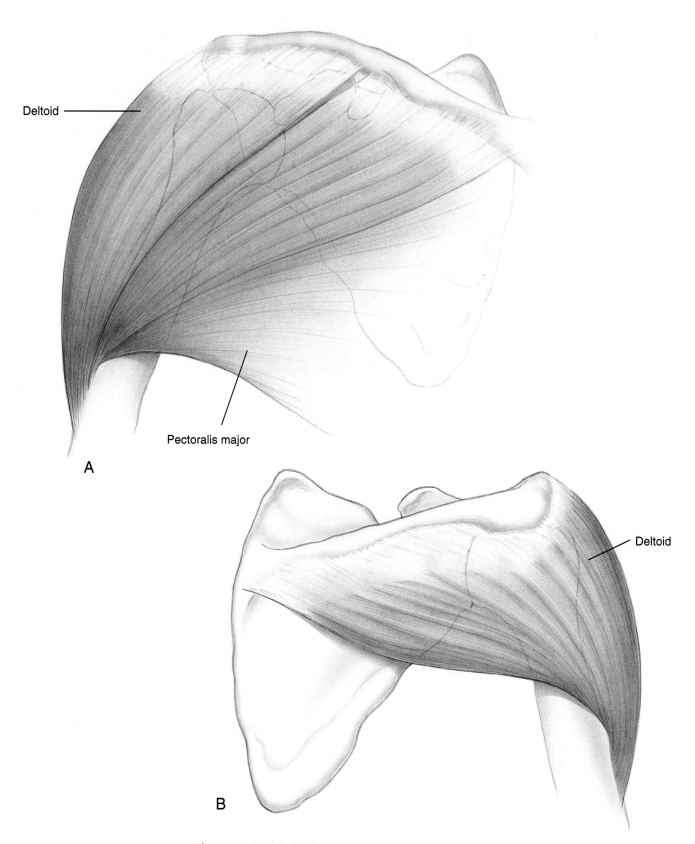

Deltoid

Pectoralis major

A

B

Deltoid

Figure 1.16. **(A)** The deltoid (anterior view) and the pectoralis major. **(B)** Posterior view of the deltoid.

The supraspinatus stabilizes the glenohumeral joint and assists the deltoid in elevating the arm (26, 27). It receives innervation from the suprascapular nerve, which enters the middle portion of the muscle, after passing through the scapular notch, which can vary in shape (8, 119). The notch is bridged by the transverse scapular ligament, which may be bifid (119).

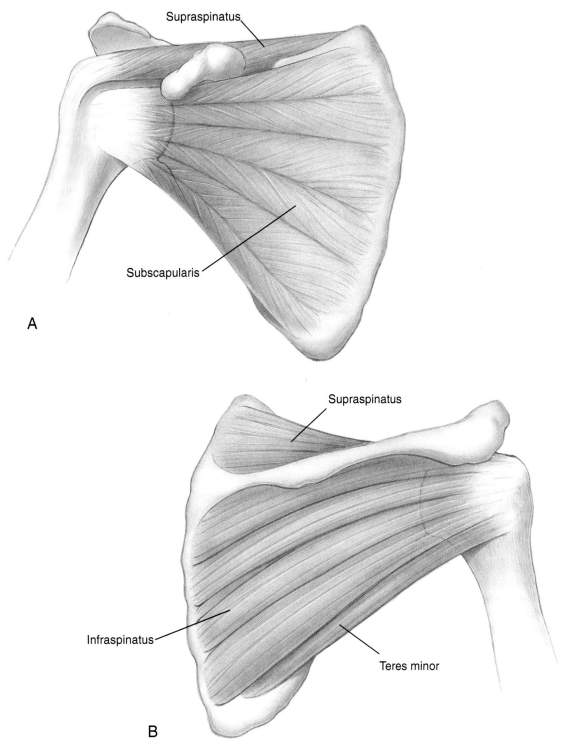

Figure 1.17.   The four rotator cuff muscles (the subscapularis, supraspinatus, infraspinatus, and teres minor) arise from the scapula to insert on the greater tuberosity. **(A)** Anterior view. **(B)** Posterior view.

Infraspinatus Muscle

The infraspinatus muscle takes origin from the infraspinatus fossa and the fascia overlying the muscle (Fig. 1.17). It extends anterolaterally to its tendinous insertion on the middle facet of the greater tuberosity. The tendon blends into the posterior joint capsule and into the tendinous insertions of the supraspinatus muscle above (19, 20). There is a distinct interval between the tendon of the supraspinatus and the infraspinatus posteriorly, somewhat analogous to the rotator interval anteriorly.

The infraspinatus and the teres minor are the primary external rotators of the shoulder and also stabilize the glenohumeral joint against posterior subluxation (27, 93, 94). After the suprascapular nerve traverses the scapular notch, it descends into the infraspinatus fossa with the suprascapular artery, providing innervation and blood supply to the infraspinatus muscle. Auxiliary circulation to the infraspinatus muscle comes from the circumflex scapular artery (60).

Teres Minor

The teres minor muscle takes its origin from the mid to upper region of the axillary border of the scapula and the infraspinatus fascia. It extends obliquely and superiorly to its insertion on the most inferior facet of the greater tuberosity (Fig. 1.17). It is an external rotator and stabilizer of the glenohumeral joint (27).

The teres minor is innervated by the axillary nerve and receives its blood supply from the posterior humeral circumflex artery (58).

Subscapularis

The subscapularis muscle represents the anterior portion of the rotator cuff. It originates form the subscapular fossa to extend laterally to its tendinous insertion on the lesser tuberosity of the humerus (Fig. 1.17). The tendon of the subscapularis is intimately associated with the anterior glenohumeral joint. The subscapularis bursa separates this musculotendinous unit from the neck of the scapular and the overlying coracoid process. The axillary nerve and the posterior humeral circumflex artery pass along the inferior border of the subscapularis muscle. The muscle is innervated by the upper and lower subscapular nerves (77). The blood supply is usually derived from the subscapular artery, but there can also be circulation from the anterior humeral circumflex artery, especially to the upper portion of the subscapularis (20, 57, 60).

The subscapularis muscle is an important internal rotator of the shoulder and the only significant internal rotator when approaching full internal rotation. It also stabilizes the glenohumeral joint by resisting anterior subluxation and by helping to compress the humeral head into the glenoid fossa (59, 93, 94).

Other Shoulder Muscles

Teres Major

The teres major comes off the dorsal surface of the scapula at the inferior angle near the axillary border of the scapula. During its course, the muscle undergoes a 180° rotation so that the former posterior fibers at its origin are now located anteriorly, at its insertion into the medial lip of the intertuberosity groove of the humerus (60). Its tendinous insertion is intimately associated with the insertion of the latissimus dorsi tendon, which lies slightly superiorly. These tendons may be separated by a bursa.

The teres major receives its innervation from the lower subscapular nerve and its blood supply from branches of the subscapular and thoracodorsal arteries. It is primarily an internal rotator and adductor of the shoulder and an extensor of the arm (20, 60).

Coracobrachialis

The coracobrachialis comes off the coracoid process to insert on the anteromedial aspect of the humerus. It flexes and adducts the glenohumeral joint. The musculocutaneous nerve and its branches can penetrate the coracobrachialis from 1.5 to 8 cm below the coracoid (2, 40) (Fig. 1.18).

Pectoralis Major

There are three portions of the pectoralis major muscle. The upper portion originates from the medial aspect of the clavicle. The tendon of the

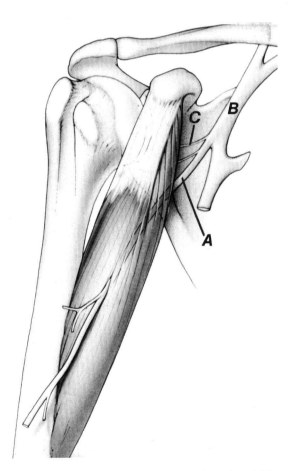

Figure 1.18. The musculocutaneous nerve **(A)** comes off the lateral cord **(B)** to penetrate the coracobrachialis. There may be small twigs **(C)** even higher. (Reproduced with permission from Flatow EL, Bigliani LU, April EW. An anatomical study of the musculocutaneous nerve and its relationship to the coracoid. Clin Orthop 1989;244:166–172).

sternal portion thus winds up slightly deep and proximal to the tendon of the clavicular portion. Unlike the multipennate clavicular portion, the sternal portion can be swung up (e.g., to reinforce the anterior glenohumeral joint after damage to the subscapularis) or down (e.g., along the chest wall to the inferior part of the scapula after serratus palsy) as a transfer in difficult reconstructions. The sternal portion originates form the manubrium sternum and the fifth and sixth ribs. Both portions of the muscle twist as they converge to insert on the lateral lip of the bicipital groove (Fig. 1.16). Innervation is provided by the lateral and medial pectoral nerves. Blood supply to this muscle is abundant; it can come from the thoracoacromial artery, the pectoral artery, the internal mammary, and the lateral thoracic arteries (20, 60).

Biceps Muscle

The biceps muscle has two heads. The long head originates from the supraglenoid tuberosity of the glenoid and the posterior superior aspect of the glenoid labrum; the short head originates from the coracoid, with the coracobrachialis and pectoralis minor (Fig. 1.15). The muscle inserts distally on the bicipital tuberosity of the radius. The long head of the biceps tendon exits the glenohumeral joint to travel in the bicipital groove under the transverse glenohumeral ligament and inferior to the pectoralis major tendon. Proximally, the tendon is located in the rotator interval between the supraspinatus and subscapular tendons. The biceps receive its innervation from the musculocutaneous nerve and its blood supply from the brachial artery (20).

QUADRILATERAL AND TRIANGULAR SPACES

Anteriorly, the quadrilateral space is bordered by the subscapularis muscle superiorly, the teres major muscle inferiorly, and the long head of the triceps medially. The lateral border is the medial aspect of the humeral shaft. The triangular space is defined by the subscapularis muscle superiorly, the teres major muscle inferiorly, and the long head of the triceps laterally. The circumflex scapular artery traverses this space. Posteriorly, the borders that define the quadrilateral space remain the same except that the teres minor is now the superior border (20).

NEUROANATOMY

The innervation of the shoulder complex is derived from the brachial plexus (C5–T1) (Fig. 1.19) with contributions from the third and fourth cervical nerves (55, 63, 76). In the supraclavicular region, the roots coalesce to form the trunks. The C5 and C6 roots form the upper trunk, the C8 and T1 roots form the lower trunk, and the C7 root forms the middle trunk. The following four terminal branches arise from the plexus above the clavicle: 1) the dorsal scapular nerve (C4, C5), which is purely motor, innervating the rhomboids minor and major and the levator scapulae; 2) the long thoracic nerve (C5, C6, C7), which is also purely motor, innervating the serratus anterior; 3) the suprascapular nerve (C5, C6), which innervates the supraspinatus and infraspinatus muscles, with sensory branches to the glenohumeral and acromioclavicular joints (76); and 4) the nerve to the subclavius (C5, C6), which in-

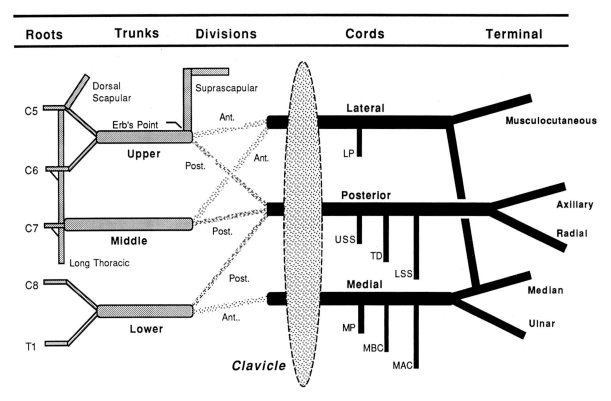

Figure 1.19. Schematic of the brachial plexus showing the relationship of the plexus relative to the clavicle. LP, lateral pectoral nerve; USS, upper subscapular nerve; TD, thoracodorsal nerve; LSS, lower subscapular nerve; MP, medial pectoral nerve; MBC, medial brachial cutaneous nerve; MAC, medial antebrachial cutaneous nerve. (Reproduced with permission from Hollingshead WH. The shoulder. In: Anatomy for surgeons. 3rd ed. Philadelphia: Harper Row, 1952;3:300–337).

nervates the subclavius muscle (33, 55, 76). After traumatic injuries to the brachial plexus, lack of these specific muscle functions can localize the level of injury, which is an indicator of future recovery (18, 70).

Distal to the clavicle, the tree trunks divide into the medial, lateral, and posterior cords. Their names reflect their positions relative to the axillary artery. The lateral pectoral nerve is the first peripheral nerve to come off the lateral cord (C5, C6, C7). It also provides motor innervation to the clavicular and sternal portion of the pectoralis major muscle and sensory innervation to the acromioclavicular joint. The terminal branches of the lateral cord are the musculocutaneous nerve, supplying motor innervation to the elbow flexors and sensation to the lateral aspect of the forearm (lateral antebrachial cutaneous nerve), and the lateral root of the median nerve.

Three peripheral nerves arise from the medial cord. The medial pectoral nerve innervates the pectoralis minor and the inferior aspect of the sternal portion of the pectoralis major. The medial brachial cutaneous and medial antebrachial cutaneous nerves provide sensation to the medial aspect of the upper arm and forearm, respectively. The medial cord terminates in the ulnar nerve and the medial root of the median nerve.

The posterior cord (C5–C8) gives rise to the upper subscapular nerve (C5), innervating the superior portion of the subscapularis muscle, and the lower subscapular nerve (C5, C6), innervating the lower portion of the subscapularis muscle and the teres major. The thoracodorsal nerve (C7, C8) originates between them, providing innervation to the latissimus dorsi. The posterior cord terminates in the radial nerve (C5–C8) and the axillary nerve (C5, C6).

Before the axillary nerve enters the quadrilateral space, it sends articular branches to the glenohumeral capsule (47). It may also send a branch that accompanies the anterior humeral circumflex artery into the bicipital groove. Additional branches to the capsule may come off the nerve when it enters the quadrilateral space. As the nerve traverses the quadrilateral space,

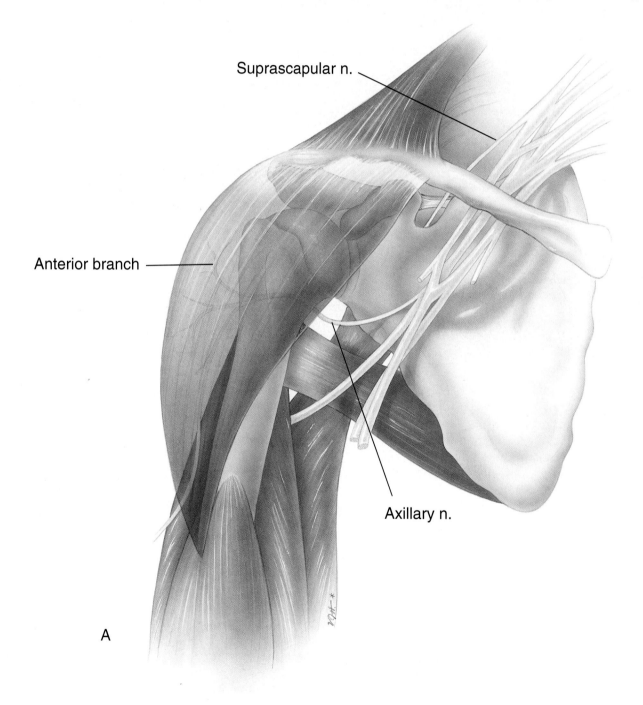

Suprascapular n.

Anterior branch

Axillary n.

A

Figure 1.20.   Peripheral nerves about the shoulder. **(A)** Anterior view. (Redrawn from Duralde XA, Bigliani LU. Neurologic disorders. In: Hawkins RJ, Misamore GW, Eds. Shoulder injuries in the athlete. New York: Churchill Livingstone 1995:243–265).

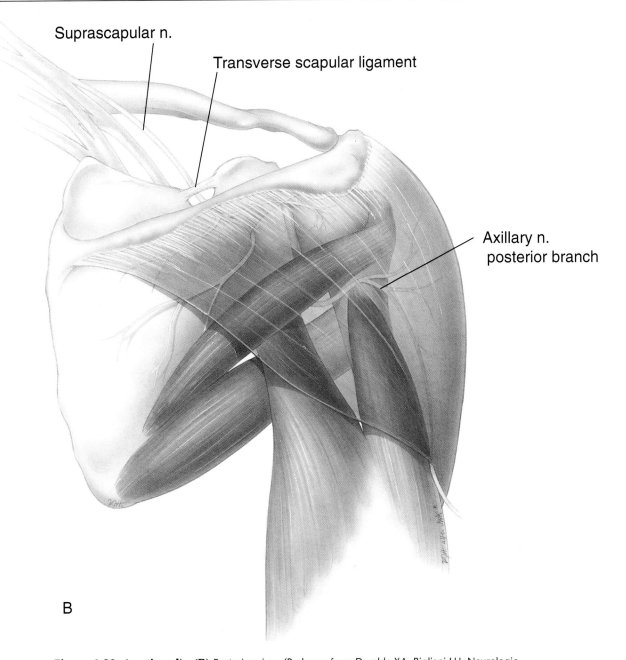

Suprascapular n.

Transverse scapular ligament

Axillary n.
posterior branch

B

Figure 1.20. *(continued)* **(B)** Posterior view. (Redrawn from Duralde XA, Bigliani LU. Neurologic
disorders. In: Hawkins RJ, Misamore GW, Eds. Shoulder injuries in the athlete.
New York: Churchill Livingstone 1995:243–265).

it wraps around the proximal humerus while lying on the deep surface of the
deltoid muscle (Fig. 1.20). It ramifies into three major branches that supply
motor innervation to the teres minor and the overlying deltoid muscle. The
lateral brachial cutaneous nerves represent the sensory branches that penetrate the deltoid muscle to provide sensation to the overlying skin.

The posterior cord continues distally as the radial or musculospiral nerve.
It may send an articular branch to the capsule, but its main function is to innervate the triceps proximally and the dorsal muscles of the forearm and
hand distally (55).

The articular branches to the shoulder joint come primarily from the axillary, suprascapular, and lateral anterior thoracic nerves (47). Branches also come from the posterior cord, and the sympathetic ganglion provides some innervation (47). These nerve fibers penetrate the outer surface of the joint capsule to form plexi in the synovium, overlying the inner aspect of the joint capsule. The contribution from the individual nerve branches can be variable (1, 47, 55).

Innervation of the acromioclavicular joint comes from the suprascapular, axillary, and pectoral nerves, with sensory innervation from the posterior branches of the supraclavicular nerves. The medial supraclavicular nerve provides sensory innervation to the sternoclavicular joint, with contributions from the nerve to the subclavius (34, 60).

VASCULAR ANATOMY

Arterial Supply

The arterial blood supply to the shoulder comes off the axillary artery, which is the continuation of the subclavian artery at the lateral border of the first rib (Fig. 1.21). There can be significant variation in the origin and distribution of these vessels as they branch from the axillary artery with extensive

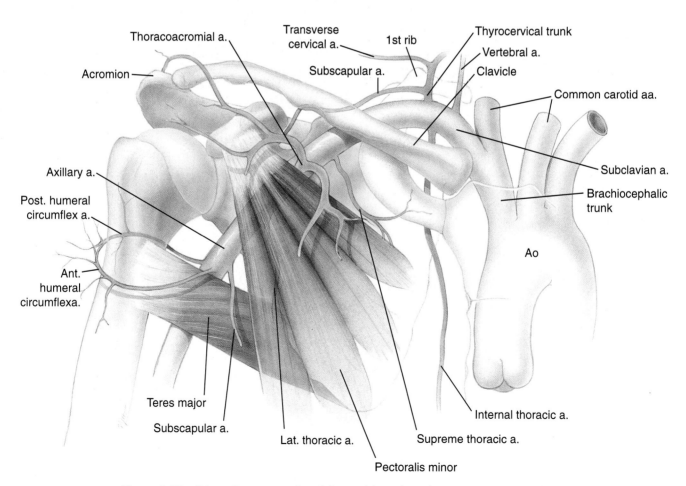

Figure 1.21. Schematic representation of the arterial supply to the upper extremity. (Redrawn from Anderson JE, ed. Grant's atlas of anatomy. 8th ed. Baltimore: Williams & Wilkins, 1983).

anastomoses, which contribute to the excellent collateral circulation around the shoulder (98). The most consistent and commonly described variations are documented below (58).

The thyrocervical trunk ascends from the subclavian artery proximal to the first rib and gives rise to the suprascapular and transverse cervical arteries. The transverse cervical artery divides into a superficial and a deep branch (the dorsal scapular artery) supplying the trapezius and rhomboid muscles, respectively. The dorsal scapular artery can also come off the subclavian artery directly.

The axillary artery continues as the brachial artery where the vessel crosses the latissimus dorsi. Traditionally, the axillary artery has been divided into three portions relative to the pectoralis minor muscle. The first portion is between the lateral border of the first rib and the superior border of the pectoralis minor. The second portion lies below the pectoralis minor, and the third portion is between the inferior border of the pectoralis minor and the latissimus dorsi.

The superior thoracic artery comes off the first portion of the axillary artery. Branches from this vessel supply the first three intercostal spaces.

The following two branches arise from the second portion of the axillary artery: the thoracoacromial artery and the lateral thoracic artery. There are four branches from the thoracoacromial artery: 1) the pectoral branch to the sternal portion of the pectoralis major muscle, 2) the deltoid artery to the clavicular head of the pectoralis major and the anterior deltoid, 3) the acromial artery to the acromioclavicular joint, and 4) the clavicular artery to the sternoclavicular joint (55, 100).

The lateral thoracic artery is the second branch from the second portion of the axillary artery. It provides circulation to the pectoralis minor, serratus anterior, and third to fifth intercostal spaces (100).

The three branches that come off the third portion of the axillary artery are the subscapular artery as well as the anterior and posterior humeral circumflex arteries. The subscapular artery travels along the subscapularis muscle, which it supplies, and continues as the thoracodorsal artery to the latissimus dorsi and teres major muscles. The circumflex scapular artery arises from the subscapular artery to traverse the triangular space, sending branches to the inferior angle of the scapula and the infraspinatus fossa (55).

At the inferior border of the subscapularis tendon, the anterior humeral circumflex artery comes off the axillary artery. After sending a twig to the tendon, the artery divides into two major branches—an ascending branch (the arcuate artery), which travels up the bicipital groove to supply the humeral head and the supraspinatus tendon (68, 105). The second branch represents the lateral continuation of the anterior humeral circumflex artery, which anastomoses with the posterior humeral circumflex artery (55).

The posterior humeral circumflex artery follows the axillary nerve into the quadrilateral space, where it ramifies with the nerve to supply the overlying deltoid muscle. It sends small branches to the acromion and the glenohumeral joint and anastomoses with the anterior humeral circumflex and thoracodorsal arteries (35, 55).

VEINS

The two most significant veins in the shoulder are the cephalic and axillary veins. The axillary vein is the proximal continuation of the basilic vein. It begins at the inferior border of the latissimus dorsi and becomes the subclavian vein at the lateral border of the first rib. The cephalic vein lies more superficially in the deltopectoral interval and penetrates the clavipectoral fascia proximally to empty into the axillary vein (55, 100). It is usually reflected laterally during the deltopectoral approach to the glenohumeral joint, as it rarely receives medial branches from the pectoralis major. This vein may be absent in approximately 4% of individuals (60).

SKIN

The anatomy of the skin is important when planning shoulder procedures. Suboptimally placed incisions can leave unattractive and prominent scars (86). Transection of the cutaneous nerves can result in areas of hypesthesia and dysesthesia, especially over the lateral aspect of the upper arm and over the clavicle. The skin over the shoulder is relatively mobile, so relatively small skin incisions can be elevated subcutaneously and retracted to allow adequate exposure during surgery.

The concept of the relaxed skin tension line (RSTL) refers to the skin lines that are perpendicular to the line of action of the pull of the underlying muscles. Incisions made along the RSTL tend to minimize scar formation (15, 29).

Sensation over the shoulder is provided mainly by the supraclavicular nerves (C3, C4), the dorsal rami of the cervical spinal nerves, and the sensory branches of the axillary nerves. There can be significant variation in the distribution and course of these sensory nerves. Overlapping of the zones supplied by different nerves is the rule rather than the exception (Allen AA, Flatow EW, unpublished data).

Biomechanics

MOVEMENT

Muscle Forces

The coordinated action of many muscles and several articulations (glenohumeral, acromioclavicular, sternoclavicular, subacromial, and scapulothoracic) is required to achieve purposeful shoulder movement. This is a complex, three-dimensional activity that can be only crudely modeled in static, two-dimensional descriptions. Nevertheless it is helpful to think in such terms to gain an overview of muscle function. In general, groups of muscles can be thought of as having two principle functions, stabilizing and rotating.

The scapula is stabilized by the parascapular muscles, especially the trapezius and serratus anterior. Without this effect, a load applied to the arm will tend to wing the scapula away from the chest wall. These muscles also rotate the scapula up to elevate the arm in coordination with glenohumeral elevation. Again, a loss of one or both muscles will impair the ability to raise the arm.

Glenohumeral motion is largely accomplished by a combination of deltoid and rotator cuff action. This can be resolved into a joint compression force and a couple, tending to rotate the humerus while compressing it into the socket (113). Muscle imbalances usually occur due to either neurologic injury or mechanical disruption (e.g., a rotator cuff tear).

KINEMATICS

Although subluxations can be induced by passive manipulations (50), the head closely follows ball-in-socket kinematics with little subluxation when the arm is positioned in space by muscle forces with intact stabilizing structures (62).

Pathologic kinematics are often related to loss of either the static or dynamic stabilizers or both. With a large rotator cuff tear, the head is no longer stabilized dynamically by the missing muscles-tendon unit(s); in massive tears, the head can boutonniere up through the tendon defect. When there is disruption or laxity of the anterior capsule and ligaments, the head may sublux or dislocate anteriorly when the muscles are surprised or caught at the limits of their mechanical effectiveness. Altered kinematics can also result from an imbalance in the system without an actual loss of stabilizers. For example, when the normally lax capsule is tightened, the head may be subluxed away from the tight side (9, 51). This can be seen clinically after overly tight anterior repairs (74). It has also been suggested that posterior-inferior capsular tightness (as is present in patients with mild loss of internal rotation and horizontal adduction) may cause anterosuperior humeral translation (potentially contributing to subacromial impingement) (75). Some of the important stabilizing mechanisms are reviewed below.

Stability

ARTICULAR GEOMETRY

Version

Many studies have looked at the relationship between glenoid and humeral version and clinical instability (65). Most have concluded that abnormal version is only rarely a factor in clinical instability (99), usually when a fracture malunion has resulted in severely abnormal humeral version or in cases of congenital glenoid hypoplasia.

Articular Conformity and Surface Area

The glenohumeral joint has highly conforming articular surfaces, although the subchondral bone, visible on radiographs, is flatter on the glenoid side (112). However, the pliant cartilage surface does have some "give" at the edges where the cartilage is thickest. The stabilizing effect of articular conformity is magnified by compressive loading.

The labrum and the "dynamized" cuff tendons form a "soft tissue" socket beyond the edge of the articular surface, increasing the functional articular surface area (54). Loss of conformity (e.g., wear of the articular cartilage of the anteroinferior glenoid from repeated dislocations) (75) or surface area (e.g., fractures involving a significant portion of the glenoid surface) (115) can decrease stability.

Atmospheric Pressure and Cohesion

Any subluxation of the glenohumeral surfaces increases the joint volume, which is contained by the capsule. This results in a vacuum that tends to resist further subluxation, much as a vacuum develops in a stoppered syringe when the plunger is pulled back. This effect has been extensively studied (17, 48, 52, 67, 124). This stabilizing effect is of low magnitude but is likely significant in supporting the arm at rest, when the muscles relax. The inferior subluxation seen after fractures may be caused in part by the loss of intraarticular suction due to a hemarthrosis.

Cohesion results from the close approximation of wet surfaces, as when two wet microscope slides stick together. This force is of low magnitude but begins instantly with the initiation of subluxation, well before tension could develop in ligaments, for example. A further stabilizing effect may come when the glenoid labrum forms a peripheral seal so that the glenoid adheres to the head as a suction cup.

MUSCLE FORCES

The rotator cuff muscles stabilize the humerus in the glenoid by compressing the head into a conforming socket, by having lines of action that tend to center the head in the glenoid and by "dynamizing" the ligaments in the glenohumeral capsule with which the cuff tendons blend (Fig. 1.22). Muscle stabilization may be coordinated by proprioceptive information from nerve endings in the capsule and ligaments (12, 71). The long head of the biceps tendon wraps around the humeral head and is tethered to the

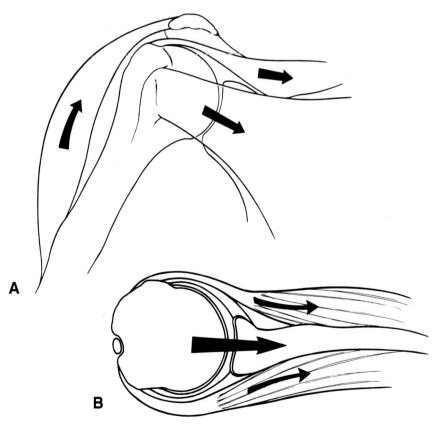

Figure 1.22. The glenohumeral muscles stabilize the shoulder by centering the head in the socket and by compressing it into a conforming socket. This forms a dynamic fulcrum for the deltoid. **(A)** Scapular plane view. **(B)** Transverse view.

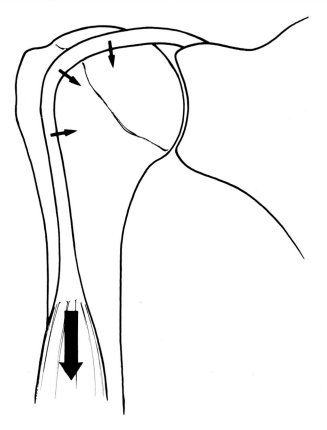

Figure 1.23. Stabilizing effect of biceps.

humerus as it passes through the biceps notch. Tension in the tendon, produced by muscle contraction, tends to stabilize the humerus into the socket (Fig. 1.23).

Furthermore, coordination of scapulohumeral rhythm repositions the glenoid under the moving humerus, adding to stability. Loss of this mechanism, for example in a patient with serratus palsy and winging of the scapula, can contribute to clinical instability.

GLENOHUMERAL LIGAMENTS

The structure, anatomy, and stabilizing function of the glenohumeral ligaments have been described earlier in this chapter. However, a proper understanding of the actual role of the ligaments in stabilizing the shoulder requires not just a qualitative description of them, but knowledge of their precise structure and strength. Unfortunately, much of our initial understanding of shoulder ligaments was limited to that derived from descriptive anatomy and surgical observations. Some distortion is, however, inevitably introduced. For example, arthroscopic inspection of ligamentous and capsular structures only observes the surface of the synovial side of the capsule. Thin, flimsy synovial tissue can appear robust and impressive if pleated or folded by arm rotation. Conversely, a significant capsular thickening may be indistinguishable from the surrounding capsule. Until recently, there were few studies of the precise structure, composition, and material properties of these structures.

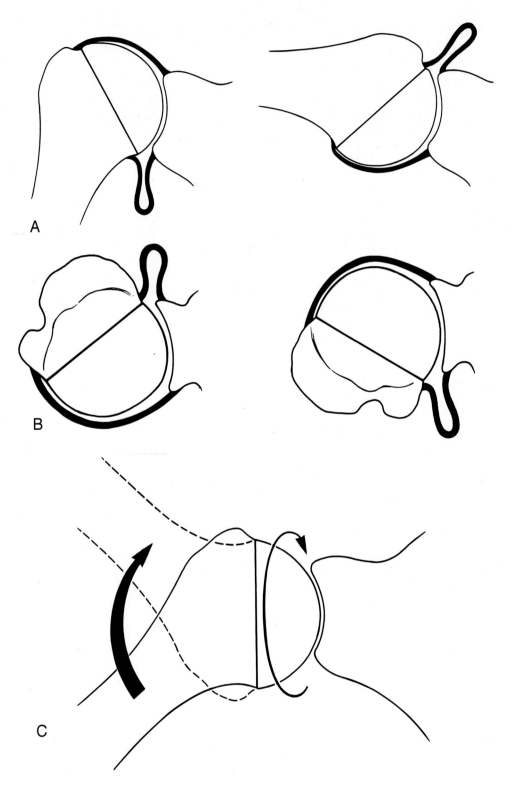

Figure 1.24. Different portions of the capsule come into play depending on arm position. **(A)** With the arm at the side, the inferior capsule (pouch) is lax while the superior capsule is drawn tight. This is reversed with arm elevation. **(B)** External rotation tends to tighten the anterior capsule, while internal rotation tightens the posterior capsule. **(C)** "Spinning" of the articular surface of the head can raise the arm and circumferentially wind-up the capsule.

Recent studies of the material properties of shoulder ligaments have found their strength in tension to be far lower than that of knee ligaments, emphasizing that in the shoulder the ligaments must load share with the muscles and other stabilizing mechanisms (11). In laboratory studies, the predominant modes of failure of the inferior glenohumeral ligament in tension were at the glenoid insertion (analogous to a Bankart avulsion) and in midsubstance (as might be expected to result in capsular stretching and laxity) (11). However, there was significant midsubstance ligament strain before failure even in the specimens that ultimately failed at the glenoid insertion. This suggests that plastic deformation of the capsule may result, especially if there is submaximal repetitive trauma (114).

Studies at different speeds of loading have shown that regions of the inferior glenohumeral ligament become stronger and stiffer at higher strain rates (118). This suggests a functional adaptation to stabilize the head during high-speed athletic use.

Different portions of the capsule become taut at different positions, and in many positions the entire capsule is lax. The relationship between arm position and which ligaments are tight is not simple, because the version and varus tilt of the head cause a coupling of rotations. For example, rotating the humeral articular surface in the glenoid can raise the humeral shaft while tightening the capsule all around the head (Fig. 1.24). This is probably the reason that acquired laxity, as in gymnasts or butterfly swimmers, is often multidirectional; each of many minor injuries stretches out only that portion of the capsule that was taut in the particular position at which the arm was when injured. The cumulative effect of multiple minor traumas in varying arm positions is a globally lax capsule. A single, violent trauma, on the other hand, would tend to focus the worst damage more on a specific region (e.g., Bankart avulsion with anteroinferior capsular stretch after a traumatic anterior dislocation) (3, 117).

CORACOACROMIAL ARCH

In the past, the coracoacromial arch was often seen only as an offending structure, causing impingement and wear on the rotator cuff. However, recent laboratory studies have shown that significant contact occurs between the arch and the underlying humerus and rotator cuff, much of it on regions uninvolved clinically in impingement (41, 42). Furthermore, the arch may be the last restraint left holding the head down when the dynamic head-centering effect of the rotator cuff is lost in massive tears (43, 69, 80, 125).

Recognition of this stabilizing effect has led us to be more conservative with bone removal during anterior acromioplasty. It has also led us to repair the coracoacromial ligament after acromioplasty in shoulders undergoing repair of massive rotator cuff tears when the muscles are atrophied and unlikely to recover a great deal of force (43).

REFERENCES

1. Arnoczky SP, Altcheck DW, O'Brien SJ. Anatomy of the shoulder. In: McGinty JB, ed. Operative arthroscopy. New York: Raven Press, 1991:425–440.
2. Bach BR, O'Brien SJ, Warren RF, et al. An unusual complication of the Bristow procedure. J Bone Joint Surg 1988;70A:458–460.

3. Bankart ASB. The pathology and treatment of recurrent dislocation of the shoulder-joint. Br J Surg 1939;26:23–29.
4. Basmajiian JV, Bazant FJ. Factors preventing downward dislocation of the adducted shoulder joint. J Bone Joint Surg 1959;41A:1182–1186.
5. Bearden JM, Hughston JC, Whatley GS. Acromioclavicular dislocation: method of treatment. J Sports Med 1973;4:5–17.
6. Bearn JG. Direct observations on the function of the capsule of the sternoclavicular joint in clavicular support. J Anat 1967;101:170–189.
7. Beaton LE, Anson BJ. Variation of the origin of the m. trapezius. Anat Rec 1942;83:41–46.
8. Bigliani LU, Dalsey RM, McCann PD, et al. An anatomical study of the suprascapular nerve. Arthroscopy 1990;6:301–305.
9. Bigliani LU, Flatow EL, Kelkar R, et al. The effect of anterior capsular tightening on shoulder kinematics and contact. J Shoulder Elbow Surg 1994;3:S65.
10. Bigliani LU, Morrison DS, April EW. The morphology of the acromion and its relationship to rotator cuff tears. Orthop Trans 1986;10:228.
11. Bigliani LU, Pollock RG, Soslowsky LJ, et al. The tensile properties of the inferior glenohumeral ligament. J Orthop Res 1992;10:187–197.
12. Blasier RB, Carpenter JE, Huston LJ. Shoulder proprioception: effect of joint laxity, joint position, and direction of motion. Orthop Rev 1994;23:45–50.
13. Boileau P, Walch G, Mazzoleni N, et al. In vitro study of humeral retrotorsion (abstract). J Shoulder Elbow Surg 1993;2:S12.
14. Boileau P, Walch G. The combined offset (medial and posterior) of the humeral sphere (abstract). J Shoulder Elbow Surg 1993;3:S65.
15. Borges AF. The relaxed skin tension lines (RSTL) vs. other skin lines. Plast Reconstr Surg 1984;73:144–150.
16. Bosworth BM. Complete acromioclavicular dislocation. N Engl J Med 1949;241:221–225.
17. Browne AO, Hoffmeyer P, An KN, et al. The influence of atmospheric pressure on shoulder stability. Orthop Trans 1990;14:259.
18. Burge P, Rushworth G, Watson N. Patterns of injury to the terminal branches of the brachial plexus. J Bone Joint Surg 1985;67B:630–634.
19. Clark J, Sidles JA, Matsen FA. The relationship of the glenohumeral joint capsule to the rotator cuff. Clin Orthop 1990;254:29–34.
20. Clemente CD, ed. Gray's anatomy. 30th ed. Philadelphia: Lea & Febiger, 1984:233–235, 370, 375 512–528.
21. Codman EA. The shoulder, rupture of the supraspinatus tendon and other lesions in or about the subacromial bursa. Boston: Thomas Todd, 1934:65–107.
22. Codman EA. The shoulder, rupture of the supraspinatus tendon and other lesions in or about the subacromial bursa. Boston: Thomas Todd, 1934:313–331.
23. Codman EA, Akerson TB. The pathology associated with rupture of the supraspinatus tendon. Ann Surg 93:354–359.
24. Cofield RH. Tears of the rotator cuff. American Academy of Orthopaedic Surgeons Instructional Course Lectures 1981;30:258–273.
25. Cofield RH. Current concepts—review of rotator cuff disease of the shoulder. J Bone Joint Surg 1985;67A:974–979.
26. Colachis SC Jr, Strohm BR. Effects of suprascapular and axillary nerve block on muscle forces in the upper extremity. Arch Phys Med Rehabil 1971;52:22.
27. Colachis SC Jr, Strohm BR, Brecher VL. Effects on axillary nerve block on muscles in the upper extremity. Arch Phys Med Rehabil 1969;645–647.
28. Cooper DE, Arnoczky SP, O'Brien SJ, et al. Histology and vascularity of the glenoid labrum—an anatomic study. J Bone Joint Surg 1992;74A:46–52.
29. Courtiss EH, Longaire JJ, Destafano GA, et al. The placement of elective skin incisions. Plast Reconstr Surg 1963;31:31–44.
30. Das SP, Ray GS, Saha AK. Observations on the tilt of the glenoid cavity of the scapula. J Anat Soc India 1966;15:114–118.

31. Debevoise NT, Hyatt GW, Townsend GB. Humeral torsion in recurrent shoulder dislocations: a technic of determination by X-ray. Clin Orthop 1971;76:87–93.

32. Dempster WT. Mechanisms of shoulder movement. Arch Phys Med Rehabil 1965;46A:49–70.

33. DePalma AF. Degenerative lesions of the shoulder joint at various age groups which are compatible with good function. American Academy of Orthopaedic Surgeons Instructional Course Lectures 1950;7:168–180.

34. DePalma AF. Surgical anatomy of the acromioclavicular and sternoclavicular joint. Surg Clin North Am 1963;43:1540–1550.

35. DePalma AF. Surgery of the shoulder. 2nd ed. Philadelphia: JB Lippincott, 1973: 35–64.

36. DePalma AF, Calley G, Bennett GA. Variational anatomy and degenerative lesions of the shoulder joint. American Academy of Orthopaedic Surgeons Institutional Course Lectures 1949;6:255–281.

37. Dines DM, Warren RE, Inglis AE, et al. The coracoid impingement syndrome. Orthop Trans 1986;10:229.

38. Dines DM, Warren RF, Inglis AE, et al. The coracoid impingement syndrome. J Bone Joint Surg 1990;72B:314–316.

39. Flatow EL. The biomechanics of the acromioclavicular, sternoclavicular, and scapulothoracic joints. In: Heckman JD, ed. Instructional course lectures. Rosemont, IL: American Academy of Orthopaedic Surgeons, 1993;42:237–245.

40. Flatow EL, Bigliani LU, April EW. An anatomical study of the musculocutaneous nerve and its relationship to the coracoid. Clin Orthop 1989;244:166–172.

41. Flatow EL, Colman WW, Kelkar R, et al. The effect of anterior acromioplasty on rotator cuff contact: an experimental and computer simulation. J Shoulder Elbow Surg 1995;4:S53–S54.

42. Flatow EL, Soslowsky LJ, Ticker JB, et al. Excursion of the rotator cuff under the acromion: patterns of subacromial contact. Am J Sports Med 1994;22:779–788.

43. Flatow EL, Weinstein DM, Duralde XA, et al. Coracoacromial ligament preservation in rotator cuff surgery. J Shoulder Elbow Surg 1994;3:S73.

44. Flood V. Discovery of a new ligament of the shoulder joint. Lancet 1829;1:672–673.

45. Freedman I, Munro R. Abduction of the arm in the scapular plane: scapular and glenohumeral movements. J Bone Joint Surg 1966;48A:1503–1510.

46. Fukuda K, Craig EV, An K, et al. Biomechanical study of the ligamentous system of the acromioclavicular joint. J Bone Joint Surg 1986;68A:434–439.

47. Gardener E. Innervation of the shoulder joint. Anat Rec 1948;102:1–18.

48. Gibb TD, Sidles JA, Harryman DT III, et al. The effect of capsular venting on glenohumeral laxity. Clin Orthop 1991;268:120–127.

49. Hall MC, Rosser M. The structure of the upper end of the humerus with reference to osteoporotic changes in senescence leading to fractures. Can Med Assoc J 1963;8:290–294.

50. Harryman DT III, Sidles JA, Clark JM, et al. Translation of the humeral head on the glenoid with passive glenohumeral motion. J Bone Joint Surg 1990;72A: 1334–1343.

51. Hawkins RJ, Angelo RL. Glenohumeral osteoarthrosis: a late complication of Putti-Platt repair. J Bone Joint Surg 1990;72A:1193–1197.

52. Helmig P, Sojberg JO, Sneppen O, et al. Glenohumeral movement patterns after puncture of the joint capsule: an experimental study. J Shoulder Elbow Surg 1993;2:209–215.

53. Hill JA, Tkach L, Hendrix RW. A study of glenohumeral orientation in patients with anterior recurrent shoulder dislocations using computerized axial tomography. Orthop Rev 1989;18:84–91.

54. Himeno S, Tsumura H. The role of the rotator cuff as a stabilizing mechanism of the shoulder. In: Bateman JE, Welsh RP, eds. Surgery of the shoulder. Philadelphia: B.C. Decker, 1984:17–25.

55. Hollingshead WH. The shoulder. In: Anatomy for surgeons. 3rd ed. Philadelphia: Harper Row, 1952;3:300–337.

56. Horwitz MT, Tocantis LM. Isolated paralysis of the serratus anterior (magnus) muscle. J Bone Joint Surg Am 1938;20A:720–725.

57. Howell SM, Imobersteg AM, Seger DH, et al. Clarification of the role of the supraspinatus muscle in shoulder function. J Bone Joint Surg Am 1986;68A:398–404.

58. Huelke DF. Variation in the origins of the branches of the axillary artery. Anat Rec 1959;135:33–41.

59. Inman VT, Saunders JB, Abbott LC. Observations on the function of the shoulder. J Bone Joint Surg 1944;26:1–30.

60. Jobe CM. Gross anatomy of the shoulder. In: Rockwood CA, Matsen FA, eds. The shoulder. Philadelphia: WB Saunders, 1990:34–97.

61. Johnson LL. The shoulder joint: an arthroscopists perspective of anatomy and pathology. Clin Orthop 1987;223:113–125.

62. Kelkar R, Newton PM, Armegnol J, et al. Three-dimensional kinematics of the glenohumeral joint during abduction in the scapular plane. Trans Orthop Res Soc 1993;18:136.

63. Kerr AT. The brachial plexus in man: the variation in its formation and branches. Am J Anat 1918;23:285–394.

64. Krahl VE. The torsion of the humerus: its localization, cause, and duration in man. Am J Anat 1947;80:275–319.

65. Kronberg M, Brostrom LA. Humeral head retroversion in patients with unstable humeroscapular joints. Clin Orthop 1990;260:207–211.

66. Kronberg M, Brostrom LA, Soderlund V. Retroversion of the humeral head in the normal shoulder and its relationship to the normal range of motion. Clin Orthop 1990;253:113–117.

67. Kumar VP, Balasubramianium P. The role of atmospheric pressure in stabilizing the shoulder. J Bone Joint Surg 1985;67B:719–721.

68. Laing PG. The arterial supply of the adult humerus. J Bone Joint Surg 1956;38A:1105–1116.

69. Lazarus MD, Yung S-W, Sidles JA, et al. Anterosuperior humeral displacement: limitation by the coracoacromial arch. American Academy of Orthopaedic Surgeons, Sixty-Second Annual Meeting, Orlando, Florida, February 1995.

70. Leffert RD. Brachial plexus injuries. Orthop Clin North Am 1970;1:399–417.

71. Lephart SM, Warner JJP, Borsa PA, et al. Proprioception of the shoulder in healthy, unstable, and surgically repaired shoulders. J Shoulder Elbow Surg 1994;3:371–380.

72. Lewis OJ. The coracoclavicular joint. J Anat 1959;93:296–303.

73. Liberson F. Os acromiale—a contested anomaly. J Bone Joint Surg 1937;19:683–689.

74. MacDonald PB, Hawkins RJ, Fowler PJ, et al. Release of the subscapularis for internal rotation contracture and pain after anterior repair for recurrent anterior dislocations of the shoulder. J Bone Joint Surg 1992;74A:734–737.

75. Matsen FA III, Lippitt SB, Sidles JA, et al. Practical evaluation and management of the shoulder. Philadelphia: WB Saunders, 1994:59–109.

76. McCann PD, Bindelglass DF. The brachial plexus—clinical anatomy. Orthop Rev 1991;20:413–419.

77. McCann PD, Kadaba M, Wooten M, et al. An anatomic study of the subscapular nerves—a guide for EMG analysis of the subscapularis muscle. Presented at the American Shoulder and Elbow Surgeons, Eighth Open Meeting, Washington, DC, February 1992.

78. McCluskey GM, Bigliani LU: Surgical management of refractory scapulothoracic bursitis. Orthop Trans 1991;15:801.

79. Milch H. Snapping scapula. Clin Orthop 1961;20:139–150.

80. Moorman CT, Deng X-H, Warren RF, et al. Role of the coracoacromial ligament, coracohumeral veil, and anterior acromion in stabilizing the glenohumeral

joint. American Academy of Orthopaedic Surgeons, Sixty-Second Annual Meeting, Orlando, Florida, February 1995.

81. Mortenson OA, Wiedenbauer M. An electromyographic study of the trapezius muscle. Anat Rec 1952;112:366–367.

82. Moseley HF, Overgaard B. The anterior capsular mechanism in recurrent anterior dislocation of the shoulder: morphological and clinical studies with special reference to the glenoid labrum and glenohumeral ligaments. J Bone Joint Surg 1962;44B:913–927.

83. Neer CS II. Articular replacement for the humeral head. J Bone Joint Surg 1955; 37A:215–228.

84. Neer CS II. Anterior acromioplasty for the chronic impingement syndrome in the shoulder. J Bone Joint Surg 1972;54A:41–50.

85. Neer CS II. Impingement lesions. Clin Orthop 1983;173:70–77.

86. Neer CS II. Shoulder reconstruction. Philadelphia: WB Saunders, 1990:1–39.

87. Neer CS II, Satterlee CC, Dalsey RM, et al. The anatomy and potential effects of contracture of the coracohumeral ligament. Clin Orthop 1992;280:13–16.

88. Norris TR, Fischer J, Bigliani LU, et al. The unfused acromial epiphysis and its relationship to impingement syndromes. Orthop Trans 1983;7:505.

89. Nuber GW, Jobe FW, Perry J, et al. Fine wire electromyographic analysis of the shoulder during swimming. Am J Sports Med 1986;14:7–11.

90. Nutter PD. Coraclavicular articulation. J Bone Joint Surg 1941;23:177–179.

91. O'Brien SJ, Arnoczky SP, Warren RF, et al. Developmental anatomy of the shoulder and anatomy of the glenohumeral joint. In: Rockwood CA, Matsen FA, eds. The shoulder. Philadelphia: WB Saunders 1990:1–33.

92. O'Brien SJ, Neves MC, Rozbruck RS, et al. The anatomy and histology of the inferior glenohumeral complex of the shoulder. Am J Sports Med 1990;18: 449–456.

93. Oveson JO, Nielsen S. Stability of the shoulder joint: cadaveric study of stabilizing structures. Acta Orthop Scand 1985;56:149–151.

94. Oveson JO, Nielsen S. Anterior and posterior instability: a cadaveric study. Acta Orthop Scand 1986;57:324–327.

95. Parsons TA. The snapping scapula and subscapular exostoses. J Bone Joint Surg 1973;55B:345–349.

96. Petersson CJ, Redlund-Johnell I. The subacromial space in normal shoulder radiographs. Acta Orthop Scand 1984;55:57–58.

97. Pieper H-G. Shoulder dislocation in skiing: choice of surgical method depending on the degree of humeral retrotorsion. Int J Sports Med 1985;6:155–160.

98. Radke HK. Arterial circulation of the upper extremity. In: Strandness DE Jr, ed. Collateral circulation in clinical surgery. Philadelphia: WB Saunders, 1969: 294–307.

99. Randelli M, Gambrioli PL. Glenohumeral osteometry by computed tomography in normal and unstable shoulders. Clin Orthop 1986;208:151–156.

100. Reid CD, Taylor GI. The vascular territory of acromiothoracic axis. Br J Plast Surg 1984;37:194–212.

101. Reiss FP, De Camargo AM, Vitti M, et al. Electromyographic study of the subclavius muscle. Acta Anat 1979;105:284–290.

102. Richardson AB. Arthroscopic anatomy of the shoulder. Tech Orthop 1988;26: 1–7.

103. Rockwood CA, Williams CR, Young DC. Inquiries to the acromioclavicular joint. In: Rockwood CA, Green DP, Bucholz RW, eds. Fractures. Philadelphia: JB Lippincott, 1975;3:1181–1251.

104. Rothman RH, Marvel JP Jr, Heppenstall RB. Anatomic considerations in the glenohumeral joint. Orthop Clin North Am 1975;6:341–352.

105. Rothman R, Parke W. The vascular anatomy of the rotator cuff. Clin Orthop 1975;6:341–352.

106. Saitoh S, Nakatsuchi MD, Latta L, et al. Distribution of bone mineral density and bone strength of the proximal humerus. J Shoulder Elbow Surg 1994; 3:234–242.

107. Sakellarides, HT. Injury to the spinal accessory nerve with paralysis of the trapezius muscle and treatment by tendon transfer. Orthop Trans 1986;10:449.

108. Sarrafian SK. Gross and functional anatomy of the shoulder. Clin Orthop 1983;173:11–19.

109. Schlemm F. Ueber die verstarkung bander aur schulter gelenk. Arch Anat 1853:45–48.

110. Sidles JA, Harryman DT, Matsen FA III. Glenohumeral and scapulothoracic contributions to shoulder motion. Orthop Trans 1991;15:762.

111. Soderlund V, Kronberg M, Brostrom L-A. Radiologic assessment of humeral head retroversion: description of a new method. Acta Radiolgica 1989;30:501–505.

112. Soslowsky LJ, Flatow EL, Bigliani LU, et al. Articular geometry of the glenohumeral joint. Clin Orthop 1992;285:181–190.

113. Soslowsky LJ, Flatow EL, Bigliani LU, et al. Quantitation of in situ contact areas at the glenohumeral joint: a biomechanical study. J Orthop Res 1992;10: 524–534.

114. Speer KP, Deng X, Torzilli PA, et al. A biomechanical evaluation of the Bankart lesion. J Bone Joint Surg 1994;76A:1819–1826.

115. Steinman S, Bigliani LU, McIlveen SJ. Glenoid fractures associated with recurrent anterior dislocations of the shoulder. American Academy of Orthopaedic Surgeons, Fifty-Seventh Annual Meeting, New Orleans, Louisiana, February 1990.

116. Strizak AM, Danzig L, Jackson DW, et al. Subacromial bursography—an anatomical and clinical study. J Bone Joint Surg Am 1982;64:196–201.

117. Thomas SC, Matsen FA III. An approach to the repair of avulsion of the glenohumeral ligaments in the management of traumatic anterior glenohumeral instability. J Bone Joint Surg 1989;71A:506–512.

118. Ticker JB, Bigliani LU, Soslowsky LJ, et al. Viscoelastic and geometric properties of the inferior glenohumeral ligament. Orthop Trans 1992;16:304–305.

119. Ticker JB, Djurasovic M, April EW, et al. Incidence of ganglion cysts and other variations in anatomy along the course of the suprascapular nerve. American Academy of Orthopaedic Surgeons, Sixty-Second Annual Meeting, Orlando, Florida, February 1995.

120. Tillet E, Smith M, Fulcher M, et al. Anatomic determination of humeral head retroversion: the relationship of the central axis of the humeral head to the bicipital groove. J Shoulder Elbow Surg 1993;2:255–256.

121. Turkel SJ, Parrio MW, Marshall JL, et al. Stabilizing mechanisms preventing anterior dislocation of the glenohumeral joint. J Bone Joint Surg 1981;63A: 1208–1217.

122. Tyurina TV. Age related characteristics of the human acromioclavicular joint. Arkh Anat Gistol Embriol 1985;89:75–81.

123. Warner JJP, Deng X-H, Warren RF, et al. Static capsuloligamentous restraints to superior-inferior translation of the glenohumeral joint. Am J Sports Med 1992;20:675–685.

124. Warner JJP, Deng X-H, Warren RF, et al. Superior-inferior translation in the intact and vented shoulder. J Shoulder Elbow Surg 1993;2:99–105.

125. Wiley AM. Superior humeral dislocation: a complication following decompression and debridement for rotator cuff tears. Clin Orthop 1991;263:135–141.

126. Wooten ME, Kadaba M, Ramakrishman H, et al. On the measurement of scapulohumeral rhythm. Orthop Trans 1991;15:570.

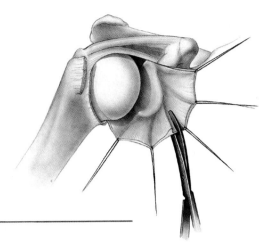

CHAPTER
2

Proximal Humerus Fractures

LOUIS U. BIGLIANI

Introduction

Although most fractures of the proximal humerus are minimally displaced and can be treated nonoperatively (3, 25, 31, 42), displaced fractures and fracture-dislocations are more complex and often require operative treatment. The goal of surgery in these more complex displaced fractures is to achieve a painless and stable shoulder so that maximum function can occur, allowing early and continued rehabilitation. As with all periarticular fractures, careful and thorough evaluation and treatment are necessary to achieve these goals. The Neer four-segment classification first published in 1970 (3, 30) provides an organized approach for the diagnosis and treatment of displaced proximal humeral fractures (Fig. 2.1). The majority of displaced fractures can be successfully treated using various techniques of ORIF or prosthetic replacement. This chapter outlines some of the more common operative procedures for displaced proximal humeral fractures.

Incidence and Etiology

Fractures of the proximal humerus are not uncommon, especially in older patients. They have previously been reported to account for approximately 4 to 5% of all fractures, but this figure may be low (3, 26, 30). Rose et al. (37) found that proximal humeral fractures occur at nearly 70% of the reported rate of proximal femur fractures, all ages considered. In older individuals, the percentage of humeral fractures significantly increases. Osteoporosis is believed to be a major factor. Also, there is a higher incidence of proximal humeral fractures in women than men by a ratio of 2 to 1.

The most common mechanism of injury for proximal humeral fractures is a fall onto an outstretched hand from a standing height or less. In most instances, severe trauma does not play a significant role. Rather, the trauma need only be minor to moderate because of the osteoporosis that may be present. In younger patients, high-energy trauma is more frequently involved, and the resulting fracture is often more serious. These patients usually have

Displaced Fractures

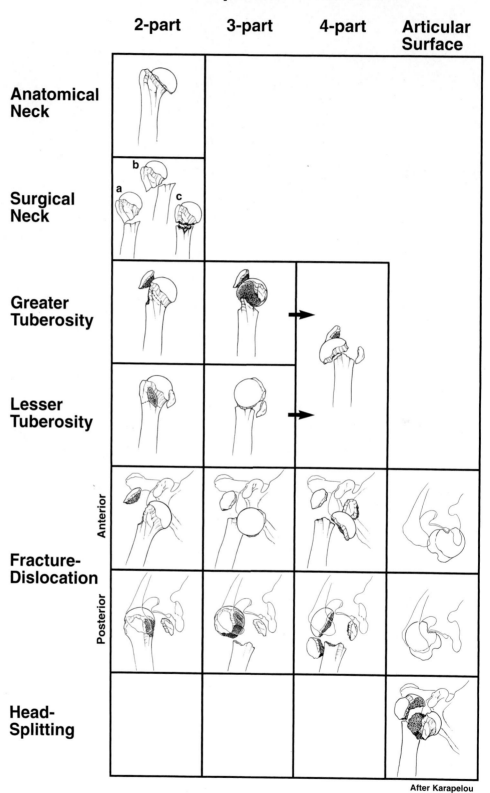

After Karapelou

Figure 2.1. The Neer four-part classification. The revised Neer classification; the six type groupings were deleted to emphasize the differentiation into fracture segments. The articular surface heading was placed at the top of the classification and head-splitting fractures were added to more clearly depict articular surface fractures.

fracture-dislocations with significant soft tissue disruption and multiple trauma.

Classification

In 1970, Neer (30) reported his four-part classification of proximal humerus fractures, which remains the standard classification for these injuries and the one most widely used in the orthopaedic literature (Fig. 2.1). The description of this classification was based on Codman's contribution of the understanding that fractures occur along the anatomic lines of epiphyseal union and 26 years of clinical experience in the treatment of proximal humerus fractures. It considers anatomy, biomechanical forces, and the resultant amount of displacement of fracture fragments and relates these to diagnosis and treatment. This classification system was described as a concept rather than a numerical classification and sets forth guidelines that are designed to be helpful in the recognition and treatment of displaced fractures (Fig. 2.1). In this classification, the four parts are the same as those described by Codman: the articular segment, the greater tuberosity, the lesser tuberosity, and the humeral shaft. When any of the four segments is displaced more than 1 cm or angulated more than 45°, the fracture is considered to be displaced. A segment may have several nondisplaced components; these should not be considered as separate parts because they are held in continuity by soft tissue. The central focus of this fracture classification is the status of the blood supply to the humeral head and the relationship of the humeral head to the displaced parts and the glenoid. The classification has been modified through the years to deemphasize the six categories on the left side of the classification and emphasize the four-segment aspect as well as articular fractures (3).

History and Physical Examination

The majority of fractures of the proximal humerus present acutely; therefore, the most common symptoms are pain, swelling, and tenderness around the shoulder, especially in the area of the greater tuberosity. Palpation of the bony contours of the shoulder is often difficult in this setting. In most instances, patients find it difficult to initiate active motion, and the arm is held closely against the chest wall. Crepitus may be present upon motion of the shoulder if fracture fragments are in contact. The elicitation of crepitus is not recommended, however, due to the pain involved and the potential risk of iatrogenic neurovascular injury. Ecchymosis generally occurs within 24 to 48 hours of the injury and may spread to the chest wall and flank and distally down the extremity. The diagnosis of a proximal humerus fracture, however, is made radiographically, and the history and physical signs only corroborate radiographic findings.

A detailed neurovascular evaluation is essential in all fractures of the proximal humerus. The brachial plexus and axillary artery are just medial to the coracoid process, and injury to these structures is not uncommon. The most common nerve injury seen with fractures around the shoulder is injury to the axillary nerve (3, 41). Sensation should be tested over the deltoid muscle in the axillary nerve distribution, because testing for deltoid activity or weakness may be very difficult due to pain. The ability of the patient to actively set the deltoid muscle in an isometric contraction, however, should be assessed. There is often inferior subluxation of the humerus in the immediate postfracture or postoperative period. In the majority of instances, this is secondary to deltoid fatigue or atony rather than to an injury to the axillary nerve. The arm should be supported in a sling, and gentle isometric exercises will help recover deltoid tone. If the situation is severe and persists for more than 4 weeks, it must be differentiated from a true axillary nerve palsy.

In addition to axillary nerve function, the motor function and sensory distribution of the musculocutaneous nerve as well as other peripheral nerves should be specifically examined. Stableforth (41) reported that nerve lesions occurred with an incidence of 6.1% after four-part anterior fracture-dislocations of the shoulder. Neer and McIlveen (33) reported on 44 consecutive patients with four-part proximal humeral fractures treated with humeral head replacement. Twelve patients had nerve injuries (27%), five of which were after attempts at closed reduction and before prosthetic replacement. Neurologic injuries associated with closed reduction methods are difficult to distinguish from those injuries that occur at the time of injury or those that occur at the time of surgery, due to the difficulty in accurately assessing nerve function in the acutely injured, swollen, and painful shoulder. Thus, the importance of an initial meticulous neurologic examination is emphasized.

Closed injury to the brachial plexus or peripheral nerves requires documentation and may be treated expectantly. Electrodiagnostic evaluation is of limited value until sufficient time has elapsed after nerve injury to demonstrate denervation potentials (3 or 4 weeks after injury). Neurologic injury should not delay the definitive management of the fracture, as most nerve injuries are neurapraxias and will resolve sufficiently to allow adequate function (3). Complete lesions that do not resolve can be evaluated and treated appropriately between 3 and 6 months after the injury.

Injury to the axillary artery occurs particularly in fracture-dislocations, but may also occur in less severe injuries (9, 23, 31, 41) and can be limb-threatening. It is important to assess peripheral pulses and question the patient concerning paresthesias in the distal extremity with all proximal humerus fractures. If there is a demonstrable diminution of the radial pulse in the presence of a proximal humerus fracture or fracture-dislocation, vascular surgery consultation may be indicated for further Doppler and/or angiographic evaluation.

Medical evaluation should be expeditious but thorough, and the possibility of associated occult injuries must be considered. Although attention is usually centered around radiographs in this setting, the patient is as important, if not more important, than the fracture type itself in regards to treatment, rehabilitation, and prognostic implications. Functional demands, activities of daily life, and patient expectations should all be determined. The patient's mental status must be assessed to determine whether he or she will be able to understand and complete the rigorous and extensive postoperative rehabilitation program required after prosthetic replacement. Although patients who mentally or physically cannot participate in or cooperate with this postoperative rehabilitation may achieve satisfactory pain relief, functional outcome will be substantially adversely affected. Thus, it is important to be aware of these factors preoperatively for proper patient and family counseling regarding surgical and postoperative expectations.

Imaging

The fracture pattern must be clearly delineated to determine whether ORIF or humeral head replacement is the best treatment option for a displaced proximal humeral fracture. This is best accomplished with the radiographic trauma series of the shoulder, consisting of three views at right angles to each other (31), anteroposterior (AP) and lateral radiographs in the plane of the scapula, and (if motion and pain permit) an axillary view (Fig. 2.2). The AP and lateral radiographs can be taken without removing the patient's extremity from the sling (Fig. 2.2A,B). The axillary view is useful to identify correctly a fracture-dislocation and to evaluate the articular surfaces of the glenoid and the humerus. This view is often ignored even though its importance has been stressed for years by several authors (3, 6, 8, 30, 39). The arm can be held gently in slight (~30°) abduction by a knowledgeable person so that further displacement of the fracture does not occur. A Velpeau axillary view (6) can be obtained without removing the patient's sling (Fig. 2.2C). The patient is seated and tilted obliquely backward approximately 40 to 45°; the plate is placed below the shoulder, and the x-ray tube comes in from above. This view is extremely helpful in those patients with significant pain that limits even the slight abduction necessary to obtain a routine axillary film. It has the additional advantage of not shifting the fracture position, as a portion of the motion required for abduction of the shoulder in the routine axillary view may occur through the fracture site (11).

Although accurate radiographs allow consistent identification of displaced segments by the experienced shoulder surgeon, computed tomography (CT) is occasionally helpful to assess tuberosity displacement and articular surface involvement (39). The head may be split or have a significant

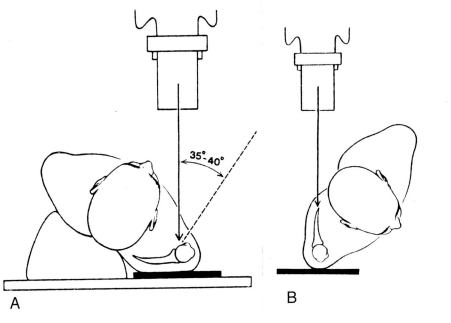
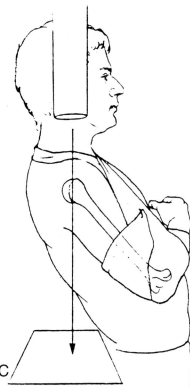

Figure 2.2.   Views for evaluation of displaced fractures of the proximal humerus. **(A)** True AP view of the glenohumeral joint. **(B)** True lateral view in scapular plane at the glenohumeral joint. **(C)** Velpeau axillary view of the glenohumeral joint.

impression defect, both of which are well visualized with CT. Morris et al. (29) have reported a series of patients in which CT was helpful in judging the amount of displacement of tuberosity fractures, and others have advocated CT in the evaluation of complex fractures and fracture-dislocations (3, 10, 22, 38, 39).

Surgical Indications

Open reduction and internal fixation (ORIF) may be required for the treatment of displaced two-part and three-part fractures and fracture-dislocations that do not respond to closed reduction and immobilization. The choice of technique and device depends on several factors, including the type of fracture, quality of the bone and soft tissue, and age and reliability of the patient. The goal with internal fixation should be a stable reduction allowing for early motion of the shoulder. The current trend is toward limited dissection of the soft tissue around the fracture fragments and the use of minimal amount of hardware required for stable fixation (8, 11).

Two-part surgical neck fractures may require ORIF, either because interposition of soft tissue prevents a closed reduction or the reduction is not stable. Various devices have been proposed for fixation, including intramedullary nails or rods, plates and screws, staples, wire, nonabsorbable sutures, multiple pins, and combinations of these. The author prefers figure-of-eight sutures or wire between the head and shaft fragment and the use of Enders rods if necessary for longitudinal stability.

Two-part greater tuberosity fractures that are displaced more than 5 mm may require ORIF, because the posterior and superior displacement will cause impingement beneath the acromion. Screws, wires, and suture material have all been proposed as types of fixation for the greater tuberosity. The author prefers nonabsorbable sutures for both the tuberosity and rent in the rotator cuff.

ORIF is indicated for most three-part fractures because closed reduction is very difficult (18). Wires, sutures, rods, screws, and plates and screws have been described. The author prefers no. 2 or no. 5 nonabsorbable suture material or if extra stability is needed, 18-gauge wire (11). It is important to use the rotator cuff for fixation, as this may be stronger than the osteoporotic bone in older patients. Enders rods may be needed for longitudinal stability. Plate and screw fixation is a reasonable option if adequate purchase can be achieved by the screw in the humeral cortex.

The indications for hemiarthroplasty for acute proximal humerus fractures are four-part fractures and fracture-dislocations, anatomic neck and head-splitting fractures that cannot be anatomically reduced and secured, and impression fractures involving greater than ~40% of the articular surface. Although ORIF is the treatment of choice for most three-part fractures (2, 3, 8, 20, 21, 35, 36), it has yielded much less satisfactory results in older patients with osteopenic bone and/or comminution precluding the establishment of a stable construct (3, 4, 8, 10, 16, 40, 43). Thus, hemiarthroplasty is also indicated in these selected three-part fractures. Some surgeons advocate ORIF of four-part fractures in young patients who have good bone stock (12–14, 20, 21, 24, 28, 35). The high risk of malunion and avascular necrosis (AVN) is acknowledged, with the understanding that late arthroplasty may be necessary (7). Esser (13, 14) and others (12, 28) have reported excellent results for ORIF in four-part fractures; other surgeons, however, have not been able to duplicate their results. In a review of the 123 four-part fractures and fracture-dislocations treated with internal fixation (ORIF) in the literature from 1970 to 1996, 56 (46%) had satisfactory results and 67 (54%) were unsatisfactory. This is in comparison to 78% excellent or satisfactory results with hemiarthroplasty. A direct prospective comparison of ORIF versus hemiarthroplasty for four-part fractures has not been performed.

The timing of hemiarthroplasty is also an important consideration. Surgery should be performed as soon as the patient is medically stable, preferably within the first 7 to 10 days after the injury. Expeditious surgery may avoid the problems of early tuberosity healing in a malunited position, muscle atrophy, soft tissue contractures, and the development of heterotopic ossification. Neer and McIlveen (33) reported ectopic bone formation in 7 of 61 patients (16%), and this complication usually developed in shoulders when surgery was delayed for longer than 10 days. Surgery is technically easier in the acute setting, and functional outcome is more predictable.

Technique

Preoperatively, the shoulder and axilla must be kept clean, and skin maceration (e.g., from a tight sling) should be avoided. General or regional (interscalene brachial plexus block) anesthesia may be used. The author prefers long-acting interscalene block anesthesia because it is safe, effective, and improves postoperative comfort. The patient is placed in the beach-chair position, with the head supported by a well-padded headrest and the injured limb supported by a short arm board. All bony prominences, including the heels, must be padded. The patient is positioned at the edge of the table with the injured arm hanging over the edge. This allows free extension of the arm, which facilitates exposure of the humeral canal if necessary. A small roll or pad is placed under the vertebral border of the scapula to stabilize it laterally. The preparation includes the shoulder, lateral neck, axilla, chest wall, front and back toward the midline, and ipsilateral arm to the wrist. The shoulder is draped with the arm free to allow positioning during surgery. Intravenous, prophylactic, broad-spectrum antibiotics are administered preoperatively and continued for 24 to 48 hours depending on the type of procedure.

SURGICAL APPROACHES

There are two basic surgical approaches for the treatment of proximal humeral fractures. The first is the superior deltoid approach (2) (Fig. 2.3B). The skin incision is made in Langer's lines just lateral to the anterolateral aspect of the acromion. Through this approach, the deltoid can be split from the edge of the acromion distally for approximately 4 to 5 cm. The deltoid origin is not removed, allowing exposure of the superior aspect of the proximal humerus. This approach is useful for internal fixation of greater tuberosity fractures and helpful for the insertion of a proximal intramedullary rod. Rotation, flexion, or extension of the humerus or all three greatly enhance exposure of the underlying structures.

The second approach is a long deltopectoral approach (2) (see Fig. 2.5B). In this approach, both the deltoid origin and insertion are preserved. The skin incision is started just inferior to the clavicle and extends across the coracoid process and down to the area of insertion of the deltoid. The cephalic vein

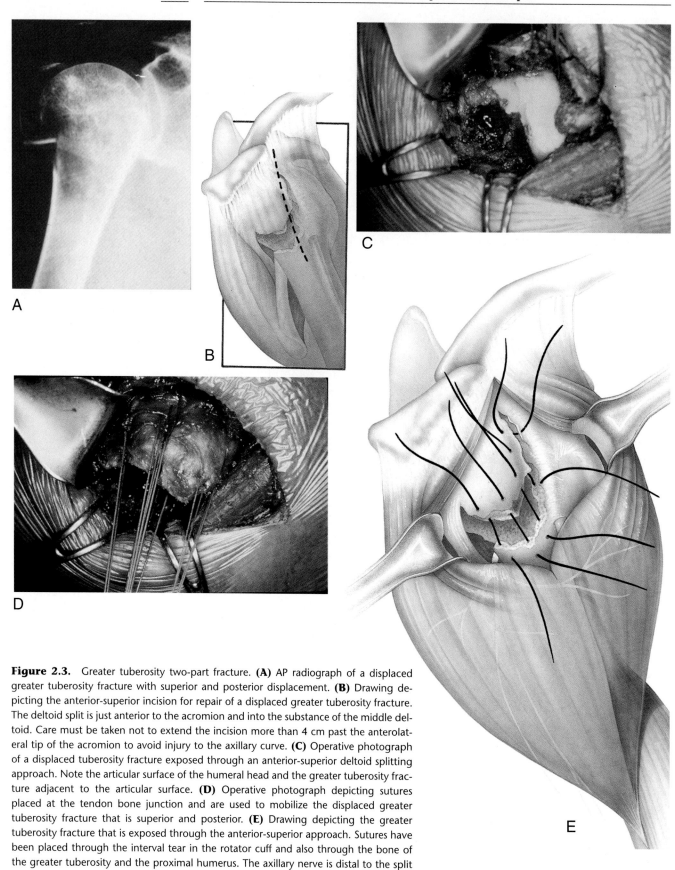

Figure 2.3. Greater tuberosity two-part fracture. **(A)** AP radiograph of a displaced greater tuberosity fracture with superior and posterior displacement. **(B)** Drawing depicting the anterior-superior incision for repair of a displaced greater tuberosity fracture. The deltoid split is just anterior to the acromion and into the substance of the middle deltoid. Care must be taken not to extend the incision more than 4 cm past the anterolateral tip of the acromion to avoid injury to the axillary curve. **(C)** Operative photograph of a displaced tuberosity fracture exposed through an anterior-superior deltoid splitting approach. Note the articular surface of the humeral head and the greater tuberosity fracture adjacent to the articular surface. **(D)** Operative photograph depicting sutures placed at the tendon bone junction and are used to mobilize the displaced greater tuberosity fracture that is superior and posterior. **(E)** Drawing depicting the greater tuberosity fracture that is exposed through the anterior-superior approach. Sutures have been placed through the interval tear in the rotator cuff and also through the bone of the greater tuberosity and the proximal humerus. The axillary nerve is distal to the split in the deltoid.

should be preserved and retracted either laterally or medially, depending on which is the easiest direction. The deltopectoral interval is dissected proximally and distally. If more exposure is needed, the superior part of the pectoralis major tendon insertion can be divided and reattached at the end of the procedure. This approach is useful for two-part surgical neck as well as three-part and four-part fractures.

Procedures that split or remove the lateral part of the acromion are unnecessary and may lead to complications. Both of these approaches are extremely worthwhile because they preserve deltoid function, which allows a more rapid rehabilitation in the postoperative period. Removal of the deltoid origin is unnecessary because it seriously affects the function of this important muscle and slows the postoperative rehabilitation program. Splitting the middle deltoid beyond 5 cm from the edge of the acromion presents a high risk of injury to the axillary nerve.

GREATER TUBEROSITY FRACTURES

In most instances, the greater tuberosity is displaced superiorly and posteriorly by the unopposed pull of the supraspinatus, infraspinatus, and teres minor muscle (Fig. 2.3A). If left to heal in this displaced position, it will block forward elevation and external rotation, especially if less than 90° of abduction. The approach that is necessary for this type of fracture is the superior approach, because it allows adequate exposure for mobilization and fixation of the displaced fracture (Fig. 2.3B).

After the approach has been made, the hemorrhagic bursa and inflamed soft tissue should be carefully cleared so that the bony edges of the displace fragment and the bed of fracture on the proximal humerus can be clearly visualized (Fig. 2.3C). Internal rotation of the arm may be needed to expose the displaced greater tuberosity. The leading edge of the lateral extension of the coracoacromial ligament may need to be resected to improve exposure. Also, downward traction on the arm will open up the subacromial space and also improve exposure.

Heavy no. 2 or no. 5 nylon sutures on large Swedged-on needles can be placed at the proximal edge of the fracture in the rotated cuff to facilitate traction on the displaced greater tuberosity (Fig. 2.3D,E). It is important not to place sutures into the bone, as there may be fissures and significant osteoporosis that may cause fragmentation of the tuberosity. The tendon may be stronger than the bone. The anterior and posterior fracture edges on the humerus must be exposed. The status of the biceps tendon must also be evaluated to rule out a dislocation anteriorly or posteriorly. The rotator cuff must be evaluated for a tear or rent in the rotator interval. Fracture hematoma and reactive bursa tissue may be cleared from the tuberosity fragment and the bed of the humerus to allow a proper fit of the displaced fracture. Anterior and posterior bursal adhesion should then be lysed to improve motion. Furthermore, a determination should be made if there is a significant impingement lesion, either a prominent acromion or a subacromial spur. Anterior acromioplasty should only be performed if there is a mechanical subacromial impingement lesion present; it is not a routine part of the procedure.

Drill holes are then made in the greater tuberosity, and four to five no. 2 nonabsorbable nylon sutures are placed anteriorly, laterally, and posteriorly in the fragment (Fig. 2.3E). Drill holes should be made in the appropriate positions at the edge of the fracture in the proximal humeral. There is often an

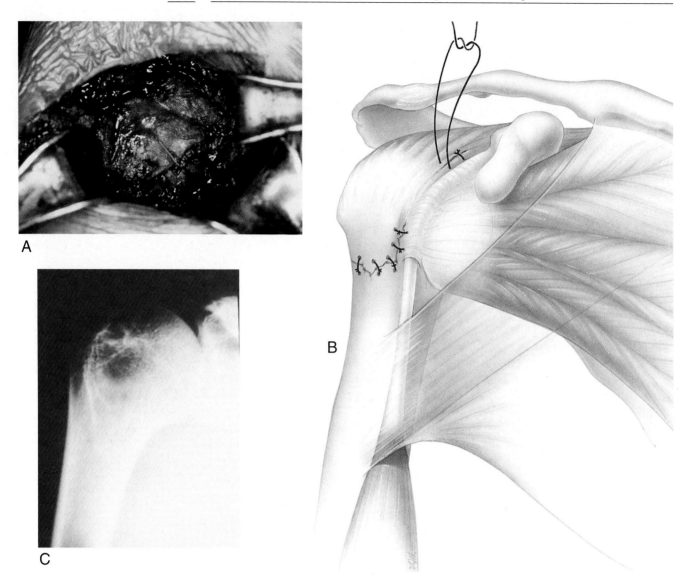

Figure 2.4.   Greater tuberosity two-part fracture. **(A)** Operative photograph showing repair of displaced greater tuberosity fractures through a superior approach. **(B)** Drawing of repair noting the rotator interval closure and the bone sutures. **(C)** Radiograph of healed greater tuberosity fracture at 1 year after surgery.

island of bone between the fracture and the posterior aspect of the bicipital groove into which sutures can be placed. The first step should be to close the rotator interval with several zero nonabsorbable nylon sutures. This stabilizes the greater tuberosity fragment which avoids posterior and superior retraction. This removes a great deal of tension from the bone repair. In addition, if there is a rent in the posterior aspect of the cuff, a suture in this rent will also help stabilize the cuff and fracture fragment. The sutures in the greater tuberosity are then placed through the drill holes in the proximal humerus, and the repair is completed (Fig. 2.4A,B). The arm is then placed through a range of motion to check stability. This should provide excellent fixation, allowing early range of motion of the proximal humerus. The arm should also be gently tested for any impingement during elevation or block to rotation (Fig. 2.4C). Lesser tuberosity fractures are quite rare, and ORIF is indicated when the fragment is large and blocks rotation or involves a significant part of the articular surface. A limited deltopectoral approach should be used. The fracture should be fixed with no. 2 nonabsorbable sutures.

SURGICAL NECK

An unimpacted or displaced two-part surgical neck fracture may require ORIF because of interposition of the biceps tendon, capsule, or subscapularis that prevents closed reduction (Fig. 2.5). Furthermore, there may be

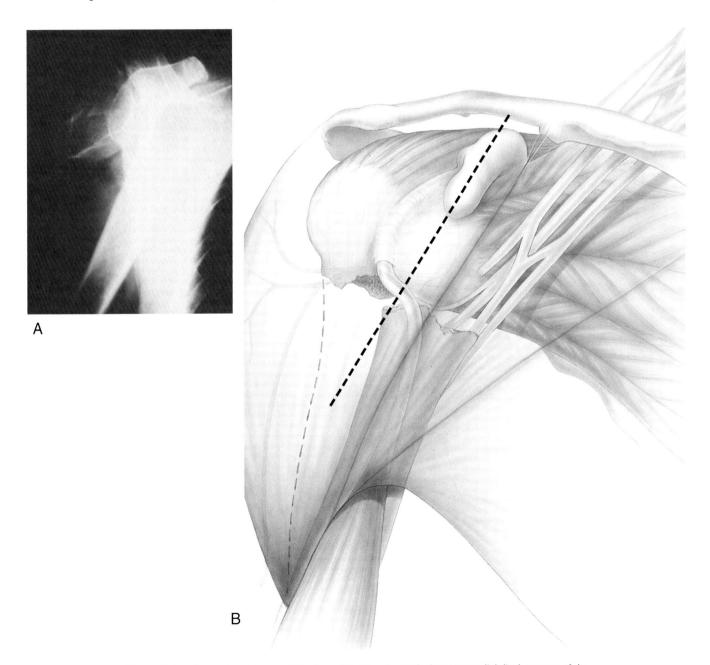

A

B

Figure 2.5. Surgical neck two-part fracture. **(A)** AP radiograph showing medial displacement of the shaft and neutral version of the humeral head because the pull of the internal and external rotators is balanced. **(B)** Drawing depicting the approach and pathology of a displaced surgical neck two-part fracture of the proximal humerus. The pectoralis major pulls the shaft medially. The long head of the biceps, capsule, and subscapularis can be interposed between the fracture. These structures may prevent a satisfactory closed reduction.

significant comminution at this area that does not allow a stable closed reduction. A long deltopectoral approach is the preferred method for exposure of this fracture (Fig. 2.5B). After the superficial exposure, it is important to identify the coracoid and strap muscles, the short head of the biceps, and coracobrachealis. Dissection medial to these is not recommended because it may result in damage to the neurovascular structures. It is important to identify the long head of the biceps because this structure may be interposed in the fracture fragment. Furthermore, this structure can be followed proximally and will allow identification of the lesser and greater tuberosities as well as the bicipital grooved area. Traction may be placed on the humerus to improve exposure. Small pieces of bone may be removed but should not be discarded and may be used for bone graft in situ following adequate ORIF. The fracture site should be carefully inspected for interposition of soft tissue, and the two ends of the fracture should be freed of soft tissue interposition so that a reduction can be achieved. At this time, it is important to determine the stability of the reduction and the need for longitudinal fixation.

Heavy nonabsorbable sutures may be placed through the rotator cuff to provide traction to improve exposure. The leading edge of the anterolateral aspect of the coracoacromial ligament may also be resected to improve exposure in the subacromial space. Internal fixation is accomplished with heavy, nonabsorbable sutures (no. 2 or no. 5) or wire incorporating the tuberosities and rotator cuff tendon (Fig. 2.6C). Sutures through the strong rotator cuff tendon insertion are usually more secure than other types of fixation in soft osteoporotic bone. Wires provide greater immediate stability but may be an irritant to the subacromial space. They may also break and migrate. Therefore, heavy nonabsorbable sutures are preferred when possible.

For surgical neck fractures that can be reduced and impacted, heavy sutures incorporating the rotator cuff may be used for fixation. For comminuted surgical neck fractures, longitudinal fixation is supplemented with intramedullary rods placed adjacent to the articular surface just inside the greater and lesser tuberosities (Fig. 2.6A,B). Small longitudinal incisions in the rotator cuff tendon are used to place these nails. A second superior split in the deltoid to facilitate nail insertion may be made through the same skin incision. The deltoid is subcutaneously exposed through. The Enders rods augment longitudinal stability and enhance the rigidity of the fixation. Originally, the author used Rush pins. However, they afforded little rotation stability and often migrated superiorly, impinging against the acromial undersurface. Enders nails were used in the latter part of the series (11). These nails are superior to straight rods because they provide three-point fixation (Fig. 2.6D). The figure-of-eight wire or suture is then passed through the eyelets of the nail, helping to prevent superior migration. However, the slot is long, and an appreciable amount of the metal can protrude proximally. The author and coworkers have modified the Enders nails with an additional hole above the slot for suture or wire incorporation. This allows insertion of the nail deeper into the head so that its proximal tip is below the surface of the tendons. The suture or wire is passed deep to the tendon, preventing proximal migration of the nail (Fig. 2.6A,B). The shoulder is then put through a range of motion, and the stability of the fixation is assessed. The rotator cuff incision and deltopectoral interval and skin are closed over suction drains.

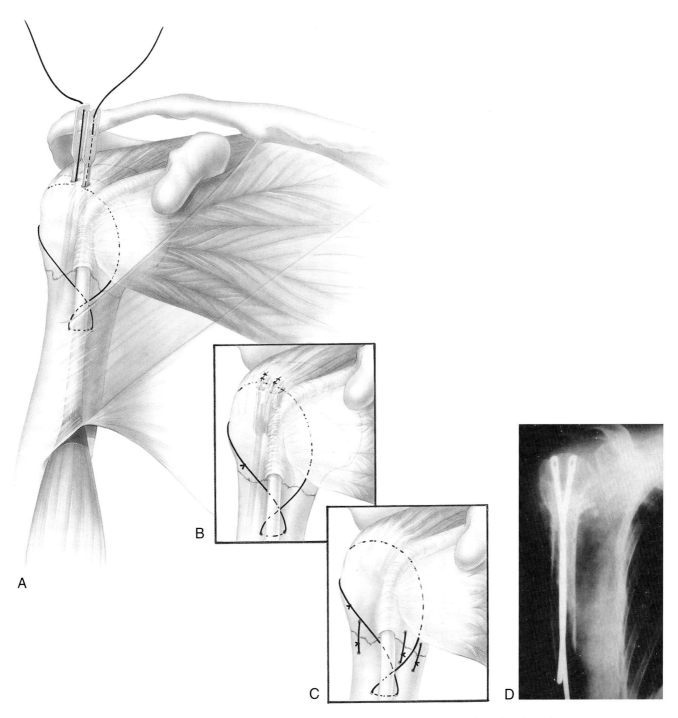

Figure 2.6. Operative repair of surgical neck two-part fracture. **(A)** Drawing depicting the reduction of a surgical neck fracture with the insertion of two Enders rods for longitudinal stability. **(B)** A no. 5 nonabsorbable nylon suture or wire can be placed through the rods as well as through the rotator cuff and the proximal shaft. The figure-of-eight configuration promotes stability. **(C)** A figure-of-eight no. 5 nylon suture or 18-gauge wire is used without Enders rods if there is minimal comminution and good longitudinal stability in the fracture. **(D)** AP radiograph of an operative repair of a displaced two-part surgical neck fracture with two Enders rods and no. 5 nonabsorbable suture.

THREE-PART FRACTURES

Closed reduction is generally less successful in the treatment of displaced three-part fractures (Fig. 2.7). These fractures are unstable because there is shaft displacement and the displaced tuberosity fragment. Repeated attempts at closed reduction should be avoided, because the fractures are often in osteoporotic bone and further fragmentation and displacement of the fragments can occur. Many methods of ORIF have been described, but the preferred method is one that uses minimal but secure internal fixation with limited soft tissue dissection.

After a long deltopectoral approach (Fig. 2.5B), the short head of the biceps and coracobracheolis should be identified. It is important not to dissect medial to these structures to avoid injury to the neurovascular structures. It is also important to determine the fracture pattern, either greater tuberosity (Fig. 2.7B) or lesser tuberosity three-part fracture (Fig. 2.7C). The more common type is the greater tuberosity three-part fracture. The fracture hematoma should be cleared from the subacromial space and the lesser tuberosity. The leading edge of the anterolateral aspect of the coracoacromial ligament can be resected to improve exposure of the subacromial space. Heavy nylon sutures may be placed through the rotator cuff, supraspinatus, and subscapularis to provide traction for increased exposure. Longitudinal traction may also be placed in the shaft of the humerus to improve exposure.

In three-part fractures, the displaced tuberosity is repaired to the head and the other tuberosity first, and then these fragments together are repaired with figure-of-eight sutures to drill holes in the shaft (Fig. 2.8A–C). Heavy (no. 2 or no. 5) nonabsorbable nylon sutures or wire are the preferred methods of fixation. Several no. 2 or no. 5 sutures or 18-gauge figure-of-eight wires provide adequate fixation in most cases. The sutures should be passed through the rotator cuff and the bone because the rotator cuff may be stronger and provide better fixation than the osteoporotic bone. A large 14- or 16-gauge spinal needle or plastic catheter is helpful in passing sutures or wire through the cuff. If longitudinal fixation is needed, an Enders rod may be placed through the head and tuberosity fragment (depending on the fracture) (Fig. 2.8A) to improve fixation and should then be tested for secure fixation through a range of motion. The rotator interval is closed. The subcutaneous tissue and skin are carefully closed (Fig. 2.8D).

PROSTHESES

A long deltopectoral approach is preferred for placing a prosthesis for a four-part fracture (Fig. 2.9A–C). After the coracoid process is identified, the clavipectoral fascia is incised lateral to the coracoid muscles, which are gently retracted medially. The hemorrhagic bursa and fracture hematoma are irrigated and debrided, and the subacromial space is cleared. The leading anterior edge of the coracoacromial ligament is usually excised to enhance superior exposure. Subacromial decompression is not a formal part of this procedure, but if the subacromial space is tight and there is mechanical impingement, an anterior acromioplasty may be performed to prevent postoperative impingement and facilitate range of motion.

Identification of the four major segments of the proximal humerus in fracture surgery is critical and may be difficult. The long head of the biceps tendon, found under the upper edge of the pectoralis tendon, is a useful guide proximally to the rotator interval between the lesser and greater tuberosities

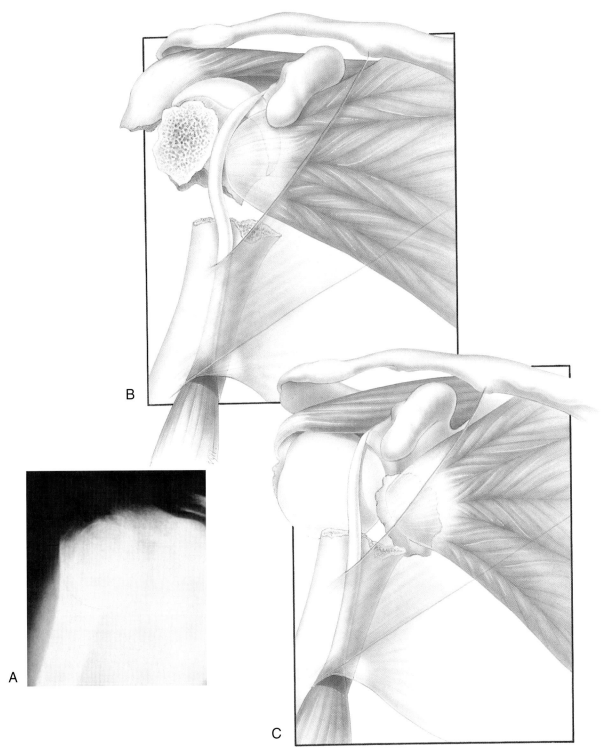

Figure 2.7. Three-part fracture. **(A)** AP radiograph of a greater tuberosity three-part fracture. There is displacement of the greater tuberosity, shaft, and head fragment with lesser tuberosity. **(B)** Drawing of a three-part greater tuberosity fracture. The humeral head is rotated inward due to the unopposed pull of the subscapularis. The shaft is displaced medially, secondary to the pull of the pectoralis major. The greater tuberosity is displaced superiorly and/or posteriorly secondary to the pull of the external rotators. **(C)** Drawing depicting the pathology of a lesser tuberosity three-part fracture. The head is rotated outward so the articular surface is facing anteriorly due to the unopposed pull of the external rotators. The lesser tuberosity fragment is displaced medially because of the pull of the subscapularis. The shaft is pulled medially because of the pull of the pectoralis major.

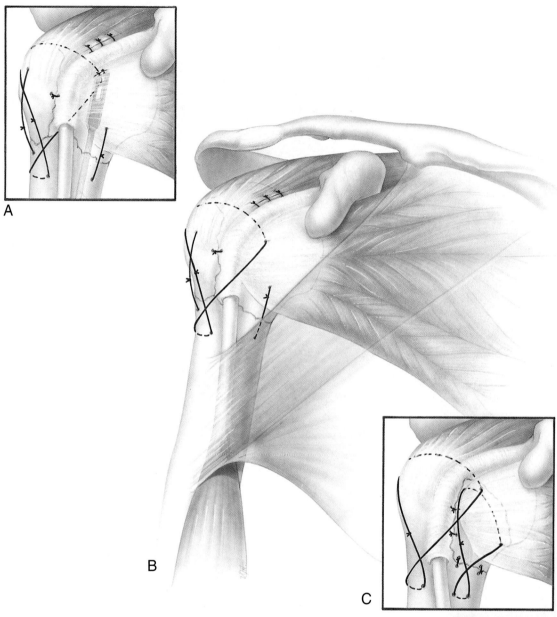

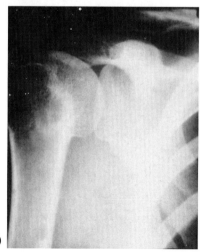

Figure 2.8. Operative repair of three-part fractures. **(A)** Drawing depicting an operative repair of a three-part greater tuberosity fracture with heavy no. 5 nonabsorbable sutures or wire. The greater tuberosity fragment is repaired both to the head and lesser tuberosity fragment as well as to the shaft. The lesser tuberosity and head fragment is also repaired to the shaft. An Enders rod has been inserted into the lesser tuberosity for longitudinal stability. **(B)** Drawing depicting a three-part greater tuberosity fracture repaired by figure-of-eight sutures without an Enders rod because there is longitudinal stability. If there is a rent in the rotator interval, this is also repaired with nonabsorbable zero nylon sutures. **(C)** Drawing depicting an operative repair of a three-part lesser tuberosity fracture. The lesser tuberosity fragment is repaired both to the head and greater tuberosity fragment as well as to the shaft. If longitudinal stability is needed, an Enders rod can be placed in the greater tuberosity fragment. **(D)** AP radiograph of a healed three-part greater tuberosity fracture at 1 year after surgery. An Enders rod was not needed for longitudinal stability.

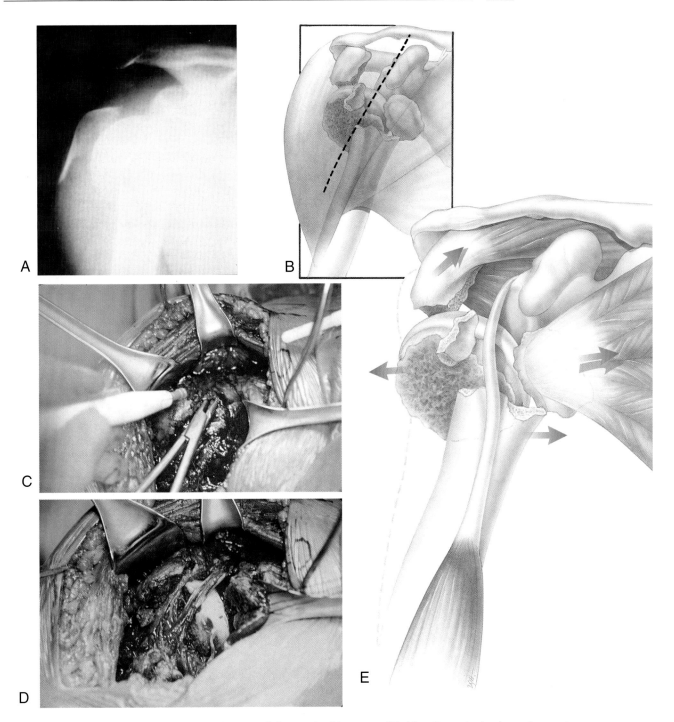

Figure 2.9. Four-part fracture of the proximal humerus. **(A)** AP radiograph showing a four-part fracture of the proximal humerus. The head is subluxated laterally. The greater tuberosity is superior, and the lesser tuberosity is medial. **(B)** Drawing depicting the long deltopectoral approach needed to expose a four-part fracture. **(C)** Operative photograph showing the rotator interval being opened. The biceps tendon is inferior to this incision, and the biceps is used to find the glenohumeral joint. **(D)** Operative photograph of the exposed humeral head with greater tuberosity superior, lesser tuberosity medial, and the long head of the biceps over the articular surface. **(E)** Drawing depicting a four-part fracture of the proximal humerus with the greater tuberosity being pulled superiorly and posteriorly, the head subluxating laterally, the lesser tuberosity being displaced medially, and the shaft also being displaced medially. The head is a free-floating fragment secondary to the lack of soft tissue attachment.

(Fig. 2.9C). The biceps tendon should be preserved throughout the procedure and can be retracted anteriorly or posteriorly. The bicipital groove may be fractured as an intermediate fragment between the tuberosities or attached to one of the displaced tuberosities. The lesser tuberosity is usually displaced medially from the pull of the subscapularis, and the greater tuberosity may be displaced superiorly (beneath the acromion), posteriorly, or both from the pull of the supraspinatus and infraspinatus (Fig. 2.9D,E). If the greater tuberosity is far posterior, traction and extension and dissection with a blunt elevation are helpful to retrieve the tuberosity. Number two heavy nylon stay sutures are placed around the tuberosities at the level of the tendon-bone attachment (Fig. 2.10). This allows mobilization of the fragments and their associated muscles. Fracture lines and comminution within the tuberosities should not be disrupted as the intact soft tissue sleeve will assist in tuberosity healing. It should be emphasized that the subscapularis tendon should not be taken down from its attachment on the lesser tuberosity; it should be mobilized as a bone/tendon unit (to preserve blood supply) through the fracture line at the base of the tuberosity. During mobilization of this lesser tuberosity/subscapularis unit, care must be taken to identify and protect the axillary nerve and anterior humeral circumflex vessels. This is especially pertinent in procedures performed 2 to 3 weeks after injury and in elderly patients with friable, atherosclerotic vessels. In addition, further comminution of osteoporotic tuberosity fragments through vigorous retraction should be avoided.

If the tuberosities are separated by the fracture, the lesser tuberosity is retracted medially and the greater laterally; the head fragment is then removed and preserved as a source of potential bone graft. However, if the tuberosities remain attached to each other with an intact rotator interval but cover the displaced head fragment, their anatomic relationship may be preserved. They may be lifted up like a hood to enable extraction of the head fragment. This technique has the advantage of reducing the risk of postoperative tuberosity displacement. If this cannot be done, the head is extracted in the standard fashion after opening the interval and separating the tuberosities.

Caution should be exercised with anterior fracture-dislocations, because the humeral head may be difficult to extricate from under the coracoid muscles and may lie in close proximity to the axillary artery and brachial plexus. Usually the subscapularis tendon and muscle provide a protective barrier, but the head may be dislocated below the subscapularis. After the position of the neurovascular structures are identified, the head fragment is carefully and atraumatically removed.

The arm is then extended, adducted, and externally rotated, delivering the humeral canal and shaft. The medullary canal is prepared with sequential reamers. Proper stem size is determined by preoperative templating radiographs and by the humeral trials, determining which stem best fills the medullary canal. Because cement fixation is indicated in all cases of hemiarthroplasty for proximal humerus fractures, there is no need to obtain a tight press-fit of the prosthetic humeral shaft into the canal. Using too large a stem and cement risks intraoperative humeral shaft fracture, especially in osteopenic bone. Proper head size is estimated by evaluating the removed head fragment, measuring with templating, and using the contralateral shoulder if available. Head size is ultimately determined by assessing tuberosity and rotator cuff tension after insertion of the trial prosthesis and reapproximation of the tuberosities and cuff (Fig. 2.11, see Fig. 2.14B and Fig 2.15A).

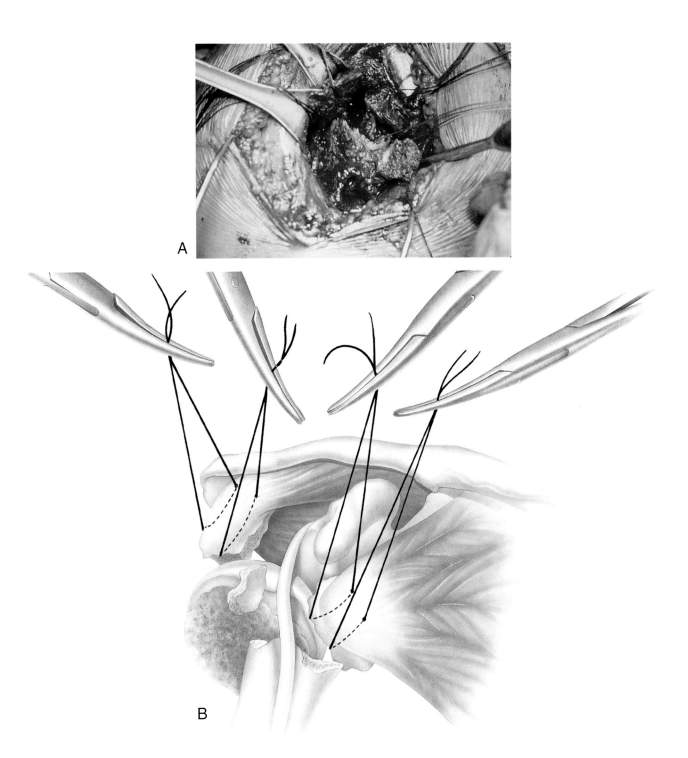

Figure 2.10. Operative exposure of four-part fracture. **(A)** Operative photograph depicting the four-part fracture of the proximal humerus. The head has been removed. Sutures placed at the tendon bone junction help to retract the greater and lesser tuberosities. The shaft has been exposed in the inferior aspect of the wound. **(B)** Drawing also depicting the fracture pathology with sutures in the tendon bone junction for exposure. The biceps tendon is in the middle of the field but can be retracted anteriorly or posteriorly, whichever is easier.

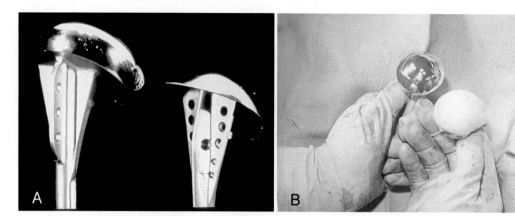

Figure 2.11. The proximal humeral prosthesis. **(A)** The original Neer prosthesis (right), which was designed in 1951, and the new design (left), which was modified in 1973. Currently, modular prostheses are also available. **(B)** Humeral head size is estimated by removing the head fragment and measuring against the prosthesis with templates or using the contralateral shoulder radiograph if available. However, the ultimate decision concerning head size is determined by the assessment of the tuberosity and rotator cuff tension after insertion of the trial prosthesis and reapproximation of the tuberosities and cuff.

A careful determination regarding the proper height of the prosthesis must be made. Through the achievement of proper height and anatomic humeral head retroversion, satisfactory length and tension will be restored to the myofascial sleeve and allow placement of the tuberosities beneath the prosthetic head against the shaft of the proximal humerus. If the prosthesis is placed deep into the remaining shaft and not left appropriately proud, especially in fractures with significant comminution and loss of bone substance at the level of the surgical neck, the myofascial sleeve will be too lax and inferior subluxation and/or dislocation will occur. However, a prosthesis that is placed too proud will effectively "overstuff" the joint, place excessive tension on the soft tissues, and lead to postoperative stiffness. The tension in the biceps tendon can sometimes be helpful in establishing the proper height of the prosthesis. If necessary, a portion of the humeral head may be used as a bone graft to support the prosthesis at the appropriate height. Several large pieces of the head may be used, or a U-shaped or doughnut-shaped graft can be fashioned from the humeral head.

The proper version of the prosthesis is important for postoperative stability and function. It should be positioned at approximately 30 to 40° of retroversion in routine acute fracture cases (Fig. 2.12A,B). This position can be identified by comparing the head position with the distal epicondylar axis of the humerus and usually involves placing the fin just posterior to the bicipital groove. Slight anterior placement of the prosthetic fin increases retroversion, and posterior placement decreases retroversion. Version should be appropriately decreased or increased in procedures for anterior or posterior fracture-dislocations, respectively. The exact amount of version alteration in these complex cases depends on associated bony and soft tissue injuries as well as the chronicity of the dislocation. The humeral shaft following a fracture usually does not have enough bony support to allow a trial reduction of a prosthesis. However, if a sponge is placed down the shaft, this provides enough support for insertion of a prosthesis, allowing a trial reduction to evaluate anterior and posterior stability. The prosthesis should be stable in the limits of external rotation (60°) and internal rotation (30°) with the arm at the side.

Secure fixation of the prosthesis within the medullary canal of the proximal humerus routinely requires polymethylmethacrylate fixation. The canal should be prepared by removing loose bone, blood, and debris (Fig. 2.13A). Cement is necessary to provide rotational stability and will prevent possible

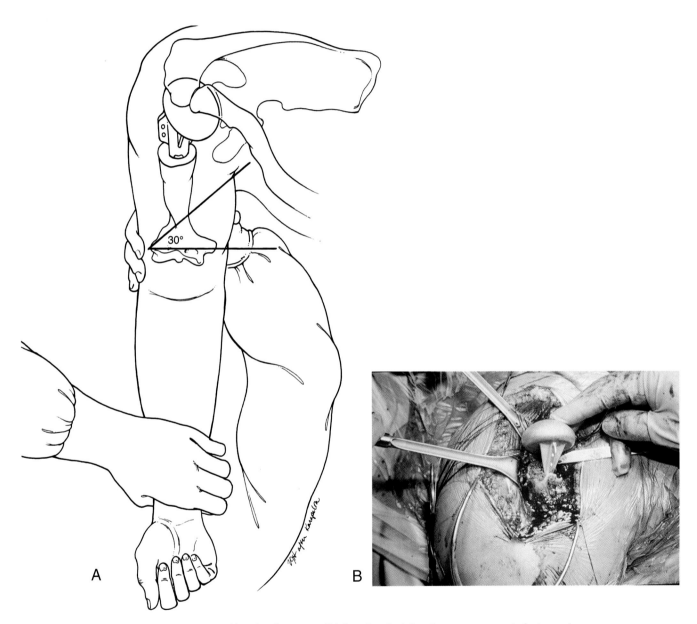

Figure 2.12. Humeral head replacement. **(A)** Drawing depicting the proper amount of retroversion (approximately 30–40°). This position can be identified by comparing the head position with the distal epicondylar axis of the humerus. Usually, the fin is placed just posterior to the bicipital groove. Slight anterior placement of the lateral fin increases retroversion, and posterior placement decreases retroversion. **(B)** Operative photograph showing testing of a trial prosthesis for version as well as proper height and length tension. Proper height is determined by estimating the length of the tuberosities and approximating them to the shaft. It is important that the tuberosities are fixed below the humeral head. The humeral shaft is prepared for cement insertion using a thrombin-soaked sponge to improve hemostasis.

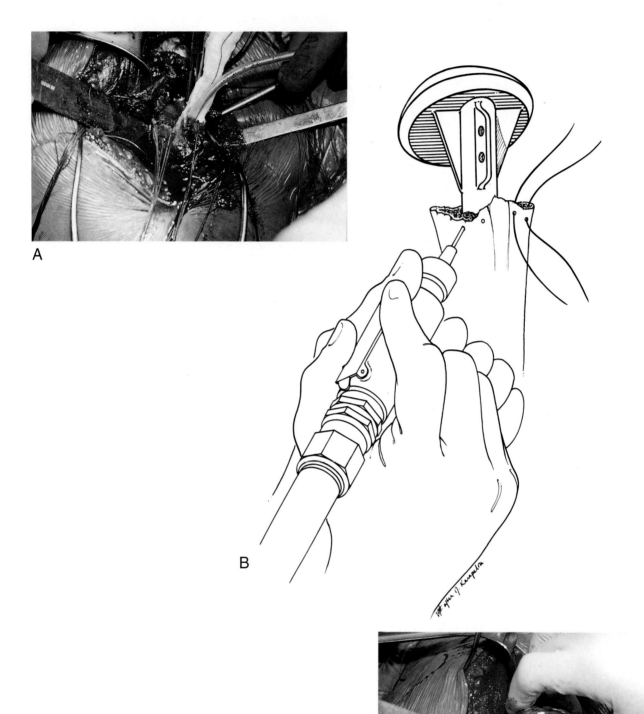

A

B

C

Figure 2.13. Operative repair of four-part fracture. **(A)** Operative photograph showing canal preparation with a thrombin-soaked sponge and suction tip. **(B)** A trial prosthesis is used as a guide for placement of the holes for the tuberosity repair. It is important to perform this before the cementing so the sutures can be passed. Generally, three to four heavy nonabsorbable nylon sutures are placed for the greater tuberosity, and two to three are placed for the lesser tuberosity. **(C)** The humeral head has been cemented into position in the appropriate amount of retroversion.

subsequent prosthetic rotation and/or subsidence within the osteoporotic humeral shaft, with resulting loss of version and stability. Before cementing, drill holes are made in the proximal shaft and nonabsorbable no. 2 or no. 5 sutures are placed (Fig. 2.13B). These sutures are used during tuberosity reconstruction to prevent their superior displacement; three to four sutures are used for the greater tuberosity and two to three are used for the lesser tuberosity (Fig. 2.13B). The prosthesis is then cemented in place with proper height and retroversion reestablished (Fig. 2.13C). A distal cement restrictor can be used to prevent the intramedullary extravasation of cement toward the elbow. However, care must be taken to avoid pressurization of the humeral canal with doughy cement and a large prosthesis, especially in patients with thin, osteoporotic bone, as this can cause the humeral shaft to fracture. Excess cement is then carefully removed at the site of the surgical neck to allow the bone-to-bone contact necessary to achieve tuberosity union. There should be overlap between the tuberosity fragments and the humeral shaft.

The proper head diameter will achieve stability and also allow closure of the rotator cuff around the prosthesis without undue tension (Fig. 2.14A).

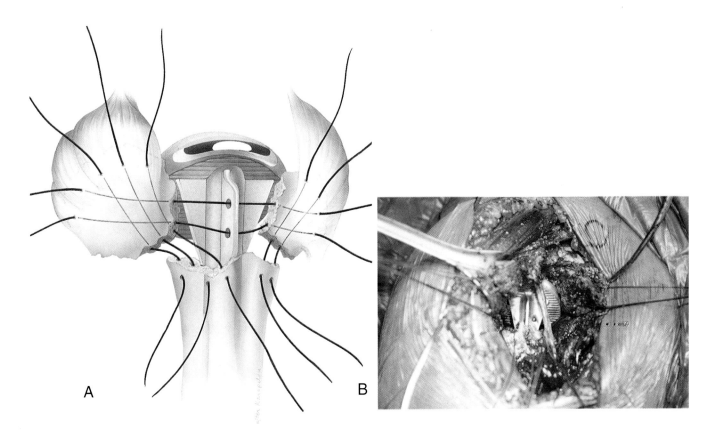

A   B

Figure 2.14. Operative repair of the tuberosities and four-part fractures. **(A)** Drawing depicting the procedure for reattachment of the tuberosities to both the prosthesis and the humeral shaft. **(B)** Operative photograph showing relocation of the biceps tendon and preparation for repair of both tuberosities. The tuberosities must be secured below the head of the prosthesis to avoid impingement. The greater tuberosity is repaired first, followed by repair of the lesser tuberosity. Finally, the sutures to the fin of the prosthesis in both tuberosities are tied. Cancellous bone graft from the humeral head may be used as bone graft beneath the tuberosity fragments as necessary. Again, it is important that the edges of the tuberosities overlap with the edge of the humeral shaft to ensure proper tuberosity healing.

Since the advent of modular humeral prostheses, more choices are available to the surgeon regarding head sizes to fit the prosthesis to a particular patient and condition. Various trial head sizes are available and should be compared to establish maximum stability and range of motion. When debating between two different head sizes that both maintain stability, it is usually preferable to err toward the smaller size to allow improved range of motion. Too large a head occupies the majority of the capsular volume and does not allow adequate excursion of the posterior/inferior capsule necessary for elevation. In addition, the smaller head size facilitates tuberosity reattachment. The previously placed stay sutures in the greater and lesser tuberosity/cuff units that aided in mobilization are used to reduce the tuberosities to the humeral shaft beneath the prosthetic head (Fig. 2.14A,B).

Once the prosthesis has been cemented within the humeral shaft and the proper head size selected, attention is focused on secure tuberosity reconstruction and rotator cuff repair. The biceps tendon is placed back in its groove, and the previously placed large nonabsorbable sutures are now used to reduce the tuberosities and secure them to the fin of the prosthesis, to each other, and to the proximal humeral shaft (Fig. 2.15). The tuberosities must be secured below the prosthetic head to avoid subsequent impingement. The greater tuberosity is repaired first, followed by repair of the lesser tuberosity. Finally, the sutures through the fin of the prosthesis and both tuberosities are tied (Fig. 2.15C). Cancellous bone graft from the humeral head may be used as bone graft beneath the tuberosity fragments as necessary. Again, it is important that the edge of the tuberosities overlap with the edge of the humeral shaft to ensure proper tuberosity healing.

The rotator cuff interval between the supraspinatus and subscapularis tendon is repaired, and the leading edge of the pectoralis major tendon is repaired anatomically (Fig. 2.15C). The arm is then placed through a careful range of motion, and the tuberosity repair inspected. This evaluation aids the surgeon in planning the limits of the postoperative rehabilitation program. Closed suction drains are placed under the deltoid, and the deltopectoral interval is reapproximated. Subcuticular skin closure is preferred, and the limb is immobilized in a carefully padded sling and swathe (Fig. 2.16).

REHABILITATION

Rehabilitation of the shoulder after repair for a displaced proximal humerus fracture is essential, because adequate motion is needed to optimize function. The most useful protocol is the three-phase system described by Hughes and Neer (19, 32). Each rehabilitation program is individualized for the patient, and the surgeon is intimately involved in the program throughout its course.

The surgeon determines the initial rehabilitation program at the time of surgery. Factors considered in this decision are the quality of the soft tissues and bone, status of the rotator cuff and deltoid, security of the internal fixator, tuberosity fixation to the humeral shaft and to each other (in the case of a prosthesis), intraoperative range of motion achieved, and the overall condition of the patient as well as his or her ability to participate in therapy. A sling is generally used for protection but is removed several times a day for exercises for 6 weeks or until the fracture is healed. The first goal of therapy is restoration of glenohumeral and scapulothoracic motion. The patient must clearly understand the difference between early passive motion

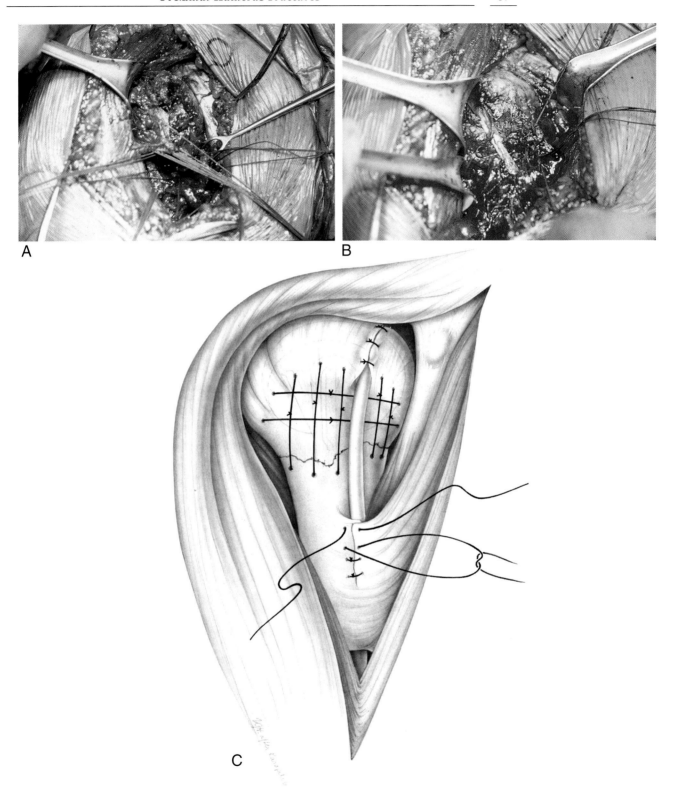

Figure 2.15. Operative repair of four-part fracture. **(A)** In this operative photograph, the tuberosities have been mobilized and pulled down beneath the head of the prosthesis. **(B)** In this operative photograph, the sutures have been tied with replacement of the biceps tendon in an anatomical position in closure of the rotator cuff. **(C)** Drawing depicting the final repair. The horizontal sutures go beneath the biceps and through the fin of the prosthesis.

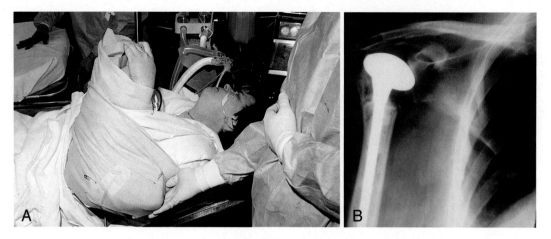

Figure 2.16. Postoperative Four-Part Fracture. **(A)** Operative photograph depicting the bulky dressing in a secure position after repair of a four-part fracture. **(B)** AP radiograph showing healed tuberosities after a humeral head prosthesis for a four-part fracture.

(performed in the immediate postoperative period) and later active motion and strengthening (performed after motion is restored and tuberosity union has occurred). The patient must be warned that too vigorous early active exercises may result in tuberosity displacement, which is a devastating complication (3, 17, 43).

Passive motion is begun on the first postoperative day. This is initially limited to passive elevation in the plane of the scapula and is performed by the surgeon or therapist. The patient is instructed in gentle gravity-assisted pendulum exercises and is encouraged to perform range of motion exercises for the ipsilateral hand, wrist, and elbow. Supine passive external rotation with a stick within defined limitations (usually less than 30°) is begun on the second or third postoperative day. Pulley-assisted elevation can involve a significant active component and is avoided until tuberosity union has occurred.

Initial exercises are performed three times daily, with each session lasting approximately 10 to 15 minutes. While hospitalized, patients are taught and assisted in their therapy programs by the physical therapist and are advised to exercise independently each day as soon as they learn how to properly perform the exercises alone. A friend or family member is instructed in performing passive elevation of the arm, so that this may be done on days when outpatient physical therapy is not available. These passive exercises are continued for approximately 6 weeks. At the time of discharge from the hospital, the patient should have a good understanding of how to perform the rehabilitation program properly and should have achieved approximately 140° of elevation and 20 to 30° of external rotation.

Assisted elevation with a pulley and isometric strengthening of the rotator cuff and deltoid are initiated when there is evidence of tuberosity healing (at approximately 6 to 8 weeks after the operation). The patient is taught to assist the elevation of the involved shoulder with the opposite extremity through the pulley system. Gradually the patient is taught to use the involved extremity muscles more actively and the contralateral extremity muscles less assistively. Shoulder extension and internal rotation stretching exercises are then initiated. Activities of daily living including performing personal hygiene tasks, eating, and washing are advanced to build muscle strength and endurance. The patient is instructed to use the arm initially at waist level and close to the body, and then gradually (in the ensuing weeks) to begin to reach outward and upward. The other arm should be used for support as necessary and as dictated by comfort and lack of pain. Gentle stretching is encouraged during this phase to ensure that motion is maintained and gradually improved. These stretches are gentle and emphasize full glenohumeral and scapulothoracic elevation.

More aggressive stretching and strengthening exercises are initiated at approximately 12 weeks after the operation. Theraband progressive resistance exercises and light weights of 1 to 3 pounds are used when the patient has achieved almost complete motion without pain. The patient requires encouragement and should be congratulated upon successful progress and perseverance. The patient must also understand that maximum benefits are often not achieved until 12 to 18 months after the operation.

RESULTS

Various techniques have been proposed to treat fractures of the proximal humerus. Results have been variable depending on a variety of different factors, including the type of fracture, quality of the bone and soft tissue, age and reliability of the patient, and fracture healing. The results from ORIF using the technique of limited internal fixation of displaced fractures has had a high percentage of acceptable results. Flatow et al. (15) reported satisfactory results in 12 patients having ORIF (with sutures) of displaced two-part fractures of the greater tuberosity of the proximal humerus. All fractures healed without postoperative displacement, and internal fixation by heavy nonabsorbable sutures provided enough stability for early passive motion. Six patients had excellent results and six had good results, with active elevation averaging 170°.

Cuomo et al. (11) reported that 96% of patients with two-part and three-part displaced surgical neck fractures of the proximal humerus had satisfactory results with ORIF. In this series, a technique of limited internal fixation was used for these displaced fractures. Eighty-two percent of patients had good or excellent results, and 14% had satisfactory results. There was only one unsatisfactory result. In these patients, there was satisfactory fixation allowing early passive motion.

The results of primary prosthetic replacement for severe fractures of the proximal humerus have been extensively reported (1, 5, 10, 16, 17, 23, 27, 31, 34). In reviewing the literature, 77% of 355 patients with proximal humerus fractures treated with hemiarthroplasty have had excellent or satisfactory results. The achievement of a relatively painless shoulder is reliable, with most studies reporting greater than 90% satisfactory pain relief. The rate of return of active motion and function, however, is more variable. This is likely due to the many factors that influence functional outcome, including the patient's age, gender, and motivation; the fracture type; and the timing of surgery. In addition, adherence to important technical factors (restoration of humeral length, anatomic reconstruction and healing of tuberosities, appropriate version, and soft tissue tensioning) and to an extended supervised rehabilitation program are necessary to maximize the patient's function.

The expected active forward elevation after hemiarthroplasty for a proximal humerus fracture ranges from 90° to 120°. The achievement of up to

150° of elevation, however, is possible with a properly performed procedure in a well-motivated patient with good rotator cuff and deltoid muscles.

REFERENCES

1. Bade MA, Warren RF, Ranawat C, et al. Long-term results of Neer TSR. In: Bateman JE, Walsh RP, eds. Surgery of the shoulder. St. Louis: CV Mosby, 1984:194–302.
2. Bigliani LU. Treatment of two- and three-part fractures of the proximal humerus. American Academy of Orthopaedic Surgeons Instructional Course Lectures. 1989;39:231–244.
3. Bigliani LU. Fractures of the proximal humerus. In: Rockwood CA, Green DP, eds. Fractures in adults. 3rd ed. Philadelphia: JB Lippincott, 1990:871–927.
4. Bigliani LU. Malunion of four-part anterior fracture-dislocation following open reduction internal fixation. Tech Orthop 1994;9:99–101.
5. Bigliani LU, McCluskey GM. Prosthetic replacement in acute fractures of the proximal humerus. Semin Arthroplasty 1990;1:129–137.
6. Bloom MH, Obata WG. Diagnosis of posterior dislocation of the shoulder with use of Velpeau axillary and angle up roentgenographic views. J Bone Joint Surg 1967;49A:943–949.
7. Brooks CH, Revell WJ, Heatley FW. Vascularity of the humeral head after proximal humeral fractures. J Bone Joint Surg 1993;75B:132–136.
8. Cofield RH. Comminuted fractures of the proximal humerus. Clin Orthop 1988;230:49–57.
9. Compito CA, Self EB, Bigliani LU. Arthroplasty and acute shoulder trauma: reasons for success and failure. Clin Orthop 1994;307:27–36.
10. Connor PM, D'Alessandro DF. Role of hemiarthroplasty for proximal humeral fractures. J South Orthop Assoc 1995;4:9–23.
11. Cuomo F, Flatow EL, Maday MG, et al. Open reduction and internal fixation of two- and three-part displaced surgical neck fractures of the proximal humerus. J Shoulder Elbow Surg 1992;1:287–295.
12. Darder A, Darder A, Sanchis I, et al. Four-part displaced proximal humeral fractures: operative treating using Kirschner wires and a tension band. J Orthop Trauma 1993;7:497–505.
13. Esser RD. Treatment of three- and four-part fractures of the proximal humerus with a modified cloverleaf plate. J Orthop Trauma 1994;8:15–22.
14. Esser RD. Open reduction and internal fixation of three- and four-part fractures of the proximal humerus. Clin Orthop 1994;299:244–51.
15. Flatow EL, Cuomo F, Maday MG, et al. Open reduction and internal fixation of two- part displaced fractures of the greater tuberosity of the proximal part of the humerus. J Bone Joint Surg 1991;73A:1213–1218.
16. Goldman RT, Koval KJ, Cuomo F, et al. Functional outcomes after humeral head replacement for acute three- and four-part proximal humerus fractures. J Shoulder Elbow Surg 1995;4:81.
17. Green A, Barnard L, Limbrid RS. Humeral head replacement for acute, four-part proximal humerus fractures. J Shoulder Elbow Surg 1993;2:249–254.
18. Hawkins RJ, Bell RH, Gurr K. The three-part fracture of the proximal humerus: operative treatment. J Bone Joint Surg 1986;68A:1410–1414.
19. Hughes M, Neer CS. Glenohumeral joint replacement and post-operative rehabilitation. Phys Ther 1975;55:850–858.
20. Jaberg H, Warner JJ, Jakob RP. Percutaneous stabilization of unstable fractures of the humerus. J Bone Joint Surg 1992;74A:508–515.
21. Jakob RP, Miniaci A, Anson PS, et al. Four-part valgus impacted fractures of the proximal humerus. J Bone Joint Surg 1991;73B:295–298.
22. Jurik AG, Albrechtsen J. The use of computed tomography with two- and three-dimensional reconstructions in the diagnosis of three- and four-part fractures of the proximal humerus. Clin Radiol 1994;49:800–804.

23. Kraulis J, Hunter G. The results of prosthetic replacement in fracture-dislocations of the upper end of the humerus. Injury 1976;8:129–131.

24. Kristiansen B. Treatment of displaced fractures of the proximal humerus: transcutaneous reduction and Hoffman s external fixation. Injury 1989;20:195–199.

25. Leyshon RL. Closed treatment of fractures of the proximal humerus. Acta Orthop Scand 1984;55:48–51.

26. Lind T, Kroner TK, Jensen J. The epidemiology of fractures of the proximal humerus. Arch Orthop Trauma Surg 1989;108:285–287.

27. Moeckel BH, Dines DM, Warren RF, et al. Modular hemiarthroplasty for fractures of the proximal part of the humerus. J Bone Joint Surg 1992;74A:884.

28. Mouradian WH. Displaced proximal humeral fractures: seven years experience with a modified Zickel supracondylar device. Clin Orthop 1986;212:209–218.

29. Morris MF, Kilcoyne RF, Shuman W. Humeral tuberosity fractures: evaluation by CT scan and management of malunion. Orthop Trans 1987;11:242.

30. Neer CS. Displaced proximal humeral fractures: part I—classification and evaluation. J Bone Joint Surg 1970;52A:1077–1089.

31. Neer CS. Displaced proximal humeral fractures: part II—treatment of three-part and four-part displacement. J Bone Joint Surg 1970;52A:1090–1103.

32. Neer CS. Shoulder rehabilitation. In: Neer CS, ed. Shoulder reconstruction. Philadelphia: WB Saunders, 1990:487–533.

33. Neer CS, McIlveen SJ. Recent results and technique of prosthetic replacement for 4-part proximal humeral fractures. Orthop Trans 1986;10:475.

34. Nicholson GP, Flatow EL, Bigliani LU. Shoulder arthroplasty for proximal humeral fractures. In: Friedman RJ, ed. Arthroplasty of the shoulder. New York: Thieme 1994:183–193.

35. Paavolainen P, Björkenheim JM, Slätis P. Operative treatment of severe proximal humeral fractures. Acta Orthop Scand 1983;54:374–379.

36. Resch H, Beck E, Bayley I. Reconstruction of the valgus-impacted humeral head fracture. J Shoulder Elbow Surg 1995;4:73–80.

37. Rose SH, Melton LJ, Morrey BF, et al. Epidemiologic features of humeral fractures. Clin Orthop 1982;168:24–30.

38. Schai P, Imhoff A, Preiss S. Comminuted humeral head fractures: a multicenter analysis. J Shoulder Elbow Surg 1995;4:319–330.

39. Sidor ML, Zuckerman JD, Lyon T, et al. The Neer classification system for proximal humeral fractures: an assessment of interobserver reliability and intraobserver reproducibility. J Bone Joint Surg 1993;75A:1745–1750.

40. Sorensen KH. Pseudarthrosis of the surgical neck of the humerus: two cases, one bilateral. Acta Orthop Scand 1964;34:132–138.

41. Stableforth PG. Four-part fractures of the neck of the humerus. J Bone Joint Surg 1984;66A:104–108.

42. Svend-Hansen H. Displaced proximal humeral fractures. Acta Orthop Scand 1974;56:359–564.

43. Tanner MW, Cofield RH. Prosthetic arthroplasty for fractures and fracture-dislocations of the proximal humerus. Clin Orthop 1983;179:116–128.

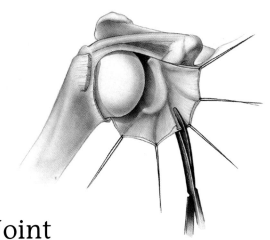

CHAPTER

3

Operative Treatment
of Degenerative and Arthritic
Diseases of the Glenohumeral Joint

MELVIN POST AND ROGER G. POLLOCK

Introduction

Reconstruction of an arthritic glenohumeral joint attempts to achieve a pain-less, functioning joint, which permits placement of the hand in a wide variety of positions that would not otherwise be possible. Although glenohumeral arthrodesis, resection arthroplasty, (71), and autogenous fibula graft (64) have places in the orthopaedic surgeon's methods of treatment, prosthetic arthroplasty is preferable in most cases, except when there is active sepsis or a flail shoulder. Arthrodesis significantly limits movement of the shoulder, drastically curtails hand placement, and requires prolonged postoperative care. Humeral head resection diminishes muscle strength and motion of the shoulder joint because the fulcrum of the shoulder is lost. Also, patients often continue to complain of localized discomfort in varying degrees. Prosthetic replacement of the humeral head yields the best results when the shoulder girdle muscles, especially those of the rotator cuff, are reasonably intact and functioning.

This chapter reviews arthrodesis, resection arthroplasty, and prosthetic replacement of the humeral head with and without glenoid surface replacement.

Clinical Evaluation

A careful history and medical evaluation are undertaken so that an accurate and complete diagnosis is known before the surgical procedure is planned. For example, rheumatoid arthritis often affects other joints and the surrounding tissues that can influence the sequence of different joint operations. If the knees and hips are severely involved with rheumatoid arthritis and require replacement, it may be best to treat the lower extremities before the shoulders. If a history of diabetes causing polyneuropathy and associated pain in the shoulder girdle is present, this may affect the decision to operate, because the overlying consideration of pain may relate more to diabetes than to any intrinsic pathology within the shoulder joint itself. Each process

73

affecting the shoulder ordinarily causes varying degrees of localized pain. Attention should be focused on its location, character, frequency, duration, variation, and distribution of radiation and intensity (123). Simply put, the surgeon should attempt to correlate the symptoms with the shoulder anatomy and physiology.

The surgeon should examine ranges of motion in all joints of both upper extremities and compare both sides. Joint stability should be assessed. Neurologic and vascular examinations are performed, and muscle strength is evaluated, especially of the shoulder girdle muscles. An evaluation of the cervical spine may be necessary, especially in a patient with rheumatoid arthritis who may demonstrate limited extension or instability that can interfere with endotracheal intubation, thereby requiring fiber-optic intubation. Shoulder motion is nearly always limited. Both active and passive ranges of motion should be recorded for combined elevation, external rotation, and internal rotation using the conventions of measurement established by the American Shoulder and Elbow Surgeons (Fig. 3.1).

Muscles should be tested with and without the elimination of gravity. An attempt is made to differentiate if a muscle group is prevented from fully contracting due to pain or to any intrinsic weakness within the muscle. The examiner should also know whether there is nerve paralysis causing weakness. A brachial plexus injury could affect the results of an arthroplasty procedure. It is also essential to examine the muscles controlling the movement of the scapula, especially if a procedure such as a glenohumeral arthrodesis is being considered.

The rotator cuff is important in providing synchronous motion of the glenohumeral joint, and the best results of prosthetic arthroplasty, specifically with respect to active motion and function, are seen when the rotator cuff is intact (39, 68, 70, 72, 86, 115, 116, 144). Thus, it is useful to assess the status of the rotator cuff preoperatively to help predict the ultimate results of reconstruction. It is unwise to repair a tear of the rotator cuff alone in the presence of significant glenohumeral arthritis (29, 60, 106). Evidence of impingement and symptomatic disease of the acromioclavicular joint are also addressed at the time of arthroplasty.

The preoperative evaluation of the soft tissues and capsule must be considered. If the joint capsule is enlarged or redundant, as in the case of a chronic subluxation or dislocation, this may need to be addressed during a procedure such as an arthroplasty. If anterior contractures are present, they must be corrected in the arthroplasty to allow motion and stability for the prosthesis. A contracture requires releasing and may require lengthening of the anterior soft tissues, including the subscapularis, and releasing the coracohumeral ligament. Other contractures must be released, and the proper tension must be obtained in the entire rotator cuff mechanism to achieve maximum function around a prosthetic device. If significant synovitis is present, it must be treated intraoperatively and an adequate synovectomy must be performed.

Plain films, including axillary and anteroposterior views of the glenohumeral joint in internal and external rotation, must be taken. To achieve a true profile of the glenohumeral joint, the anteroposterior views can be taken with the patient standing and the scapula flush against the x-ray cassette, which results in the torso being rotated 30 to 40°, thereby showing the glenohumeral space and its adjacent bony structures.

The humeral head should be studied to determine if it is flattened, sclerotic, or eroded. Large subchondral cysts must be identified and managed intraoperatively with methyl methacrylate or bone grafting (109, 123). Peripheral osteophytes are most often observed radiographically inferiorly and

SHOULDER ASSESSMENT FORM
AMERICAN SHOULDER AND ELBOW SURGEONS

Name:		Date	
Age:	Hand dominance: R L Ambi	Sex: M F	
Diagnosis:		Initial Assess? Y N	
Procedure/Date:		Follow-up: M; Y	

PHYSICIAN ASSESSMENT

RANGE OF MOTION		RIGHT		LEFT	
Total shoulder motion Goniometer preferred		Active	Passive	Active	Passive
Forward elevation (Maximum arm-trunk angle)					
External rotation (Arm comfortably at side)					
External rotation (Arm at 90° abduction)					
Internal rotation (Highest posterior anatomy reached with thumb)					
Cross-body adduction (Antecubital fossa to opposite acromion)					

SIGNS

0 = none; 1 = mild; 2 = moderate; 3 = severe

SIGN		Right	Left
Supraspinatus/greater tuberosity tenderness		0 1 2 3	0 1 2 3
AC joint tenderness		0 1 2 3	0 1 2 3
Biceps tendon tenderness (or rupture)		0 1 2 3	0 1 2 3
Other tenderness - List:		0 1 2 3	0 1 2 3
Impingement I (Passive forward elevation in slight internal rotation)		Y N	Y N
Impingement II (Passive internal rotation with 90° flexion)		Y N	Y N
Impingement III (90° active abduction - classic painful arc)		Y N	Y N
Subacromial crepitus		Y N	Y N
Scars - location		Y N	Y N
Atrophy - location:		Y N	Y N
Deformity : describe		Y N	Y N

Figure 3.1. American Shoulder and Elbow Surgeons Basic Shoulder Evaluation Form. (Data from Gerber C. Integrated scoring systems for the functional assessment of the shoulder. In: Matsen F, ed. The shoulder: a balance of mobility and stability, Rosemont, IL: American Academy of Orthopaedic Surgeons, 1993). *(continued)*

medially. The amount and location of cartilage loss should be assessed. The quality of the bone must be considered. Superior subluxation of the head often indicates severe rotator cuff tear or disease (118, 123, 126). Arthrography and magnetic resonance imaging are helpful in diagnosing full-thickness rotator cuff tears (28).

STRENGTH
(record MRC grade)

0 = no contraction; 1 = flicker; 2 = movement with gravity eliminated
3 = movement against gravity; 4 = movement against some resistance; 5 = normal power.

	Right	Left
Testing affected by pain?	Y N	Y N
Forward elevation	0 1 2 3 4 5	0 1 2 3 4 5
Abduction	0 1 2 3 4 5	0 1 2 3 4 5
External rotation (Arm comfortably at side)	0 1 2 3 4 5	0 1 2 3 4 5
Internal rotation (Arm comfortably at side)	0 1 2 3 4 5	0 1 2 3 4 5

INSTABILITY

0 = none; 1 = mild (0 - 1 cm translation)
2 = moderate (1 - 2 cm translation or translates to glenoid rim)
3 = severe (> 2 cm translation or over rim of glenoid)

	Right	Left
Anterior translation	0 1 2 3	0 1 2 3
Posterior translation	0 1 2 3	0 1 2 3
Inferior translation (sulcus sign)	0 1 2 3	0 1 2 3
Anterior apprehension	0 1 2 3	0 1 2 3
Reproduces symptoms?	Y N	Y N
Voluntary instability?	Y N	Y N
Relocation test positive?	Y N	Y N
Generalized ligamentous laxity?	Y N	

Other physical findings:

Examiner's name:

_____   _____Date

Figure 3.1. *(continued)*

PATIENT SELF-EVALUATION

Are you having pain in your shoulder? (circle correct answer)	Yes	No

Mark where your pain is on this diagram:

Do you have pain in your shoulder at night?	Yes	No
Do you take pain medication (aspirin, Advil, Tylenol etc.)?	Yes	No
Do you take narcotic pain medication (codeine or stronger)?	Yes	No
How many pills do you take each day (average)?	pills	

How bad is your pain today (mark line)?

No pain at all   0 —— 1 2 3 4 5 6 7 8 9 —— 10   Pain as bad as it can be

Does your shoulder feel unstable (as if it is going to dislocate?)	Yes	No

How unstable is your shoulder (mark line)?

Very stable   0 —— 1 2 3 4 5 6 7 8 9 —— 10   Very <u>un</u>stable

Circle the number in the box that indicates your ability to do the following activities:
0 = **Unable** to do; 1 = **Very** difficult to do; 2 = **Somewhat** difficult; 3 = **Not** difficult

ACTIVITY	RIGHT ARM	LEFT ARM
1. Put on a coat	0 1 2 3	0 1 2 3
2. Sleep on your painful or affected side	0 1 2 3	0 1 2 3
3. Wash back/do up bra in back	0 1 2 3	0 1 2 3
4. Manage toileting	0 1 2 3	0 1 2 3
5. Comb hair	0 1 2 3	0 1 2 3
6. Reach a high shelf	0 1 2 3	0 1 2 3
7. Lift 10 lbs. above shoulder	0 1 2 3	0 1 2 3
8. Throw a ball overhand	0 1 2 3	0 1 2 3
9. Do usual work - List:	0 1 2 3	0 1 2 3
10. Do usual sport - List:	0 1 2 3	0 1 2 3

Figure 3.1. *(continued)*

On the glenoid side, the amount of cartilage loss and sclerosis should be observed, and whether it is central or posterior should be noted. Peripheral osteophytes occasionally may interfere with function of the prosthetic head or placement of the glenoid component. The degree of erosion—whether central, posterior, or anterior—with flattening and narrowing of the glenoid vault helps determine whether a glenoid component can or should be inserted. If the glenoid is seriously eroded, it may require bone grafting (109, 123). This should be determined preoperatively so that adequate preoperative planning can occur. A bone graft can often be taken from the resected humeral head, making sure to incorporate some of the subchondral bone in the graft and cancellous bone.

Radiographic examination of the humeral shaft in two planes helps determine the quality of the bone, thickness of the cortices, and diameter of the intramedullary canal. Preoperative templating allows the surgeon to plan for the correct stem size.

Adequate preoperative laboratory testing should be done including hematologic, chemistry grouping, and EMG testing when indicated.

Arthrodesis of the Shoulder

In the past, tuberculosis and poliomyelitis were the conditions that most often required a need for shoulder arthrodesis (8). These problems have largely disappeared in the Western world. Moreover, the success of shoulder arthroplasty has further narrowed the indications for arthrodesis. Patients are often dissatisfied with the results of fusion and frequently complain of limited position of the hand placement. In addition, shoulder pain may not always be relieved.

INDICATIONS

Shoulder arthrodesis is still a worthwhile procedure in properly selected cases. With successful fusion, the patient can raise the hand to the mouth and head, grasp objects in front of the body, and push and pull forcefully. The procedure is recommended for 1) low-grade infections of the shoulder (such as tuberculosis) to prevent disease progression and provide a stable, painless shoulder joint and 2) specific paralytic conditions (especially poliomyelitis flail shoulder still seen in the non-Western world), irreversible brachial plexus damage, and other disorders causing paralysis of the glenohumeral muscles and severe loss of function (75). Whenever surgeons consider a shoulder fusion, they should be sure that the opposite shoulder has good function. Arthrodesis may also be performed after failed arthroplasty when the rotator cuff and deltoid have both been destroyed and nothing more can be done to salvage the shoulder joint. It may rarely be done in selected cases of failed multiply operated multidirectional instability. Cofield and Briggs (29) reported adequate pain relief and restoration of function in 75% of 71 shoulders in which arthrodesis was performed. In 68 of 71 shoulders, solid fusion was obtained in one operation. Richards et al. (133, 134) showed a high rate of fusion with a surgical procedure using a single plate and screw fixation. They found the highest patient satisfaction in those patients undergoing the operation for brachial plexus injury, osteoarthritis, and failed total shoulder arthroplasty.

The operation was much less satisfactory in those patients who were arthrodesed for failed operations for multidirectional instability, even though fusion was obtained.

PREREQUISITES

Before shoulder arthrodesis is undertaken, it is important that the patient have a stable scapula to control upper extremity movement. Good strength should be present in the trapezius and serratus anterior muscles. A good range of scapulothoracic motion must be demonstrated preoperatively. At operation, adduction contractures must be corrected.

TIMING OF PROCEDURE

Shoulder fusion can be performed successfully in children with a flail shoulder who have reached age 10, because ossification of the humeral epiphysis is usually complete by that age (29). Joint fusion is best done between 12 and 15 years of age, because enough cancellous bone is present in the humeral head, and operation will not interfere with growth of the arm (5) (Table 3.1). Makin (94) reported excellent fusions for flail shoulder in seven children aged 5 to 9 years (94). All shoulders fused and little humeral length was lost. The shoulders were fused in 80 to 90° of abduction, with the expectation that some abduction would be lost with growth. This did not occur, and abduction was excessive. Early fusion should be discouraged because of possible epiphyseal injury and growth disturbance after fusion, the tendency for change and uncertainty of the angle at the fusion site with growth, and the chance of fusion failure (140). Nevertheless, Barr et al. (6) and Makin (94) showed that arthrodesis before age 12 years allowed a better range of motion of the shoulder girdle than the same operation in the older age groups.

OPTIMUM POSITION

The final position of shoulder fusion must permit several things to occur. The hand must reach the face, head, and midline of the body in front. Lifting, pulling, and pushing must be possible, and there must be comfort of the extremity with the arm at the side. Finally, the scapula should lie flat against the chest wall.

Table 3.1. Recommended positions for shoulder arthrodesis

Author	Year	Abduction (Degrees)	Forward Flexion (Degrees)	External Rotation (Degrees)	Internal Rotation (Degrees)	Mininum Age for Fusion (Years)	Best Age for Fusion (Years)
Gill	1931	45 or less (measured from vertebral border of scapula)				10	
Brett	1933	70 (adult)	20			8	12–15
Barr et al.	1942	70–90 (arm from side of body)	15–25	25–30		6	12.5 (average)
May	1962	65	60	40			After 10
Charnley and Houston	1964	45 (clinical position to side of body)	45		45		
Rowe	1974	15 to 20 (arm from side of body)	25 to 30		45 to 50		
Beltran et al.	1975	50	20		25		

Care must be taken to avoid excessive flexion, which causes winging of the scapula. When serratus anterior strength is deficient, the angle of fusion in abduction should not be more than 30° in relation to the vertebral border of the scapula. The curve of the chest wall and the strength of the muscles must be considered when deciding the position of flexion. Excessive rotation and abduction will produce poor functional and cosmetic results (12). The best functional position for shoulder fusion has been studied by numerous investigators over the years (66). Obviously, there is no standard position. However, Rowe (138) stated that poor results occur with excessive abduction and forward flexion of the arm (Fig. 3.2). He concluded that lifting and elevating the hand to the face are achieved more efficiently without the humeral ab-

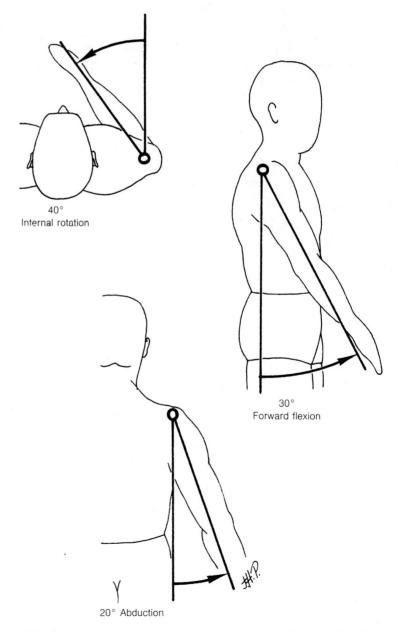

40°
Internal rotation

30°
Forward flexion

20° Abduction

Figure 3.2 Rowe's recommendation for optimum arthrodesis of the shoulder. Abduction angle is measured from the side of the body. (From Post M. The shoulder: surgical and nonsurgical management. 2nd ed. Philadelphia: Lea & Febiger, 1988).

duction. This is primarily accomplished by elbow flexion of 135°, started with the arm in neutral at the side of the body and supplemented by scapular rotation (30° of forward flexion of the shoulder). He believed that the only reason for more humeral abduction was the presence of strong scapulothoracic muscles and weak elbow flexors. In this instance, flexing of the elbow to permit the hand to reach the mouth is more easily achieved by the horizontal position of the forearm. After shoulder fusion, hand placement at any point depends primarily on the relative movements of abduction, rotation, and flexion of the fused shoulder. Cofield and Briggs (29) stated that the position of fusion had little effect on the results. For most cases, the authors prefer the Rowe method (138).

METHODS OF FUSION

Successful shoulder fusion requires effective contact between cancellous bone of the decorticated humeral head and glenoid and adequate postoperative immobilization. Fortunately, both the humeral head and vault of the scapular neck have abundant cancellous bone. Unfortunately, the small area of glenoid face and the difficulty of maintaining a desired position between the humeral head and scapula make fusion of the glenohumeral joint technically more difficult than fusion of other joints in the body. The authors prefer internal fixation methods that use compression techniques, including the use of cancellous bone screws with washers around the heads and local autogenous bone grafts. In addition, a nut at the end of a cancellous bone screw may be used to increase compression between the rawed acromion and humerus.

Since Albert's attempt (3) to perform shoulder fusion in 1881, various techniques have been devised to accomplish this operation. They may be classified as 1) intraarticular (17), 2) extraarticular (119, 127, 152), 3) combined intraarticular and extraarticular (13, 38, 96, 100, 127, 143, 146, 147, 152), and 4) compression arthrodesis (10, 19, 20).

AUTHORS' PREFERENCE

For arthrodesis attempted the first time in lean, compliant patients with good cancellous bone, the authors prefer the Moseley technique (Fig. 3.3) (100). In theory, for noncompliant patients or in those with nonunion after failed arthrodesis, a plate and screws are preferred.

The patient is placed in a semisitting or beach chair position. In this method, a longitudinal incision is made in the deltopectoral groove for 12 cm starting just lateral to the acromioclavicular joint. Full-thickness skin flaps are developed. Using electrocautery dissection, the anterior and lateral deltoid muscle is removed from its origin on the lateral 2 cm of clavicle and anterior and lateral acromion so as to expose the underlying glenohumeral joint. The anterior and lateral capsule is sharply incised and removed, leaving the posterior and posterolateral capsule intact. Using gouges, osteotomes, and rongeurs, any residual cartilage overlying the glenoid and the humeral head is removed. A power burr may be used to remove any sclerotic bone down to raw bleeding bone. In addition, the coracohumeral ligament and any tissue on the undersurface of the acromion are removed down to raw bleeding bone. After this has been achieved, the subchondral bone on the undersurface of the acromion is carefully removed, so that good bleeding bone may come in contact with cancellous bone of the humeral head.

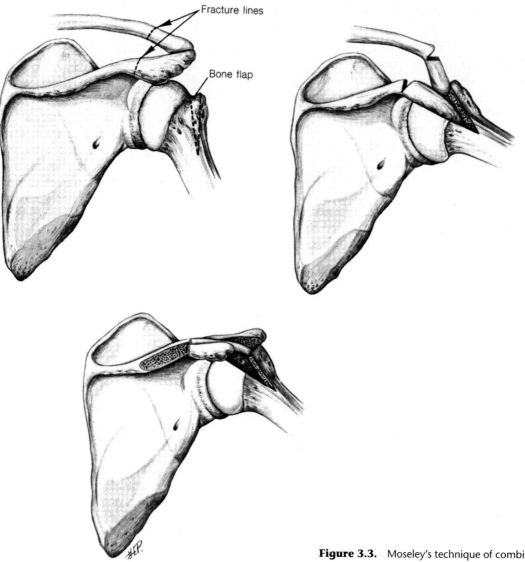

Figure 3.3. Moseley's technique of combined intraarticular and extra-articular arthrodesis.

If necessary, the lateral 1 or 2 cm of clavicle are removed to permit superior subluxation of the humeral head, so that it comes in good contact with the underlying surface of the acromion. Often, this is not necessary. The authors prefer the position of Rowe (30° of flexion, 40° of internal rotation, and 20° of abduction) (138).

Using 3.2-mm Steinmann pins and with the arm held by an assistant in the desired position and the humeral head superiorly subluxated, the pin is power driven across the glenoid perpendicularly from lateral to medial after the head has been shaped to make optimum contact between the cancellous surface of the undersurface of the acromion and the glenoid. A similar pin is driven downward from the center of the acromion into the humeral head and medial cortex of the proximal humerus. The position of the arm is checked, making certain that the hand can be passively brought to the face and moved into various desired positions. Care must be taken to avoid excessive abduction, as this causes a prominent and uncomfortable scapula when the arm is brought to the side of the body. In addition, the arm is weak when lifting away or in forward flexion with excessive abduction. In general, there is enough contact between the raw cancellous surfaces so that additional bone graft is not required. If it is needed, it may be taken locally from the humeral head or, in addition, from the ipsilateral ilium.

With the Steinmann pins in place, a 6.5-mm cancellous bone screw with a washer is threaded perpendicularly across the humeral head to its glenoid. Care must be taken to avoid having the thread positioned between the contacting bony surfaces so as to avoid a gap and distraction of the parts. When this has been achieved, a second 6.5-mm cancellous bone screw and washer are inserted through the acromion into the humeral head and proximal shaft.

The patient is placed in an adjustable rigid orthosis with the arm and elbow in the desired position. A closed system wound drain is inserted, and the skin edges are approximated. The drain is removed the next morning when the output is usually low. Radiographs are taken to check the position of the fused joint and that there has been no change at the arthrodesed site.

In cases of nonunion, patients of large mass, and noncompliant patients, the authors prefer the A.O. technique, as reported by Kostuik and Schatzker (83) and Riggins (135).

In this method, with the patient in a beach chair or semisitting position, a skin incision is made at the top of the acromion starting just medial to the posterior angle of the scapular spine and extended downward in the deltopectoral groove for 8 to 10 cm. Full-thickness skin flaps are developed. The lateral and anterior deltoid is sharply elevated from its origin using electrocautery dissection. The deltoid may be split without fear of injury to the axillary nerve, because the deltoid is not required and is not used in arthrodesis of the shoulder as a functional muscle. The anterior and lateral capsule are sharply excised, leaving the posterior capsule intact as a hinge if possible, as in the Moseley technique. The synovium is removed, along with cartilage and sclerotic bone down to bleeding bone of the humeral head and glenoid and undersurface of the acromion. The arm is placed in the desired position of abduction, forward flexion, and internal rotation (Rowe technique) and held with 3.2-mm diameter Steinmann pins inserted perpendicularly across the humeral head and through the acromion downward into the proximal shaft. A malleable metal template is used to shape the metal plate that will be used for internal fixation of the humeral head to the glenoid and undersurface of the acromion. Once a contoured malleable bone plate is shaped, it is placed over the spine of the scapula, posterior-superior aspect of the humeral head, and downward along the shaft of the humerus (Fig. 3.4A). Cancellous bone screws are used to fix the plate to the upper shaft and to the spine. Cortical bone screws are placed through the plate in more dense cortical bone. One or two 6.5-mm diameter cancellous screws are placed perpendicularly across the plate and humeral head into the glenoid. Care must be exercised to avoid the threads from distracting or creating a gap between the humeral head and glenoid to minimize the risk of nonunion. In exceptionally large patients, a posterior buttress plate may also be used to control rotaton and add stability to the arthrodesed shoulder (Fig. 3.4B–D). A second buttress plate to control rotation in exceptional cases may be added to the spine of the scapula at the posterior aspect of the humerus.

A closed drainage system is used, and the drain removed 24 hours later. The arm is immobilized for several weeks. An orthosis or plaster spica cast is not necessary with this technique. Radiographs are then taken to determine

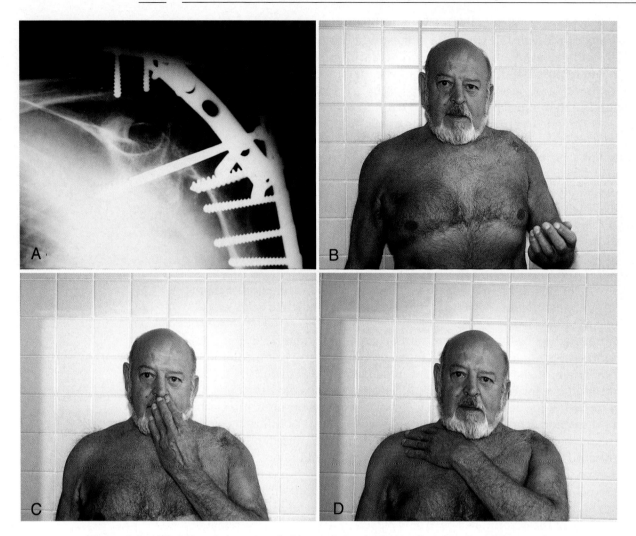

Figure 3.4. **(A)** A.O. technique. A malleable metal plate is contoured to the spine of the scapula and onto the lateral surface of the humerus. A posterior buttress plate may be used to control rotation. **(B–D)** Multiple operations for rotator cuff tear of the left shoulder had failed in a 52-year-old man. Pain was severe. A.O. technique was used to fuse his shoulder. There was a solid arthrodesis in 4 months. Note the postoperative motions 15 months later. The result was excellent.

the position. They are repeated at 1, 2, and 4 weeks thereafter and later taken every 6 to 8 weeks to be certain that healing is occurring and that the position has not changed. The internal fixation is not removed for at least 12 months or until good bony healing has occurred. When the screws are removed, care must be exercised for several months, so as not to stress the bone until there is adequate filling of the holes created by the screws (Fig. 3.5).

RESULTS

According to Cofield and Briggs (29), patient satisfaction is 80% after arthrodesis. When a cast or orthosis is removed, stretching exercises for the scapulothoracic muscles are performed. Strengthening exercises are added thereafter in a gentle manner to avoid disruption of the healing fusion site.

No matter how good the fusion is following an arthrodesis, upper extremity function is not as good as following a total shoulder arthroplasty. Hawkins et al. (67) showed that a range of acceptable positions did not com-

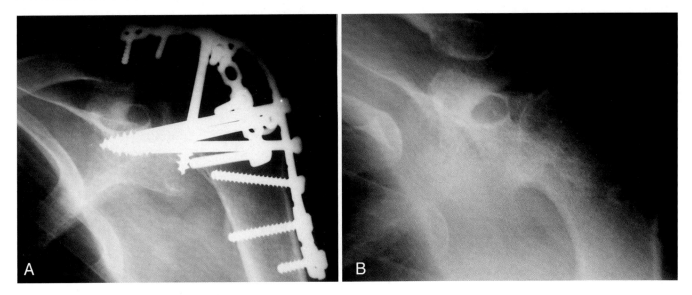

Figure 3.5. **(A)** Multiple operations for rotator cuff tearing had failed in a man aged 52 years. A.O. technique is shown. Fusion occurred in 12 weeks with excellent pain relief. **(B)** The internal fixation plates and screws were removed 14 months postoperatively. The result was excellent.

promise the functional result. These authors suggested a 25 to 40° abduction angle for the arm, 20 to 30° of flexion, and 25 to 30° of internal rotation. The side of the trunk is commonly used as the reference point, with the scapula being held in the anatomic position.

In summary, a good result is defined as the patient being able to reach the face and top of the head as well as the opposite shoulder with ease.

COMPLICATIONS OF ARTHRODESIS

Malposition of the Arthrodesed Glenohumeral Joint

The purpose of an arthrodesis is to permit a position of the fused parts to allow maximum power for lifting, pushing, and pulling. The scapular muscles must not be strained when the arm is at the side of the body or placed in an elevated position. The hand must be able to reach the face, head, and midline of the body in front of the body. If the arm is placed in excessive abduction, the patient may complain of pain around the shoulder girdle due to abnormal tension on the scapular muscles, including the serratus anterior, rhomboids trapezius, and levator scapulae (Fig. 3.6). Severe pain around the scapula may ensue due to muscle fatigue, pain, and abnormal tension on the scapular muscles and those muscles that attach to the cervical spine. The authors prefer the position recommended by Rowe (138) to avoid these problems.

Excessive external rotation will limit the ability of the patient to reach the contralateral axilla or to reach behind the back. Similarly, excessive internal rotation will decrease the ability of the patient to comb the hair, wash the face, or perform other activities concerning the head and neck. This can be most disabling.

Persistent Pain

Even when an excellent fusion has been achieved, the patient may continue to complain of pain around the shoulder girdle, especially when

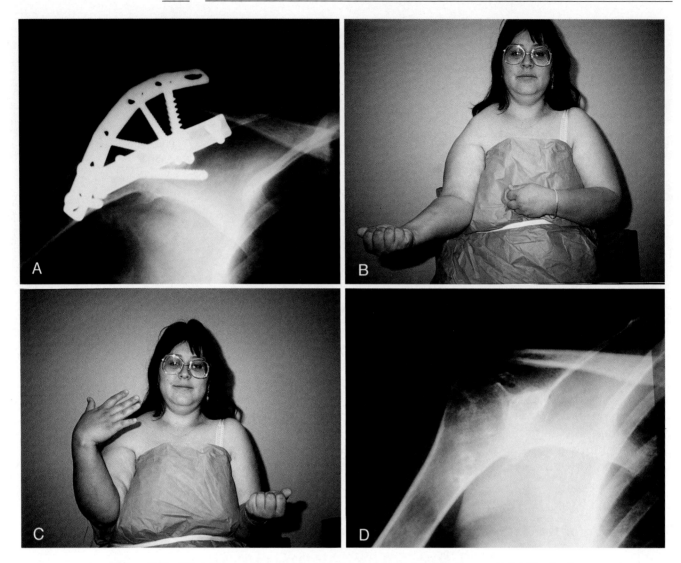

Figure 3.6. **(A)** A 24-year-old woman had a fusion for a septic right glenohumeral joint. The shoulder was fused in external rotation, and excessive abduction was noted on the postoperative radiograph. **(B,C)** The patient has shoulder girdle pain and could not reach her face or touch her body. She could not internally rotate her arm and was severely disabled. **(D)** The plate and screws were removed. The patient requires a revision.

tension in the scapular muscles is increased. This may be caused by a complication of malposition with excessive abduction, symptomatic arthritis in the acromioclavicular joint that was not addressed during the operation, general muscle ache, and other unforeseen reasons.

Nonunion

Cofield (28) found a pseudarthrosis rate of 10% in almost 500 reported cases. It is essential that good contact is made between the cancellous bone of the humeral head and that of the glenoid vault during the procedure. Contact and movement between the opposing cancellous bone surfaces should be kept to a minimum, because the upper extremity is a long lever arm that might cause tension rather than compression that may contribute to nonunion.

Failure of Fixation

Cancellous bone screws may pull out from bone that is highly demineralized, thus permitting loss of adequate contact between the raw bony surfaces of the humeral head and glenoid. A plate used for internal fixation may be unable to hold the bony parts in contact because the bone is demineralized, thereby permitting loosening of the screws. These are not recommended for internal fixation in demineralized bone because they do not provide good compression.

Fracture

While the glenohumeral joint is fusing postoperatively and especially after fusion, excessive torque or trauma on the upper extremity may cause a fracture in the humerus. Many of these fractures occur in patients with a paralytic condition (28, 29). Also, if too much bone is removed from the acromion, the thinned acromion may fracture. If so, a large cancellous bone screw is placed in the longitudinal position through the acromion and into the humerus.

Nerve Complications

If the arm is fixed in an excessive amount of abduction, the suprascapular nerve may develop neuritis, which causes shoulder pain. Ulnar neuritis or palsy may develop if the patient rests the elbow on hard objects. As in any shoulder operation, reflex sympathetic dystrophy may develop postoperatively.

Infection

Infection at the fusion site may prevent union. Care in achieving asepsis during and after the operation must be achieved to avoid this complication. As an example, the authors avoid injuring the skin during the operation and use wound drainage for at least 24 hours to avoid hematoma and the formation of a dead space.

The authors do not recommend external fixation or external pins because pin tract infections may occur. Charnley and Houston (20) have reported a 10% incidence of pin tract infection with their external compression device when used for shoulder fusion.

Resection Arthroplasty of the Humeral Head

Jones (74) demonstrated that after humeral head resection, a stable shoulder could be obtained by transplanting the rotator cuff muscles into the proximal humerus. He was among the first to state that the shoulder girdle must be in a fixed position and stabilized through the muscle action on the scapula to allow the arm to be elevated. Stabilization of the scapula and clavicle is affected by the actions of the subclavius and pectoralis minor anteriorly, the trapezius and rhomboids posteriorly, and the serratus anterior muscle acting on the vertebral border of the scapula. Working synchronously, these muscles fix the scapula against the chest wall. Although these are the most important scapular stabilizers, other muscles such as the biceps and coracobrachialis attaching to the coracoid process can act as secondary stabilizers.

After the scapula is stabilized, the proximal humerus must be fixed within the shallow glenoid before the arm can be actively elevated. This is accomplished by the subscapularis in front and the supraspinatus, infraspinatus, and teres minor behind. These "short rotator" muscles are neither small nor unimportant, as was once erroneously believed. Their combined weight was shown by Jones (74) to be greater than that of the deltoid. Acting together, all the shoulder muscles permit the meeting of prodigious work demands. Therefore, any injury or operation that disrupts the integrity of the joint or weakens the muscle action impairs the function of the arm and the whole extremity. It follows that if the short rotator muscles are in a weakened state, the function of the arm will be correspondingly decreased.

It should be stressed that replacement of a resected proximal humerus with a fibula graft as described by Rovsing (137) and Albee (2) is seldom indicated. It can be used for resectable tumors of the proximal humerus (64). However, postoperative function is usually poor, and the graft is prone to fracture.

INDICATIONS

In the past, humeral head resection was performed for resectable tumor, localized infection of the proximal humerus, severe crush injury, four-part fractures, and severe fracture-dislocations of the humeral head with obvious attendant loss of blood supply to the fragments. In recent years, improved surgical techniques and replacement procedures have greatly narrowed the indications for resection arthroplasty. The procedure is of greatest value in eliminating local infection in the proximal humerus (Fig. 3.7).

PREREQUISITES

If optimum results are to be realized, the lesion should be localized to the proximal humerus, and a functioning rotator cuff should be available for reattachment to the humeral shaft. The rest of the shoulder girdle muscles should be normal. Even when these conditions are met, the patient often will have limited motion and a varying degree of discomfort after the procedure. Failure to meet these requirements will result in poor outcome. In some instances, the surgeon may perform this operation even in the presence of a nonfunctional or highly deficient rotator cuff.

OPERATION

The patient is placed in a semisitting or beach chair position with the torso elevated 30°. A sandbag is placed behind the shoulder blade. The knees should be flexed slightly, and the lower extremities should be wrapped with elastic bandages. The upper extremity is draped free.

The upper portion of the Henry approach can be used (Fig. 3.7A). A 12.5-cm curvilinear incision is started over the superolateral acromion, then continued medially toward the acromioclavicular joint and the lateral clavicle, and gently curved downward in the direction of the deltopectoral groove on the lateral side of the coracoid tip. When a less extensive exposure is needed, a straight longitudinal incision is placed overlying the deltopectoral groove and starting just above and lateral to the coracoid.

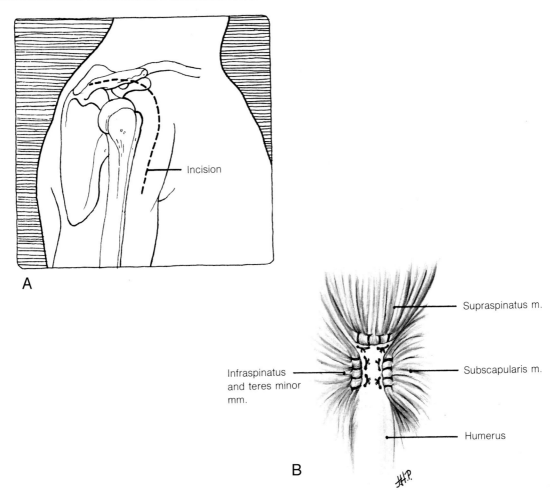

Figure 3.7. Reattachment of rotator cuff. **(A)** Dotted line indicates incision for anterior Henry approach to the shoulder. **(B)** Jones method for reattaching rotator cuff structures to the proximal humerus. The tendons of each of the muscles must be identified and attached directly to the shaft for best results. (From Post M. The shoulder: surgical and nonsurgical management. 2nd ed. Philadelphia: Lea & Febiger, 1988).

The cephalic vein is identified, its lateral muscle branches tied and cut, and the vein retracted medially. The authors prefer to retract the vein medially, especially in those patients who have previously undergone the operation, because this avoids excessive traction and possible tearing of the cephalic vein as it dips into the clavipectoral fascia. The deltopectoral groove is followed proximally toward the clavicle. The deltoid origin is usually left attached, the arm abducted, and the deltoid retracted. The strap muscles are gently retracted medially, recalling that the neurovascular branches lie just medial to these muscles. It should be recalled that the small branches of the musculocutaneous nerve may enter the coracobrachialis as high as 15 mm distal to the coracoid process (15).

The subscapularis and its underlying capsule are now seen. The capsule is opened first by transecting the tendon of the subscapularis 1.5 cm medial to the lip of the bicipital groove. The infected bone of the humeral head is then osteotomized and removed. Debridement of synovium and necrotic cuff tissue is carried out as necessary (112).

Traction is placed on the infraspinatus-teres minor, supraspinatus, and subscapularis tendons. An area on the lateral upper humeral shaft is marked as the site of attachment for these structures (Fig. 3.7B). It is important to define these structures. Merely attaching a large mass of capsule to the shaft haphazardly may give a poor result. The patient must be able to bring the arm to the side of the body without excessive tension on the muscles or the site of rotator cuff reattachment. Small slots are made in the cortex either with a narrow gouge or small burr and heavy no. 5 nonabsorbable sutures placed through the drill holes and tendons. These are tied after the surrounding surface cortex is scarified. The wound is flushed with saline solution. The deltopectoral interval is then closed over a closed wound drainage system, which is used for 24 hours to obviate hematoma formation.

AFTERCARE

The extremity is immobilized for 25 days in Velpeau position, and gentle passive and pendulum motion exercises are then started. The patient is permitted to exercise the elbow in front of the torso. After several more days, gentle active exercises are begun and gradually increased as tolerated. An optimum result is often not achieved for at least 6 months.

In recent years, the authors' preference for this operation has been limited to patients with severe localized infection and rarely with failed total shoulder replacement for which revision surgery cannot be performed.

Replacement Arthroplasty

There is now extensive experience with replacement arthroplasty of the shoulder, which is used for treating various types of arthritis involving the glenohumeral joint. The indications and techniques of prosthetic shoulder replacement have evolved over a long period. Pain relief has been achieved in a high percentage of patients treated with prosthetic arthroplasty for a variety of diagnoses (1, 21, 26, 33, 36, 45, 58, 61–63, 95, 98, 99, 128, 151, 155). Functional restoration can be more difficult to achieve and depends on the integrity of the muscles, especially the rotator cuff and deltoid at the time of arthroplasty. To achieve a successful outcome with shoulder arthroplasty, the importance of addressing and correcting soft tissue contractures and resurfacing the articular surfaces cannot be overemphasized. The choice of whether to resurface the humeral articular surface alone or both the glenoid and humeral articular surfaces is made on the basis of the extent of the articular damage, the available bone stock, and the integrity of the soft tissues (especially the rotator cuff). Likewise, the postoperative rehabilitation will depend largely on the condition of the soft tissues at surgery.

HISTORICAL REVIEW

The chief reasons for most shoulder operations are relief of pain and improvement of motion. Replacement arthroplasty may produce excellent results, providing both pain relief and increased function.

Few shoulder replacements were performed in the early part of this century because the technology was not well advanced. In 1894, Péan reported the first artificial shoulder joint replacement in a 30-year-old patient who had a destructive tuberculous process of the upper extremity (91, 113). A constrained prosthesis was implanted; its humeral component was made of iridescent platinum with a head made of a hard rubber ball crossed by two deep grooves placed at right angles to each other. Each groove contained two separate metal loops, one joining the rubber ball to the platinum stem and the other held to the glenoid by two screws. This replacement was remarkable, considering the absence of advanced technology and the lack of knowledge of asepsis at the time.

Most early prostheses were replacements of the humeral head. Richard et al. (132) used an acrylic humeral stem device, whereas Krueger (85) and Neer et al. (105) first used a cobalt-chrome humeral stem to replace the head. Later, Ducci (41) and Lynn et al. (92) used humeral stem prostheses to replace the upper end of the humerus. Casuccio (18) also used a similar device for replacement of the proximal humerus. Haraldsson (65) reported on a fenestrated humeral stem component to replace the upper humerus in a locally destructive tumor. This component allowed the tenocapsular apparatus parts to be reattached to one another through the perforations in the prosthesis. This muscle-sling fixation appeared to give good fixation. Eventually, many surgeons used hemiarthroplasty with a glenoid liner when residual short rotator muscle power was good and reconstruction of the soft tissue capsule could be performed with the expectation of restoring function (2, 23, 44, 90, 104, 140). Other shoulder replacement systems have also been tested with a variety of results (4, 9, 14, 16, 53, 55–57, 73, 77, 82, 87, 89, 97, 129, 130, 153). These prosthetic designs have ranged from completely unconstrained to constrained systems. Some prostheses, like that of Swanson (148), have used a bicentric implant containing a self-contained ball and socket component that allows movement between two moving surfaces. The outside cup allows alignment of the cup to the glenoid face. Clayton et al. (21, 22) tried a subacromial spacer, thereby avoiding abutment of the greater tuberosity against the acromion. Theoretically, this device can be used as a salvage procedure for failed total shoulder procedures. Steffee and Moore (145) have used resurfacing arthroplasty techniques in the shoulder, as in the hip. Rydholm and Sjörgren (139) used resurfacing in 72 rheumatoid shoulders with good results.

To overcome the loss of the stabilizing short rotator muscles, several authors have used various designs of constrained joints to substitute for the loss of the rotator cuff (43, 44). Clayton et al. (22) tried subacromial polyethylene spacers with Neer replacements when the integrity of the rotator cuff could not be restored. Constrained-type replacements have been tried in these severe cases, in which the rotator cuff mechanism was highly deficient (117, 124–126). Semiconstrained joints made of cobalt-chrome (Stanmore type) were reported by Coughlin et al. (32), Lettin et al. (87), and Lettin and Scales (88, 89). Their prostheses were cemented into bone. Although dislocations were reported, the humeral component could be replaced by manipulation. In these procedures, the metal glenoid is also cemented within the glenoid vault, which is skived out, possibly allowing prosthetic loosening. Macnab and English (93) used a prosthesis that replaced the humeral head with a glenoid liner whose extended superior lip provided for some fulcrum. Both components were porous and coated with sundered cobalt-chrome to allow better bony attachment of the parts. Bickle (23) used a constrained joint, whose metal glenoid component was cemented within the glenoid vault, requiring removal of much of the cancellous bone from the vault. Numerous complications occurred, including glenoid fractures, loosening of the glenoid component, prosthetic neck failure, and dislocation.

Fenlin et al. (46, 47) reported on a constrained joint whose design used a humeral stem component of reverse configuration containing a thin-walled large cup, within which articulated a large ball that extended laterally from a metal glenoid component. The latter component required considerable removal of cancellous bone from the vault and the ability to insert a metal spike within the small medullary canal located along the axillary border of the scapula. Kessel and Bayley (78, 79) and Reeves et al. (129–131) also used a smaller reverse head configuration. They believed that this provided both an acceptable range of abduction and circumduction motion and stability.

Post et al. (117, 124–126) reported on constrained replacements that used a humeral component with a small diameter head and a metal glenoid cup and polyethylene liner, permitting planned dislocation of the metal head beyond a specific torque when the motion limits of the prosthesis were exceeded (Fig. 3.8). This dislocatable feature was added to protect the fragile scapula

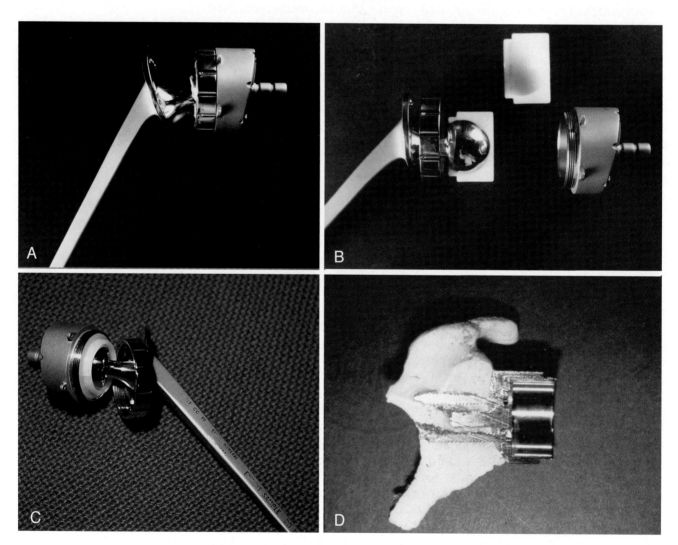

Figure 3.8. **(A)** Constrained prosthesis with dislocatable feature used by the author (M.P.) (fully assembled). **(B)** Constrained prosthesis uses the principle of surface mount of the glenoid component that avoids disruption of the glenoid vault. The components are shown disassembled. Note the locking metal ring around the neck of the stem. **(C)** Partially assembled MRTS constrained prosthesis is shown. **(D)** The glenoid component is surface mounted as shown in a cut specimen.

from fracture. Experience with this type of prosthesis has shown that scapular fracture is essentially obviated by the dislocation feature of this design. Early material failures involving breakage of the humeral neck component have not been encountered since the prosthesis was revised to a large diameter neck and using cobalt-chrome (120, 124, 126). Loosening of the metal glenoid component from the glenoid vault was not encountered in the majority of patients in the first 5 years of use. Thereafter, glenoid screws made by casting methods have broken, leading to loosening in 5 of 104 cases. Theoretically, the risk of screw breakage is lessened if the screws are partially hooded at the back of the metal glenoid component. Moreover, pullout of the glenoid component was observed in several cases over time, as the bone became demineralized in older patients, or the glenoid vault was destroyed by a metastatic lesion in one patient.

Other noteworthy constrained prostheses have been tested in humans. Kölbel et al. (80–82) used a small reversible head protruding laterally from the glenoid vault. Little disruption of the vault contents occurs because the main point of attachment is by means of a metal strut that is part of the metal neck to the base of the scapular spine. The strut is fastened with a bolt. Both Post et al. (124–126) and Kölbel et al. (80–82) were among the first to point out the value in preserving the glenoid vault and avoiding disruption of the subchondral bone of the glenoid.

Zippel (154) reported success with a constrained design. However, he experienced loosening, undoubtedly due to the necessity of disturbing the glenoid vault when inserting the glenoid component. Similarly, Gristina et al. (55, 56) tried a monospheric design and also had good results and few failures with a constrained prosthesis of trispheric design. Buechel et al. (15, 16) reported good results using a constrained joint with a floating socket design that contained a nondislocatable, dual sphere with centers offset to provide a fulcrum. Like Fenlin's design (46), the reversed configuration allowed a greater range of motion.

Prosthetic Replacement of the Humeral Head

When the proximal humeral articular surface alone is irreparably damaged, prosthetic replacement of the humeral head is a satisfactory means of relieving pain and restoring shoulder function. The most popular unconstrained prosthesis still in use, and the one used by the authors, is the Neer or Neer type design. The Neer series I humeral component, flattened on top, was first used in 1951. The series II Neer humeral components (1973) were revised so that the articular surface was no longer flattened on top (110) (Fig. 3.9). The series II humeral head sizes are 15 mm and 22 mm, and the three stem diameters are 6.3, 9.5, and 12.7 mm. The radius of curvature of the articular surface of each size head is 44 mm, which is the size of the average humeral head and matches the glenoid component. Other similar unconstrained devices, many of which have modular head components, are now available, including the Cofield unconstrained shoulder with a surface mount metal-backed glenoid (30). Rockwood and Matsen (Rockwood C, personal communication, 1992) have used the Global Total Shoulder System (DePuy, Warsaw, Indiana), which incorporates glenoid components designed with a constant 3-mm radial mismatch or nonconformance. All glenoid component radii are

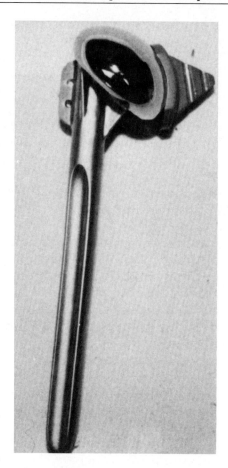

Figure 3.9. Neer II prosthesis with trial glenoid component. (From Post M. The shoulder—surgical and nonsurgical management. 2nd ed. Philadelphia: Lea & Febiger, 1988).

3 mm larger than the corresponding size of the humeral head radii. In recent years, modular humeral head prostheses have been developed that offer the potential advantages of allowing better soft tissue tensioning with greater size selection and easier revision to a total shoulder, if the glenoid later becomes eroded (Rockwood C, personal communication, 1992).

INDICATIONS FOR PROSTHETIC HUMERAL HEAD REPLACEMENT

Prosthetic humeral head replacement is most often indicated for acute fracture-dislocations or four-part displaced fractures of the humeral head in which the blood supply of the bone fragments is almost certainly lost (84, 105, 149). Other indications are posterior fracture-dislocations with a 45 to 50% impression defect or head-splitting fractures. In addition to these injuries, selected three-part fractures in older patients and selected anatomic neck fractures may require hemiarthroplasty. Avascular necrosis (36) of the humeral head is another fairly common indication for humeral hemiarthroplasty. Humeral hemiarthroplasty may also be used in patients with glenohumeral arthritis and a highly deficient rotator cuff (24, 42, 114). Finally, humeral head replacement without glenoid resurfacing may be considered in younger, more active patients with glenohumeral osteoarthritis (155) and a concentric glenoid (Fig. 3.10).

INDICATIONS FOR GLENOID COMPONENT REPLACEMENT

When the glenoid articular surface is also damaged, consideration is given to glenoid resurfacing. The indication for a glenoid component is present when the subchondral bone and underlying vault contain large bone cysts or when there is severe irregular erosion or an incongruity of the glenoid surface. If there is uneven or eccentric wear of the glenoid with posterior erosion, then humeral hemiarthroplasty alone may not yield satisfactory results, and total shoulder arthroplasty is usually performed (Fig. 3.11). Similarly, if there is severe erosion of the glenoid and lateralization of the humeral head is required (and if enough of the glenoid vault is present), a glenoid component may be inserted to restore more normal tension in the soft tissues and a more normal

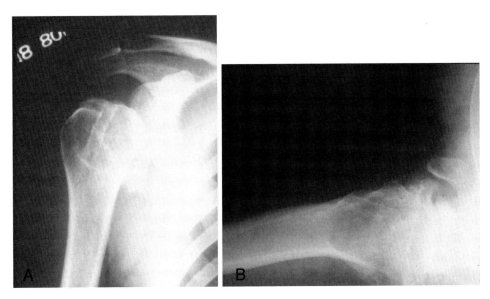

Figure 3.10. **(A,B)** Anteroposterior and axillary radiographs of an osteoarthritic shoulder with concentric glenoid wear. Humeral hemiarthroplasty might be considered in a younger, more active patient with this radiographic pattern of osteoarthritis.

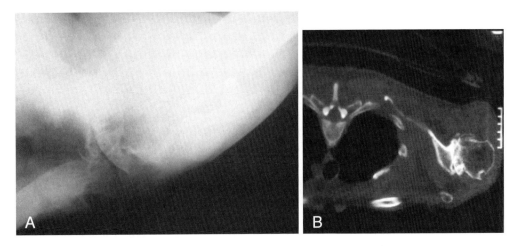

Figure 3.11. **(A,B)** Anteroposterior and axillary radiographs of an osteoarthritic shoulder with eccentric glenoid wear. Here the posterior glenoid is eroded, leading to posterior subluxation of the humeral head. Total shoulder arthroplasty is usually performed in such cases of osteoarthritis.

fulcrum of the metal humeral head. Glenoid resurfacing is usually avoided when there is insufficient bone to implant a glenoid component (e.g., in some patients with severe rheumatoid arthritis) or when the rotator cuff is severely deficient or irreparable (e.g., cuff tear arthropathy and some patients with rheumatoid arthritis) (37, 49, 50).

CONTRAINDICATIONS

Unconstrained prosthetic replacement of the humeral head should not be performed when the short rotators and deltoid are nonfunctioning (i.e., a flail shoulder) and when active infection is present.

It is essential for the surgeon to understand the chief pathology and anatomy of the various stages of each diagnostic condition (40, 150) so that preoperative planning can reduce unnecessary surprises intraoperatively and allow the surgeon to solve special intraoperative problems and achieve an optimum outcome. Each diagnostic category poses special features that should be known beforehand, if possible.

Features of Various Disease States

OSTEOARTHRITIS

The premiere features of osteoarthritis of the glenohumeral joint are joint space narrowing, subchondral sclerosis, cystic changes in the subchondral and metaphyseal regions, peripheral osteophytes, and distortion of the humeral head (104) (Figs. 3.10 and 11). The articular surface of the glenoid may be sclerotic and eburnated and devoid of cartilage. Osteophytes may encroach on the bicipital groove, block rotational motion, and even extend inferiorly and medially toward the axillary nerve. The joint capsule may be distended and contain varying amounts of clear yellow synovial fluid. Loose bodies may be present. Occasionally, when the joint subluxates posteriorly, the posterior capsule may be stretched. The synovium may be hypertrophied, friable, and inflamed not only anteriorly but posteriorly. Consideration should be given to restoring the normal tensions in the soft tissue to permit adequate stability and movement of the prosthetic head. Specifically, this requires adequate release of anterior soft tissue contractures and occasionally even formal subscapularis lengthening. The flattening of the glenoid and posterior erosion from posterior subluxation of the head must be addressed by lowering the less worn anterior side, accepting the increased glenoid retroversion, and then altering the humeral component version; in rare cases, bone grafting the deficient glenoid may be necessary (109, 110). The cuff may be attenuated but is rarely torn.

RHEUMATOID ARTHRITIS

The pathology seen in shoulders with rheumatoid arthritis varies from mild to very severe (151). Friedman and Ewald (51) have shown that unconstrained total shoulder replacements performed in patients who have rheumatoid arthritis with class IV functional capacity and who had Stage III or IV rheumatoid progression achieved excellent relief of pain and satisfactory improvement in motion (with severe rheumatoid involvement of the shoulder). When less severe rheumatoid disease was present and the soft tissues were less adversely affected, function was correspondingly better with a glenohumeral arthroplasty (52). Neer (103) classified the pattern of rheumatoid shoulder involvement as dry, wet, or resorptive, with the possibility of low grade, intermediate, or severe changes within each group. With the dry form, there is a marked tendency for loss of the joint space (Fig. 3.12), periarticular sclerosis, bone cysts, and stiffness. In the wet form, there is exuberant synovial disease with marginal erosions and protrusion of the humeral head into the glenoid. The chief feature of the resorptive type is bone resorption (Fig. 3.13).

In rheumatoid arthritis, the soft tissues and bone are affected. The subdeltoid bursa may show inflammation, fibrosis, and synovial hypertrophy.

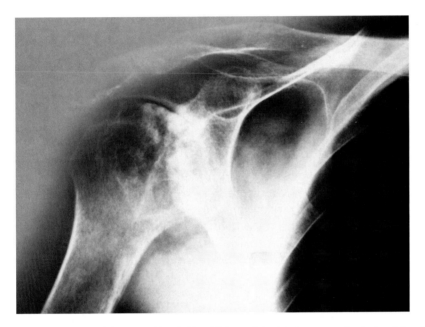

Figure 3.12. Advanced rheumatoid arthritis with loss of the joint space and anterior dislocation.

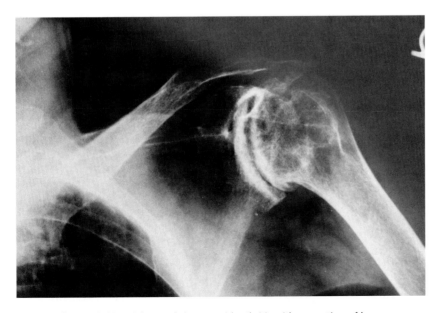

Figure 3.13. Advanced rheumatoid arthritis with resorption of bone.

The bone is osteopenic in varying degrees and may show erosions, resorption, sclerosis, cysts, and even fracture in exceptional cases. In the last situation, this may result from a severe erosion and indentation of the proximal medial humeral shaft cortex that has impinged on the inferior glenoid. The cartilage may be partially or completely lost. The rotator cuff exhibits inflammation, fibrosis, attenuation, and stretching and tearing in varying degrees. Full-thickness rotator cuff tears are seen in approximately one-fourth to one-third of these cases. The synovial lining may be inflamed, fibrotic, and show exuberant synovial hypertrophy. The shoulder capsule may be inflamed, fibrotic, attenuated, and stretched. There may be mild to severe instability of the glenohumeral joint in advanced cases. In long-standing rheumatoid arthritis of the shoulder, varying degrees of erosion of the subchondral and adjacent bony structures may occur.

TRAUMATIC ARTHRITIS

Traumatic arthritis results from previous fractures, dislocations, or fracture-dislocations. Samilson and Prieto (141) reviewed 74 shoulders with a history of a single or multiple dislocation that showed radiographic evidence of glenohumeral arthritis. The dislocations were anterior in 62 patients and posterior in 11 patients. One patient had multidirectional instability. Those patients with posterior instability had a higher incidence of moderate or severe arthritis, as did shoulders that had undergone previous surgery in which internal fixation devices compromised the joint surfaces. Zuckerman and Matsen (157) showed complications relating to the use of metallic internal fixation devices. Many of these patients had had operations for treatment of recurrent shoulder dislocations. Hawkins et al. (67) used hemiarthroplasty if a chronic posterior dislocation was greater than 6 months' duration or if the humeral head defect involved more than 45% of the articular surface. When the glenoid is destroyed, a total shoulder arthroplasty is needed. Tanner and Cofield (149) reviewed 28 cases with chronic fracture problems requiring prosthetic arthroplasty. In this series, 16 had malunions with a joint incongruity, 8 had posttraumatic osteonecrosis, and 4 had nonunion of a surgical neck fracture with a small, osteopenic head fragment. In the authors' experience, traumatic arthritis may be well treated with hemiarthroplasty if 1) the glenoid is not severely eroded and remains fairly concentric and 2) the incongruity between the joint surfaces is not great.

OSTEONECROSIS

Aside from posttraumatic osteonecrosis of the humeral head, the systemic use of steroids is another common cause of osteonecrosis of the humeral head. Various conditions that are associated with osteonecrosis include alcoholism, sickle cell disease, hemophilia, decompression sickness, hyperuricemia, Gaucher's disease, pancreatitis, familial hyperlipidemia, renal or other organ transplantations, lymphoma, and lupus erythematosus (34, 35, 136). Cruess (34) classified osteonecrosis by using a staging system. In this system, Stage I is a preradiologic stage. Radiographs are often normal. However, bone scans or magnetic resonance imaging may show changes within the humeral head. Stage II shows radiologic changes including osteoporosis, osteosclerosis, or a combination of the two. Subchondral osteolytic lesions without fracture and without a change in the humeral head shape are present. Stage III exhibits a crescent sign. This suggests a fracture through the abnormal subchondral bone. In the humeral head, this is usually located superior and centrally. There are only mild changes in the contour of the head in this stage. Stage IV shows collapse of the subchondral bone with deformity or, in some cases, a separated osteocartilaginous flap. Stage V contains the same findings as in Stage IV but also includes pathologic changes in the glenoid. The use of this classification system aids in determining a prognosis and treatment plan. The more advanced the stage, the more severe the complaints and progression of symptoms and findings. In the later stages, hemiarthroplasty often becomes necessary. For example, in a study of 18 patients who had steroid-induced osteonecrosis of the humeral head, Cruess (34) found that hemiarthroplasty produced good results in an advanced group who had severe pain and significant deformity. When the glenoid is severely involved, a total shoulder replacement is required. If pain is not a significant factor, then operative treatment will not be necessary, especially if progression does not occur.

Operation for Unconstrained Arthroplasty

GENERAL COMMENTS

Soft tissue contractures must be released, including contractures of the coracohumeral ligament, the capsule, and most notably the subscapularis, which may have to be lengthened. Enough lengthening of the subscapularis may be obtained in most cases if the insertion of the subscapularis tendon is elevated at its attachment at the lesser tuberosity and later reattached directly to the anatomic neck region. In some cases, a formal Z-plasty lengthening is advantageous (27). Large rotator cuff tears should be repaired whenever possible.

Glenohumeral instability needs to be corrected to achieve a correct amount of tension in the shoulder capsule and rotator cuff (27, 119). How this is done will change the postoperative rehabilitation program. Corrective measures for glenoid deficiencies need to be addressed.

Massive bone loss of the proximal humerus, such as with tumor resection, needs to be adequately managed. For example, a long stem prosthesis may be needed along with bone grafting of the proximal humerus.

The choice of cementing versus press-fitting the humeral component is based on bone quality, which usually corresponds to the age of the patient in osteoarthritic patients. Thus, cement fixation is usually chosen for patients with poor bone stock and older patients with osteoarthritis. Cement fixation is also used for patients with complex fractures, rheumatoid arthritis, and usually osteonecrosis. The results of a well-done press-fit shoulder arthroplasty are comparable to cemented stems (121). Surgeons should be familiar with both types of procedures, so that they can weigh the risks and benefits of each technique (59).

Operative Technique for Prosthetic Replacement

The patient is placed on the operating table in a semireclining position (60°), and the patient's head is secured to a head rest to avoid rotation or hyperextension of the cervical spine. A short arm side board is attached to the operating table at the midaspect of the humeral shaft level. Folded towels are placed beneath the ipsilateral scapula to minimize movement of the shoulder blade, and the arm is draped free so that it may be positioned off the table and can be rotated or flexed (Fig. 3.14). A broad-spectrum antibiotic is administered intravenously before surgery and is continued for 24 to 48 hours postoperatively. A 15-cm skin incision is made starting just beneath the clavicle and extending just lateral to the coracoid process toward the deltoid insertion on the lateral aspect of the humeral shaft (11, 119) (Fig. 3.15). The

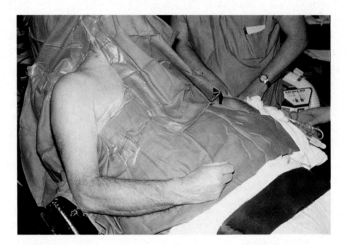

Figure 3.14.   Positioning for prosthetic shoulder replacement. The patient is placed in a semireclining position with the arm extending over the side of the operating table, supported by a short arm board.

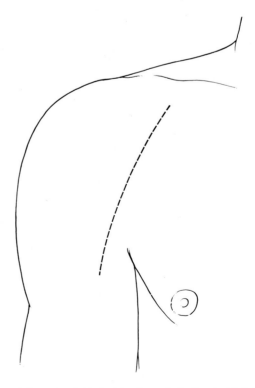

Figure 3.15.   A long deltopectoral skin incision is used, starting just inferior to the clavicle and proceeding over the coracoid process down obliquely to the region of the deltoid insertion.

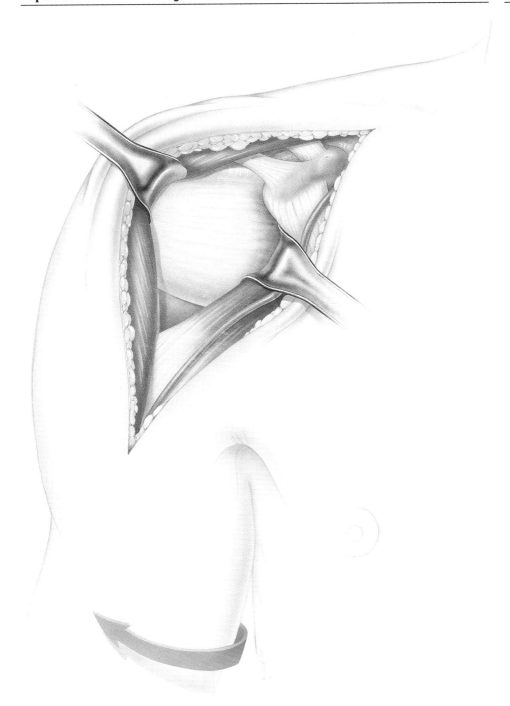

Figure 3.16. The deltopectoral interval is developed, carefully retracting the pectoralis major medially and the deltoid laterally. The cephalic vein may be retracted either laterally with the deltoid
or as shown here, or medially with the pectoralis, but should be preserved whenever possible.

cephalic vein and the deltopectoral interval are identified. The authors prefer
to retract the cephalic vein medially, especially in patients who have undergone operation previously, to avoid stretching and tearing of the cephalic
vein as it traverses the clavipectoral fascia. Venous branches from the deltoid
are identified, tied, and transected (119). The pectoralis major is retracted medially along with the conjoint tendon, while the deltoid is retracted laterally
(Fig. 3.16). In nearly all cases, the deltoid origin is left intact. If additional

exposure is needed, the sternal portion of the pectoralis major tendon can be partially divided. The pectoralis tendon is later repaired.

The clavipectoral fascia over the subscapularis tendon is incised longitudinally lateral to the coracoid. Particularly in shoulders that exhibit cuff arthropathy or poor function of the rotator cuff with a tendency to subluxate superiorly, the coracoacromial ligament and its arch should be preserved (156).

The anterior humeral circumflex vessels at the lower edge of the subscapularis tendon are identified, tied off or coagulated, and transected.

The subscapularis tendon is then transected with the underlying joint capsule at its insertion onto the lesser tuberosity (Fig. 3.17A). Before transecting the tendon, the surgeon should determine whether there is any mechanical block or soft tissue contracture that may be limiting external rotation. The authors often achieve lengthening of the subscapularis by elevating the

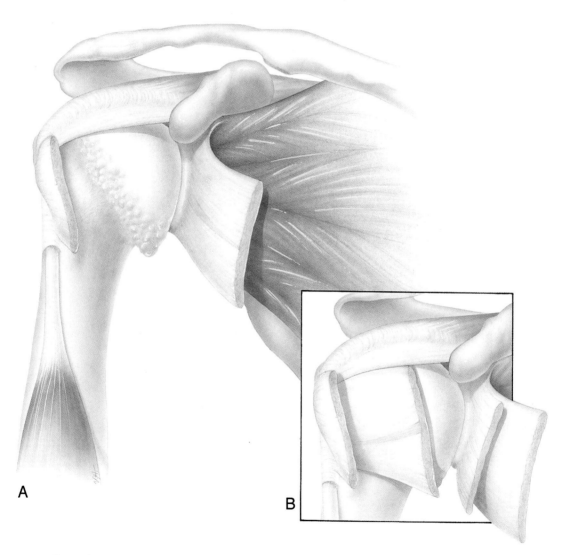

Figure 3.17. **(A)** The subscapularis tendon and the joint capsule are incised together and as far laterally as possible to preserve maximal length of these contracted anterior soft tissues. **(B)** Occasionally, a formal Z-plasty lengthening of the capsule and subscapularis must be performed for severe internal rotation contracture (such as when these tissues had been previously shortened, as in an overtightened Putti-Platt instability repair).

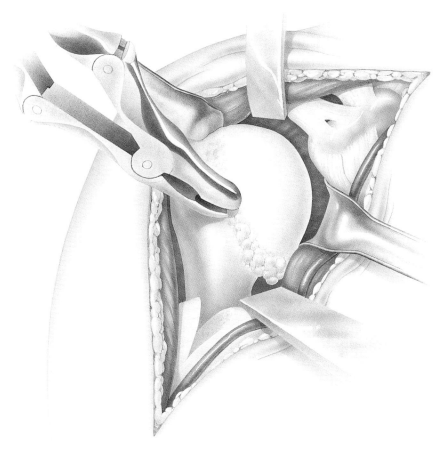

Figure 3.18. A rongeur is used to remove the peripheral osteophytes around the humeral head. In cases in which there are large osteophytes, especially inferiorly, this will facilitate dislocation of the humeral head.

subscapularis tendon laterally at its insertion and later reattaching it more medially in the anatomic neck region, just under the osteotomized area of the humeral head. The subscapularis is also released from the underlying capsule to correct the anterior soft tissue contracture. The capsule is also carefully released inferiorly and occasionally posteriorly, while protecting the axillary nerve, to balance the soft tissues. For severe soft tissue contractures of the subscapularis tendon, especially if the tendon has previously been shortened (as in a Putti-Platt repair for instability), it can be lengthened by Z-plasty (Fig. 3.17B) before fully transecting the tendon; every centimeter of length gained allows 10 to 15° of external rotation to be achieved.

Next, the humeral head is exposed. The arm is gently externally rotated to dislocate the diseased head. In osteoarthritis, if large osteophytes have locked the humeral head in the glenoid and prevent dislocation, cheilectomy of osteophytes at the inferior peripheral humeral head may first be necessary to permit dislocation of the head (Fig. 3.18). The surgeon must be careful to identify and protect the axillary nerve. If a Hohman or Darrach retractor is positioned in front of the axillary nerve to protect it, even if it is visualized, care must be taken not to stretch the nerve. In most instances, with the head intact and a trial silhouette of the humeral component to assess the correct angle (Fig. 3.19), the arm is externally rotated 35° and the diseased head is excised with an osteotome or power saw blade placed in the straight up-and-down

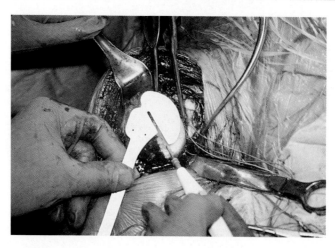

Figure 3.19.   A silhouette of the prosthesis may be used to mark correctly the amount of humeral head that should be excised. This will help to prevent the common error of resecting excessive bone and placing the prosthesis below the level of the greater tuberosity.

position (Fig. 3.20). If the head has collapsed because of osteonecrosis, for example, much less bone may need to be removed than usual. If desired, instrumentation is available for most prosthetic devices that permit humeral head resection in the desired version position.

The arm is hyperextended off the side of the table to deliver the humeral shaft into the wound. A rongeur can then be used to remove remaining portions of the peripheral osteophytes along the humeral neck (Fig. 3.21). If possible, the arm board should be shifted superiorly. The correct retroversion angle is 30 to 40° in most cases (101, 102, 110, 119). Care should be taken not to resect too much humeral head (Fig. 3.20B). In acute fractures, the humeral head is removed, and the tuberosities with the attached rotator cuff are mobilized and later reattached to the bone shaft beneath the dome of the metal humeral head using no. 5 nonabsorbable sutures. The humeral bone should be made raw using a rounded power burr. The authors prefer nonabsorbable sutures to monofilament wire fixation. If a large bone defect exists, the prosthetic stem may need to be elevated and an autogenous bone graft used to fill the defect (see Chapter 2).

The proper size stem and head are selected. The prosthesis is positioned at the appropriate height and version angle to maximize myofascial sleeve tension for stability and deltoid muscle tension for strength (Fig. 3.22). For example, proper height of the prosthesis provides soft tissue tension and allows the correct placement of the tuberosities beneath the head of the prosthesis in an acute fracture of the proximal humerus. With acute fracture of the proximal humerus, the prosthesis should not ordinarily be placed downward against the remaining humeral shaft, because the humerus is usually shortened and the proper height will not be achieved. In addition, the tuberosities will not fit beneath the head. The prosthesis is inserted at 30 to 40° of retroversion and should point backward toward the glenoid while the arm is held in the neutral position with the elbow at the side. An intact bicipital groove can be a useful guide for determining humeral head retroversion, because the lateral fin of the stem should be placed at the bicipital groove or just posterior to the groove to achieve 30 to 40° of retroversion. The more the lateral fin is placed behind the groove, the less the degree of retroversion is obtained.

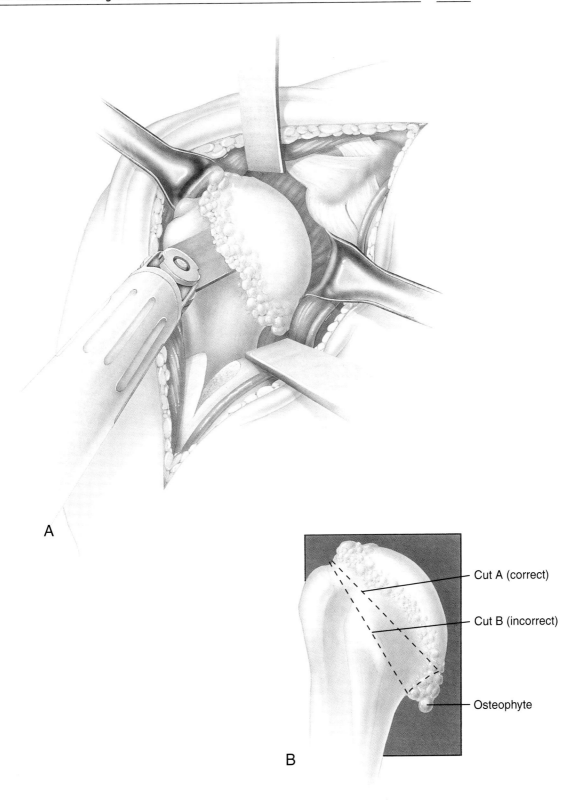

Figure 3.20.   **(A)** An oscillating saw is used to excise the humeral head while retractors protect the rotator cuff and biceps superiorly and the axillary nerve inferiorly. With the arm externally rotated to 35°, the cut is directed straight down toward the floor, yielding appropriate version. **(B)** Cut A resects only the humeral head, whereas the incorrect cut (cut B) resects excessive bone and would allow the humeral prosthesis to sit too low on the humeral neck.

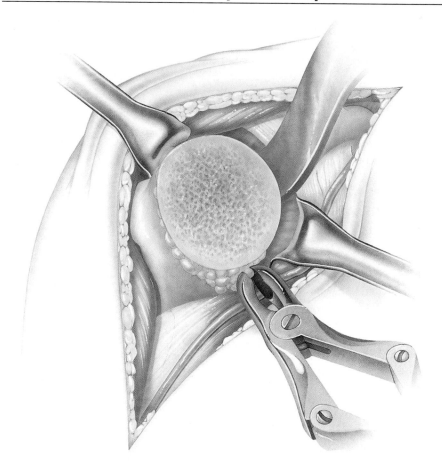

Figure 3.21. After the humeral head has been excised, a rongeur is again used to remove any remaining osteophytes from the region of the humeral neck, because these osteophytes could abut on the glenoid and limit motion.

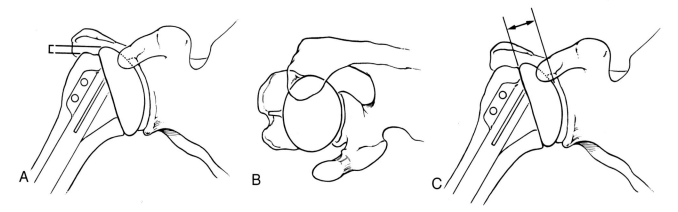

A   B   C

Figure 3.22. Several anatomic factors must be considered in the correct placement of the humeral head prosthesis. **(A)** The prosthesis should be seated slightly superiorly with respect to the greater tuberosity to prevent impingement of the tuberosity with abduction of the arm. **(B)** Appropriate version of the prosthesis should be achieved by placing the fin of the prosthesis just posterior to the biceps groove to achieve 30 to 40° of retroversion. **(C)** The head size is chosen to restore an appropriate distance between the tuberosity and the glenoid to allow an adequate fulcrum for raising the arm. This head size should allow passive translations of the prosthesis of approximately 50% of the glenoid width in the anteroposterior dimension and similar translations superoinferiorly.

The lateral fin usually points just posterior to the bicipital groove. Slight anterior placement of the fin increases retroversion, and posterior placement decreases retroversion. If the bicipital groove is absent, the humeral condyles should be palpated with the thumb and forefinger to estimate retroversion. Alternatively, the trial prosthesis can be inserted in the proper angle of version when the elbow is held at the side in the neutral position.

The humeral canal is reamed manually to the correct width and depth, taking care to avoid perforation of the humeral cortex (Fig. 3.23). The reamer is started laterally just posterior to the bicipital groove.

If a Neer II prosthesis is used, the head component is made with two length sizes, 15 and 22 mm; both are available in three stem diameters of 6.3, 9.5, and 12.7 mm. The stem lengths range from 125 to 150 mm. For special cases, extra long stem (252 mm) and extra short stem (63 mm) components are available.

In cases of acute fracture of the proximal humerus, the bony stability for the humeral component is frequently compromised. Bone cement is needed in these cases. In the authors' experience, in cases of osteoarthritis, a press-fit can be achieved in the majority of patients. Before cementing or placing the prosthesis in the humeral canal, several drill holes are made in the proximal anterior humeral shaft so that nonabsorbable no. 5 suture may be placed

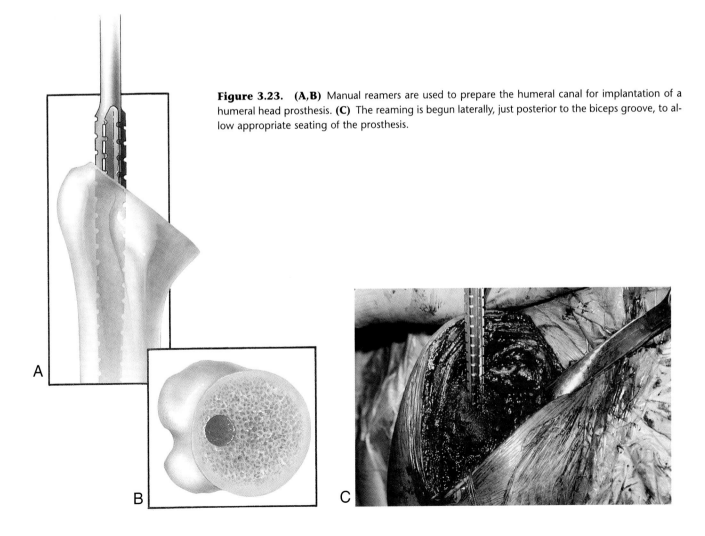

Figure 3.23. **(A,B)** Manual reamers are used to prepare the humeral canal for implantation of a humeral head prosthesis. **(C)** The reaming is begun laterally, just posterior to the biceps groove, to allow appropriate seating of the prosthesis.

through the drill holes to be later used for reattachment and reconstruction of the tuberosities and/or the rotator cuff, which may have to be reattached directly to the proximal humerus beneath the metal humeral head.

If modular components are used, especially where bone cement is employed, bone or methyl methacrylate excrescences that protrude superiorly are removed to permit proper seating of the modular component. Whether a Morse or reverse Morse taper is used, the metal parts are thoroughly dried and any blood removed to allow proper contact and obviate later loosening of the modular head. Posterior and superior parts of the prosthetic device must not reside beneath the tip or the most superior portion of the greater tuberosity, so that the complication of impingement on the undersurface of the acromion can be avoided. A large head can be used if lateralization of the humeral shaft is desired to achieve optimum tension in the capsule and leverage for the muscles. The arthroplasty should allow translation of the prosthesis of up to 50% of the diameter of the glenoid in the anteroposterior plane to avoid overtightening the joint and limiting motion. In cases in which a ballooned posterior capsule is present, such as is often seen with a chronically dislocated locked arthritic humeral head, a purse-string suture using no. 5 nonabsorbable suture can be woven into the posterior capsule to close the enlarged pouch.

In placing the trial prosthesis, the humeral canal is first located with a small, straight curette. This is important, especially when much sclerotic bone in the proximal humerus makes location of the intramedullary canal difficult. The opening of the canal is enlarged until a small T-reamer can be introduced and the canal enlarged, if possible, to receive larger size stems. It is essential that the lateral cortex is not pierced by the curette or reamer, especially in older demineralized bone. The correct stem size can be estimated by measuring the radiographs in two planes preoperatively. In osteoporotic bone, the flanges of the metal stem may be manually impacted. In dense bone, small slots may have to be cut in the proximal humerus to receive the three metal flanges and avoid fracture. Occasionally, a greater or lesser retroversion angle may be required to achieve stability. In the usual case, the trial prosthesis is positioned in 30 to 40° degrees retroversion measured with the

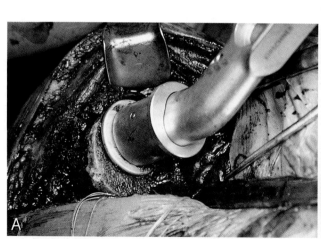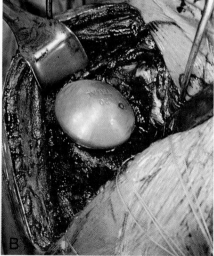

Figure 3.24. **(A)** A modular stem trial is inserted into the proximal humeral canal. **(B)** Various modular head sizes can be used in the trial fit so that the best possible fit is obtained.

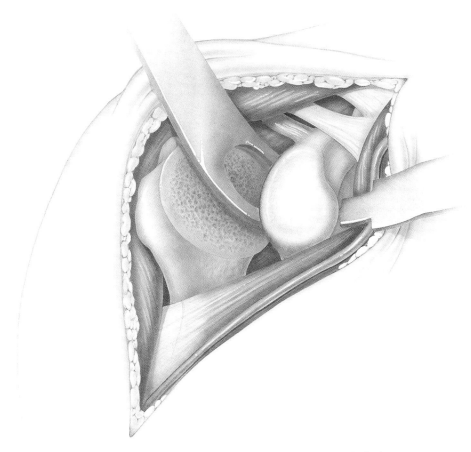

Figure 3.25. Exposure of the glenoid is obtained by using a Fukuda ring retractor to retract the proximal humerus posteriorly and a spiked Darrach retractor to expose the anterior margin of the glenoid.

patient's elbow flexed to 90° (Fig. 3.24). The prosthesis should then point backward toward the glenoid. The lateral flange of the stem is ordinarily placed just behind the bicipital groove.

Before the final humeral prosthesis is impacted or cemented, the glenoid is inspected. A Fukuda retractor is used to hold the proximal humerus away from the glenoid face (Fig. 3.25). Great care should be taken to avoid excessive retraction of the shaft, especially when the tissues are tight. If the bone is demineralized, a complication of fracture of the glenoid can result due to excessive leverage by the retractor on the posterior glenoid. If a glenoid resurfacing is necessary, a slot is started in the central glenoid with a dental drill and is then widened using a power burr (Fig. 3.26). The glenoid slot for a glenoid keel or drill holes for surface mount glenoid components must be made in the "safe zone" so that the component does not protrude beyond the cortex of the glenoid.

The authors use the glenoid component in cases of glenoid erosion, in the presence of larger glenoid bone cysts or where there is an incongruous glenoid articular surface. If the glenoid erosion is exceptionally severe, there may not be enough glenoid vault remaining to adequately hold a glenoid component. Once the bone slot is made to receive the plastic glenoid trial component, it is inserted and the stability is tested. There should be no rocking of the component. The glenoid trial component must be seated on all sides of the glenoid face and remain stable. Any peripheral osteophytes around the

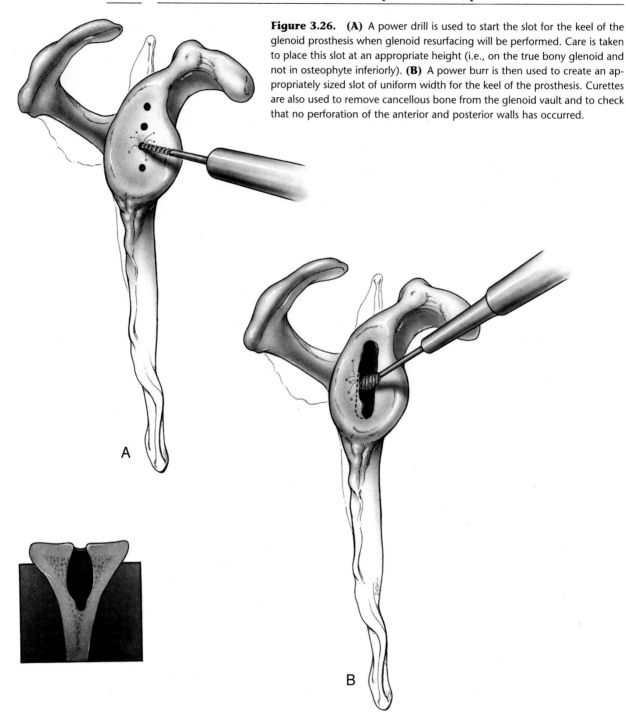

Figure 3.26. **(A)** A power drill is used to start the slot for the keel of the glenoid prosthesis when glenoid resurfacing will be performed. Care is taken to place this slot at an appropriate height (i.e., on the true bony glenoid and not in osteophyte inferiorly). **(B)** A power burr is then used to create an appropriately sized slot of uniform width for the keel of the prosthesis. Curettes are also used to remove cancellous bone from the glenoid vault and to check that no perforation of the anterior and posterior walls has occurred.

glenoid that prevent proper seating should be removed (see Fig. 3.35). With the trial humeral and glenoid components in place, the prosthetic component should not dislocate when the arm is brought to the zero anatomic position with the elbow at the side of the torso. Asymmetric wear of the glenoid is frequently seen on glenohumeral osteoarthritis, with posterior erosion or bone loss being most common (Fig. 3.27). Eccentric glenoid wear is dealt with in several ways, including with lesser wear, by lowering the high side (usually the anterior glenoid) to match the eccentrically worn posterior glenoid (Fig. 3.28), or by accepting the increased glenoid retroversion and later

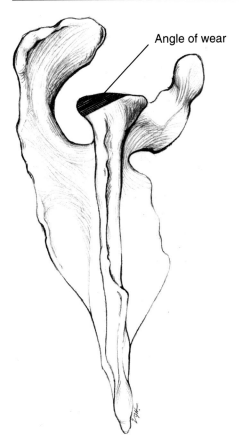

Angle of wear

Figure 3.27. Asymmetric glenoid wear is frequently encountered in osteoarthritis, as the posterior glenoid is usually eroded more than the anterior glenoid. This eccentric wear must be taken into account when performing glenoid resurfacing to prevent component loosening and instability.

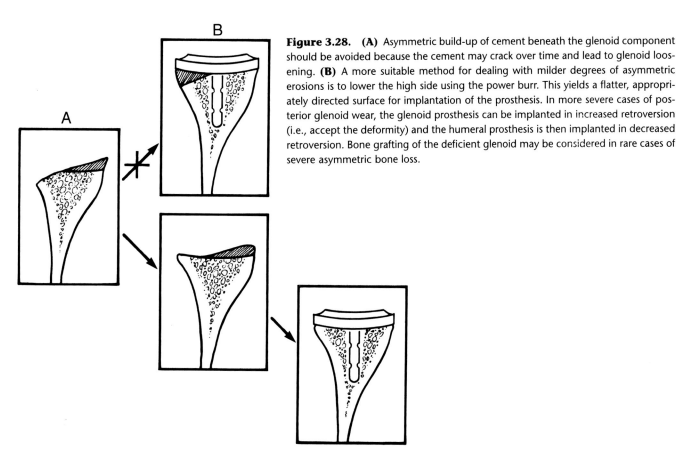

B

A

Figure 3.28. **(A)** Asymmetric build-up of cement beneath the glenoid component should be avoided because the cement may crack over time and lead to glenoid loosening. **(B)** A more suitable method for dealing with milder degrees of asymmetric erosions is to lower the high side using the power burr. This yields a flatter, appropriately directed surface for implantation of the prosthesis. In more severe cases of posterior glenoid wear, the glenoid prosthesis can be implanted in increased retroversion (i.e., accept the deformity) and the humeral prosthesis is then implanted in decreased retroversion. Bone grafting of the deficient glenoid may be considered in rare cases of severe asymmetric bone loss.

decreasing the amount of humeral retroversion; in severe cases, bone grafting the deficient side of the glenoid is used (104, 109). If a polyethylene glenoid is used, it is cemented in place after several small holes are made inside the slot to lock the cement. After the glenoid has been dried of excess blood, the cement can be injected into the slot of the glenoid by using a syringe (Fig. 3.29). Alternatively, the cement can be manually inserted or packed into the glenoid slot. The glenoid component is then implanted and held in place by the surgeon until the cement hardens to prevent shifting of the component (Fig. 3.30).

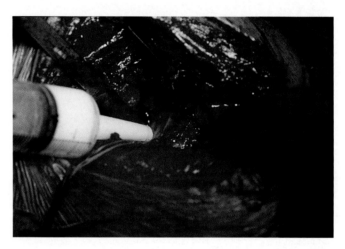

Figure 3.29.   Cement is injected into the slot using a syringe. Cement is not placed directly on the face of the glenoid. Rather, when the keel of the prosthesis is placed into the slot, a thin mantle of cement will be expelled from the slot and will cover the glenoid surface.

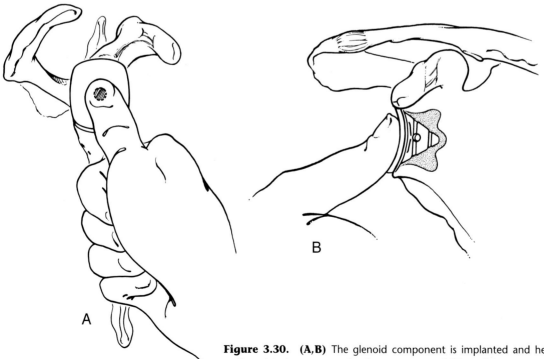

Figure 3.30.   **(A,B)** The glenoid component is implanted and held in place until methylmethacrylate bone cement hardens to prevent shifting of the component.

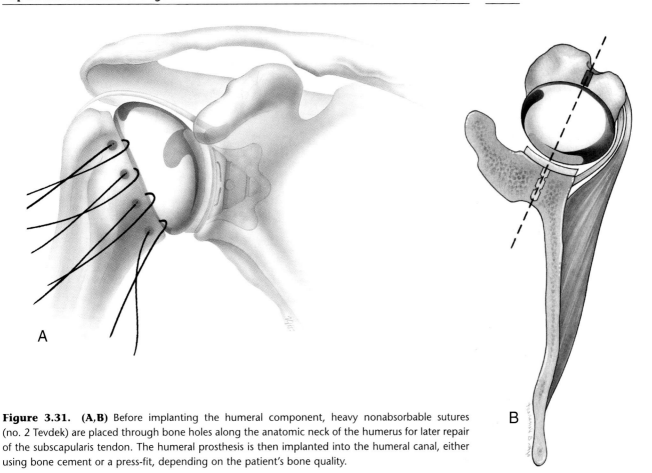

Figure 3.31. **(A,B)** Before implanting the humeral component, heavy nonabsorbable sutures (no. 2 Tevdek) are placed through bone holes along the anatomic neck of the humerus for later repair of the subscapularis tendon. The humeral prosthesis is then implanted into the humeral canal, either using bone cement or a press-fit, depending on the patient's bone quality.

Next, the humeral component is inserted. Before its insertion, nonabsorbable sutures (no. 2 Tevdek) are placed through bone holes along the anatomic neck of the humerus for repair of the subscapularis (Fig. 3.31). If cement is used, a cement restrictor is recommended whenever possible. Methylmethacrylate cement may be inserted manually in the nonsticky phase or injected in the liquid phase after the intramedullary canal is dried and a small-diameter vent tube temporarily inserted. The lower surface of the metal dome should be flush against the cut surface of the proximal humerus. Any residual osteophytes that protrude beyond the metal dome should be excised to avoid later impingement or improper seating of a modular humeral head. The subscapularis tendon is reattached with nonabsorbable heavy sutures while the arm is in the externally rotated position (Fig. 3.32).

A closed system wound drainage is used for 24 hours or longer if necessary. The subcutaneous tissues are reapproximated with absorbable sutures. Finally, the skin is closed using a subcuticular suture (Fig. 3.33). The shoulder is placed into a sling and swathe in the operating room before proceeding to the recovery room.

POSTOPERATIVE MANAGEMENT

A portable anteroposterior radiograph is taken of the shoulder (including the humeral shaft) in the recovery room, and permanent anteroposterior and axillary radiograph are taken later (Fig. 3.34). Closed suction drains are

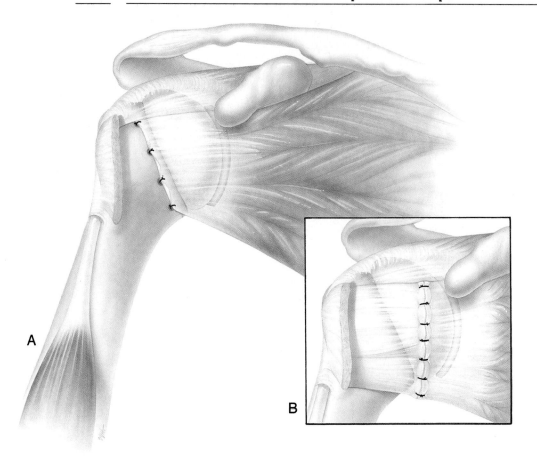

Figure 3.32. **(A)** The subscapularis is then repaired using the sutures passed through bone holes along the humeral neck. This allows effective lengthening of the contracted anterior soft tissues, as the insertion is more medial than originally. **(B)** In severe cases of anterior contracture, in which Z-plasty lengthening of the tissues has been performed, the tendon is instead repaired to the deep flap of tissue that had been created laterally.

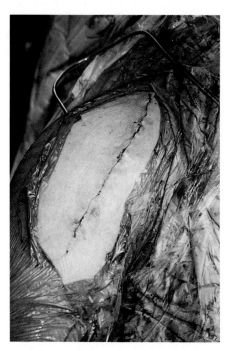

Figure 3.33. After layered repair of the deltopectoral interval and subcutaneous tissues, the skin is closed using a subcuticular suture.

removed 24 hours later. The wound is redressed. With the arm at the side, the patient is permitted to use the hand and elbow in flexion and extension. When the rotator cuff and tuberosities are intact, Phase I assistive and passive motion exercises are started. The patient is instructed in gentle pendulum rotation motions with the arm dangling at the side. Force should not be used to achieve extremes of motion (69, 108). Phase I exercises are continued for 10 days. Thereafter, very gentle isometric and gentle Phase II muscle-resistant exercises are begun using elastic bands (Theraband, yellow and red, made by Advance Rehabilitation System, Naperville, Illinois). The purpose of the Phase I and Phase II exercises is to achieve maximum combined elevation and 40° of external rotation with the arm at the side and the elbow bent to 90°. If the rotator cuff is intact and functioning, this can usually be achieved within 3 weeks. The patient may continue supervised physical therapy exercises several times each week under the care of a certified physical therapist and perform the exercises at home for 5- to 10-minute periods, five or six times per day. After 6 weeks, muscle resistance exercises to strengthen the deltoid, external rotators, and internal rotator muscles of the shoulder are increased. In most cases, a sling is not necessary after several days and light active use is permitted. After hemiarthroplasty for acute four-part fractures or after arthroplasty with a deficient rotator cuff, the program outlined above is modified to allow for tuberosity or cuff healing. In this setting, limited passive exercises are performed during the first 6 weeks and are then carefully advanced.

Operative Management of Special Problems

SOFT TISSUE CONTRACTURES

Trauma and previous operative treatment may contribute to scarring of the soft tissues. The coracohumeral ligament may be contracted. This is a defined structure and is clearly visible. It should be incised if no mechanical block exists and there is a contracture of the coracohumeral ligament, because as much as 25 to 30° of additional external rotation motion may be obtained by releasing this structure. Care should be taken to avoid injury to the coracoacromial ligament, especially in shoulders with a highly deficient rotator cuff, because this ligament may stabilize the implant against superior migration (156).

Extensive scar tissue may be present in arthritic conditions and especially in patients who have had previous operative treatment or in shoulders that have had old trauma. Excessive scar tissue must be excised. It is essential for the surgeon to examine the patient under general anesthesia to determine the true range of motion and assess whether there is a soft tissue contracture or mechanical block to external rotation and overhead motion. Adhesions between the conjoint tendon and deltoid and the underlying tissues must be freed as well as any adhesions in the subacromial region. The quality of the rotator cuff tissues, including the supraspinatus and subscapularis tendon, should be assessed. If the subscapularis tendon is of normal thickness and of good quality and external rotation motion is limited to less than zero degrees, then the Z-plasty is used to lengthen the subscapularis tendon (Figs. 3.17B and 3.32B). The authors prefer to incise the tendon just medial to the long head of the biceps and elevate a coronal portion of the entire subscapularis tendon from its insertion by sharp dissection, leaving at least half the tendon beneath and attached to the capsule. Thus, one-half to one-third of the thickness of the tendon is permitted to remain with the capsule. In some cases, to achieve an adequate dissection medially, the coracoid and its attached conjoined tendon need to be osteotomized to be reattached later. The dissection is continued medialward for at least 2 cm. With every centimeter of length that is obtained, 10 to 15° of external rotation motion is achieved. The medial rim of the Z is then completed by incising the anterior portion of the capsule and underlying subscapularis tendon that is allowed to remain with its capsule.

If the subscapularis tendon is attenuated, it is not feasible to perform a Z-lengthening. In this case, the overlapping subscapularis tendon and the coalesced underlying capsule are incised longitudinally at the insertion of the tendon at the medial bicipital lip. The capsule-tendon structure is then elevated from the anterior glenoid vault starting at the glenoid rim. Thus, enough lengthening may be obtained by elevating this structure from the one o'clock to the six o'clock position. Finally, the subscapularis tendon may be reattached to the cut anterior edge of the proximal humeral shaft to achieve a relative lengthening of the subscapularis tendon.

Anteriorly, the subscapularis tendon must be released from the underlying contracted capsule (31, 48). If the anteroinferior capsule is thickened, scarred portions of the capsule may be excised with care, extending this release posteriorly at the attachment of the capsule to the humeral neck, if needed. The surgeon should isolate and protect the axillary nerve and then extend the incision. Similarly, posterior contractures of the capsule may be released by incising the capsule along the posterior rim.

In patients exhibiting contractures of the superior portion of the glenohumeral capsule, the release can be achieved at the glenoid rim above the attachment of the labrum and the origin of the long head of the biceps. Care should be taken to avoid excessive medial dissection for fear of injuring the suprascapular nerve as it courses around the base of the spinoglenoid notch. This same release can be used to facilitate closure of a large rotator cuff tear.

After release of the contractures, the capsule can be retensioned around the implanted prosthetic components to avoid instability.

GLENOID DEFICIENCY

During the preparation of the glenoid for insertion of a glenoid component, care must be exercised not to fracture the glenoid vault while levering the proximal humerus away from the glenoid articular surface with a retractor placed behind the posterior glenoid rim. If the central portion of the glenoid contains large cysts, these must be curetted and bone grafted, usually using cancellous bone from the humeral head. If the central bony deficiency is not great, then additional methyl methacrylate bone cement may be used to fill the defect rather than bone.

If severe erosion of the entire central glenoid is present, it may not be possible to bone graft the glenoid. In this case, humeral hemiarthroplasty is prudent rather than performing a total shoulder replacement.

If the glenoid is deficient around its perimeter, then bone grafting may be required in rare cases to fill in a large asymmetric defect either anteriorly or posteriorly. If the defect is not very great, then the version of the humeral osteotomy can be changed toward a more neutral position of the glenoid, thereby creating a lesser degree of retrotorsion in the humeral component and accepting more retroversion in the glenoid component.

A large amount of methyl methacrylate by itself should not be used peripherally beneath any component and especially the glenoid to create stability.

HUMERAL DEFICIENCY

To make up for a deficiency in the proximal humerus, a longer component is often required to achieve a functioning shoulder. The resected humeral head may be reshaped and used as a bone graft, placing the metal stem through a center core of the humeral head graft before inserting it into the shaft. A problem encountered with bone grafting the proximal humerus is restoring a secure attachment of the rotator cuff to the bone beneath the dome of the humeral head.

Results of Arthroplasty

The degree of function achieved postoperatively relates primarily to the restoration of rotator cuff function and the quality of the muscles and their tendons. The best results are obtained in patients with osteoarthritis, rheumatoid arthritis, osteonecrosis, traumatic arthritis, and fracture. The poorest results, again, are achieved in patients with cuff arthropathy and failed arthroplasty procedures. The poorer results observed in traumatic arthritic cases relate to previous failed operations, scarring, and poor rotator cuff function.

Cofield (25) determined the frequency of reoperation. He found 4.5 percent of cases required revisions. After ten years of follow-up review the need for revision surgery remains under 5 percent.

Complications of Shoulder Arthroplasty

INFECTION

The incidence of infection following shoulder arthroplasty is very low (0.34% in 1168 cases). The low infection rate is due in part to careful preoperative evaluation and the excellent vascularity around the shoulder girdle. The risk of infection, however, is higher in immunocompromised patients and in patients who have undergone previous surgery (especially for fractures of the shoulder). When infection is present or there is a suspicion of infection at the time of primary revision, the usual screening blood tests (including complete blood count and erythrocyte sedimentation rate) used in conjunction with such testing as nuclear scans, aspiration, frozen sections, and imaging studies may be required.

Intraoperative Gram staining and additional culture and sensitivity studies can be performed. Imaging studies, including subtraction imaging techniques, may be helpful in identifying loose components.

When a shoulder infection is present following an arthroplasty, the infection must be eradicated. Sinus tracts with or without positive cultures must be evaluated intraoperatively using methylene blue and Renografin

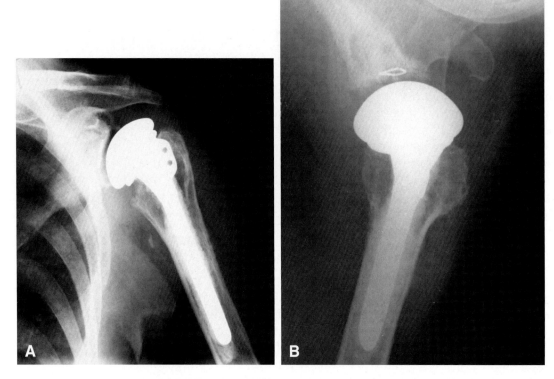

Figure 3.34. **(A)** Anteroposterior radiograph of a nonconstrained modular prosthesis.
(B) Axillary radiograph of a nonconstrained modular prosthesis.

(Bristol-Meyers-Squibb) injection into the sinus tract to determine the extent
of the infection within the deeper soft tissues.

An early infection can be managed by thorough debridement and closed
drainage with appropriate antibiotics following culture and sensitivity studies. Delayed infections should be treated with a thorough debridement of the
infected soft tissues, removal of the components and bone cement, and antibiotic coverage. In addition, antibiotic-impregnated cement spacers may be
implanted to provide local antibiotic delivery and to maintain the length of
the soft tissue sleeve. In selected cases, an experienced surgeon may elect to
perform an immediate replacement of a prosthetic device. When this is done,
the patient must be forewarned that reinfection may occur. Reimplantation
is usually performed as a staged procedure after antibiotic treatment, the duration of which will depend on factors such as the virulence of the organism.

When a septic loosening of the glenoid alone is present, the glenoid component can be removed along with any residual bone cement, and a revision
hemiarthroplasty can be performed later using a larger humeral head component. A revision arthroplasty should not be done in the presence of os-
teomyelitis.

NERVE INJURIES

Nerve injuries following shoulder arthroplasty are uncommon. Nerve injuries
associated with shoulder arthroplasty are often associated with a neur-
apraxia that can be treated expectantly. Electromyography and nerve conduction studies are useful in establishing the extent of the injury and show-

ing improvement in nerve function. The axillary nerve is most often injured, as it traverses the inferior aspect of the capsule and then curves posteriorly on the undersurface of the deltoid muscle. If the nerve is suspected of being lacerated and a complete lesion is present by electromyography with no improvement at 12 weeks, early exploration and repair is recommended. If the initial lesion is partial and improving, observation is indicated. Muscle transfers currently available for deltoid paralysis are not generally satisfactory.

On rare occasions when a prosthesis dislocates, it may contuse or compress cords of the brachial plexus. In this instance, correction of the instability to relieve compression should be done.

In very rare situations, injection of liquid cement under pressure into the medullary canal during revision surgery in bone that is highly demineralized may lead to an extravasation of cement in the midshaft, causing a thermal burn and compression of the radial nerve. Bone cement that extravasates into the soft tissues in the arm is most often caused by a perforation of the bone as it is reamed. During revision surgery, a rubber shodding should be placed next to any bone perforation to avoid cement extrusion.

FRACTURES

Intraoperative fractures are uncommon but do occur, especially in demineralized or rheumatoid bone. Fracture may occur with reaming, dislocation of the humeral head, or reduction of the prosthesis. It is essential when reaming the shaft to keep the reamers in the long axis of the shaft and to avoid allowing the tip of the reamer to roam laterally, for fear it will protrude through a thinned cortex. During revision surgery, after the prosthesis has been successfully removed, it is essential for the track of the previous stem to guide the reamer through the end of the previously placed cement at the site of the tip of the removed humeral prosthetic component. Hence, it is important to break through the most inferior part of the previous stem track with a small-diameter reamer to avoid creating a perforation in the shaft near the old tip of the prosthesis.

In other instances, the humeral shaft may fracture postoperatively, especially in demineralized bone, when too vigorous force is used to achieve extremes of motion (Fig. 3.35). In most instances, fractures will heal if treated conservatively even if cement had previously been used with good results. When fractures occur, the postoperative rehabilitation program must be modified to avoid active exercises for 8 to 12 weeks to allow sufficient fracture healing. Vigorous passive motions of the arm should be avoided.

When tuberosity fractures occur in osteoporotic bone, these can be managed the same way as a four-part fracture, with heavy nonabsorbable sutures placed through the tuberosity to allow union of the tuberosity with the shaft. The sutures should be placed through both fins of the prosthesis and through the proximal shaft. The tuberosities should not extend above the humeral head to avoid impingement on the undersurface of the acromion.

In exceptionally rare instances, fractures of the posterior glenoid may occur while a slot is being inserted in the center of the glenoid for the keel of the glenoid component. This may rarely occur when excessive traction is placed on the posterior glenoid vault by a retractor in osteoporotic bone. In these instances, it is essential to immediately insert a bone graft in the glenoid vault to create stability for the prosthetic component and obviate an additional complication of posterior dislocation of a metal humeral head.

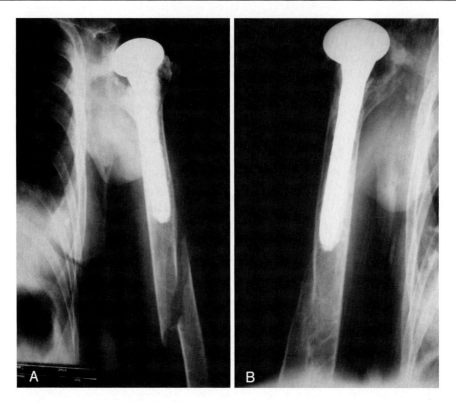

Figure 3.35. **(A)** A 65-year-old woman was undergoing rehabilitation physical therapy 6 weeks postoperatively. Excess torque was created in the humeral shaft when the arm was forced into external rotation. Note the spiral fracture in the shaft. **(B)** There was excellent union on the radiograph several months later following conservative treatment.

ROTATOR CUFF TEAR

Rotator cuff tear occurring postoperatively is one of the more frequent complications following shoulder arthroplasty, with an average incidence of 3.5%. Neer (104), reported five traumatic cuff tears in his initial report on 194 total shoulder replacements. Two underwent surgical repair, two remained weakened but without symptoms, and one produced intermittent pain but the patient refused additional surgery. Cofield (25, 31) reviewed 73 shoulder arthroplasties and noted rotator cuff tears in five patients postoperatively. One patient had significant pain and was considering additional surgery. The four other patients had anterosuperior subluxation and weakness but only minimal discomfort and refused reoperation. In the authors' experience, especially in cases having cuff arthropathy that were reconstructed, degenerative changes may occur years after shoulder arthroplasty. In these instances, most patients refuse reoperation to repair rotator cuff tears although they may complain of loss of function and perhaps pain. When weakness and/or instability occur, the rotator cuff can be repaired with good results. Lastly, when the rotator cuff is deficient anterosuperiorly, the upper portion of the subscapularis tendon may be transferred superiorly in order to correct an exposed prosthetic humeral head (111).

HEMATOMA

Most small postoperative hematomas can be treated closed and conservatively. They will absorb in most instances. When the hematoma is very large and bleeding persists and cannot be controlled, early surgical evacuation and control of bleeding is advised. Infection may occur when a hematoma breaks through the skin or wound and blood drainage continues. This is best avoided by early surgical evacuation of the hematoma.

HETEROTOPIC BONE

Heterotopic bone formation following shoulder arthroplasty is not clinically significant in most cases. Very occasionally, when it does occur and the bone formation is excessive, range of motion may be limited (Fig. 3.36).

GLENOID LOOSENING

Although radiolucent lines around the glenoid are common (30 to 83%), there is no direct evidence linking radiolucent lines and clinical loosening (7, 76). Although clinical loosening or breakage of the glenoid component is

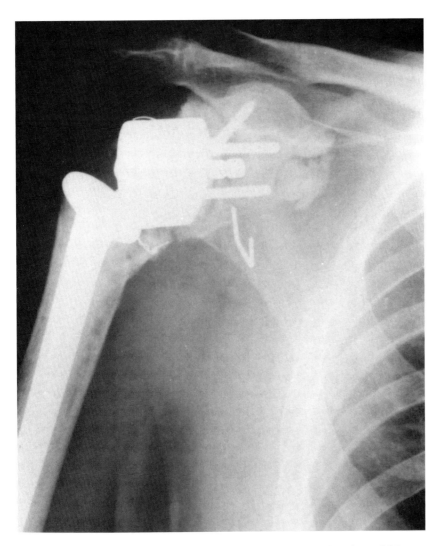

Figure 3.36.   A successful constrained total shoulder procedure (MRTS) performed 15 years previously. Over a 14-year period, motion gradually decreased with use of the shoulder as myositis ossificans around the prosthesis increased. Although motion eventually was poor, there was no pain in the shoulder.

rare, it occasionally does occur. It can be treated by either revision of the glenoid (if the remaining glenoid bone stock is satisfactory) or by simple removal of the glenoid component and placement of a larger humeral head (if the glenoid bone stock is poor).

HUMERAL LOOSENING

Humeral loosening is uncommon, but it is more likely to occur in press-fit stems, especially if the bone is osteoporotic. A good press-fit shows a thin collar of condensed bone around the stem. It is indicated when sufficient bone stock is present. Humeral loosening or subsidence is treated with revision of the humeral component to a cemented component.

IMPINGEMENT

Impingement following arthroplasty most often occurs when an excessive amount of humeral head has been removed and the humeral head component is placed too low in the shaft, thereby allowing the greater tuberosity to sit proud at the level of the apex of the dome of the component or even superior to the dome of the humeral component (Fig. 3.37). This not only limits overhead motion but often causes pain. Impingement may also result following hemiarthroplasty for fracture of the proximal humerus when the humeral component is placed too low within the shaft. When this occurs and the pain is intractable, the humeral component should be revised and placed superiorly to the tuberosities.

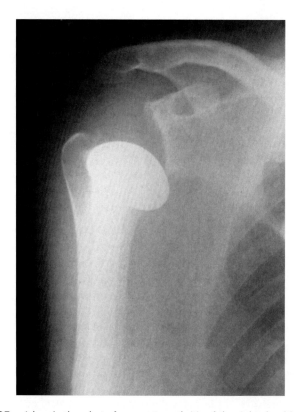

Figure 3.37.   A hemiarthroplasty for an osteoarthritis of the right shoulder. Too much head was resected. The stem was placed too low, creating a painful impingement.

REFLEX SYMPATHETIC DYSTROPHY

Reflex sympathetic dystrophy is not often observed in arthroplasty procedures. When it does occur, it should be treated conservatively. Sympathetic blocks and a variety of physical therapy modalities are used to decrease pain and maintain function in the upper extremity.

MALROTATION AND MALVERSION OF THE HUMERAL COMPONENT

Ordinarily, the humeral prosthesis is placed in 30 to 40° of retroversion to avert postoperative instability. The best reference point for the placement of the humeral component is to make certain that the lateral fin of the stem is positioned just posterior to the bicipital groove. If the anatomy is not normal or intact, the surgeon must use the distal humeral epicondyles with the arm at the side and externally rotated 35°. While in this position, a lateral fin of the humeral prosthesis should point directly at the glenoid.

In cases in which there has been chronic posterior dislocation or the posterior capsule is ballooned, the excess capsule must be reduced and perhaps a lesser degree of retroversion used to decrease the chance of instability. If the glenoid is eroded or deficient either anteriorly or posteriorly, the degree of rotation must be changed to improve stability. Often, when the glenoid is severely eroded, an autogenous bone graft should be used to increase stability of the humeral component. If malversion of the component is associated with instability of the prosthesis, the component is revised to the appropriate version and is usually cemented in revision surgery.

LOOSE MODULAR HEAD

When a modular component is used, the surgeon must be certain that the cement does not protrude superiorly as to interfere with the proper seating of the Morse taper within the modular head. In addition, all soft tissues must be retracted between the stem and the undersurface of the modular head to allow a tight fit of the head to its stem. Dissociation of the head from the stem is rare but has been reported. This problem is treated by open revision surgery to replace the dissociated head.

INSTABILITY

Postoperative subluxation or dislocation of an unconstrained arthroplasty occurs in 1 to 2% of cases. An unconstrained prosthetic device depends on the proper version of the components and correct balance of the soft tissue repair (correct tension). A functioning intact rotator cuff is essential for superior stability. The preservation of humeral length obviates inferior subluxation. Anterior and posterior instability may relate to soft tissue contracture in the direction opposite the instability. Malposition not only of the humeral but of the glenoid component may lead to instability.

Inferior instability after arthroplasty may be caused by a loss of height of the proximal humerus. Bone grafting and adequate tensioning of the rotator cuff structures with methyl methacrylate cementing along with bone grafting may obviate the inferior instability. Persistent inferior instability must be differentiated from muscle atony and injury to the axillary nerve.

If posterior glenoid wear is present, amounts of retroversion less than the usual 30 to 40° are required. However, the decrease in the retroversion should not be excessive to avoid anterior dislocation. Glenoid wear can be corrected by a combination of lowering the prominent side or changing the amount of head retroversion. In some cases, bone grafting may be required for those cases with severe glenoid deficiency. When the glenoid is severely eroded, it may not be possible to replace the glenoid component. Closed reduction and bracing may be used to treat the initial episode of instability if the implant is stable after reduction. A revision of a subluxed or dislocated prosthesis may require a combination of correcting the prosthetic malposition, bone grafting, and soft tissue balancing to achieve a correct balance.

Constrained Total Shoulder Replacement

A small number of patients who require shoulder arthroplasty will not fare well with an unconstrained procedure, because the stability needed by these devices and provided by the soft tissues for satisfactory results cannot be achieved. In a highly select group of patients, a fixed-fulcrum or constrained prosthesis may be considered. Because a constrained device is so highly dependent on its fixation directly to bone and does not rely on the soft tissues, the complications and failures are substantially higher than with unconstrained arthroplasty. It must be emphasized that a constrained total shoulder replacement should be used only when other worthwhile standard operations will not suffice.

The chief complications cited in this section relate to one type of constrained prosthesis, the Michael Reese Total Shoulder (MRTS) prosthesis. A hemispheric metal humeral head component is fixed into a polyethylene socket that is assembled from two components (Fig. 3.8). The internal diameter of the polyethylene cavity and that of the humeral ball are identical, but the diameter of the polyethylene peripheral lip is slightly smaller. It is not possible to force the metal head inside the polyethylene cavity once the plastic halves are assembled. The polyethylene parts fit precisely within the metal glenoid component.

A self-locking metal ring is first placed around the neck of the humeral component and tightened around the glenoid component after the polyethylene halves are inserted into the metal glenoid, thereby completing the assembly (Fig. 3.8). The metal glenoid has a truncated conical cup that is used exclusively; this permits the arm to hang away from the side slightly, so that impingement of the metal humeral neck on the plastic rim inferiorly is minimized. If the metal glenoid is incorrectly inserted, the metal head will become dislocated.

INDICATIONS

Intractable and disabling pain is the chief reason for a constrained replacement when the rotator cuff is completely destroyed and an unconstrained device cannot be implanted.

CONTRAINDICATIONS

The contraindications include the following: 1) previous infection, 2) complete paralysis of the shoulder caused by a neural lesion such as a stroke or a paralytic cerebral palsy, 3) loss of sufficient amounts of scapula bone substance so

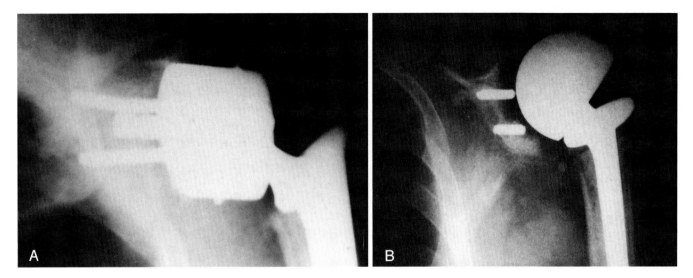

Figure 3.38. **(A)** A middle-aged man had an MRTS prosthesis inserted. Six years later, after vigorous use of the extremity, the glenoid component loosened. When one screw bent, revision surgery was recommended. The patient deferred treatment until later when both screws broke. **(B)** The glenoid component was removed, and the 22-mm humeral head was capped with a 44-mm bipolar acetabular cup.

that the metal component cannot be attached, 4) psychiatric disorders such as senility and uncontrolled alcoholism, and 5) a Charcot lesion of the joint.

COMPLICATIONS

The complications of constrained arthroplasty are the same as for unconstrained arthroplasty. However, constrained devices tend to loosen much more frequently than unconstrained devices. Moreover, the MRTS device is designed to dislocate when extremes of torque are exceeded to avoid fracture of the glenoid vault. When this latter complication occurs, revision surgery is required. When the glenoid is deficient, it is necessary to bone graft the defect before completing an arthroplasty. Post et al. (122, 126) reported eight revisions with bent or broken humeral necks for 4-mm diameter stainless steel stems in series I MRTS replacements. Broken implants were successfully revised. When the humeral neck diameter was increased to 8 mm, there was no additional bending, breakage, or material failure in the humeral neck. Other material failure has occurred, including traumatic dislocations, infection, traumatic loose stem, fractures of the humeral shaft, loose glenoids, and broken screws (5 cases in 104 patients). These significant complications relate primarily to the stress of the constrained device on the bone. There is a lesser chance of loosening in nonosteoporotic bone than in weak osteoporotic bone.

Clinical results of semiconstrained and constrained total shoulder arthroplasty have shown adequate pain relief. Post et al. (125) reported 96% pain relief with a constrained prosthesis (MRTS) in 28 shoulders and a 50% complication rate at the end of 5 years. They also showed that as the postoperative period progresses, the complication rate rises (125). Hence, constrained arthroplasty should be considered only in very select cases.

When loosening of the glenoid component occurs either by bone that has been demineralized or screws that are broken, the glenoid component can be removed and a 40- to 44-mm bipolar hip prosthesis inserted over the 22-mm humeral head (Fig. 3.38).

REFERENCES

1. Arntz CT, Jackins S, Matsen FA III. Prosthetic replacement of the shoulder for the treatment of defects in the rotator cuff and the surface of the glenohumeral joint. J Bone Joint Surg 1993;75A:485–491.
2. Albee FH. Restoration of shoulder function in cases of lost head and upper portion of humerus. Surg Gynecol Obstet 1921;32:1–19.
3. Albert E. Chirurgische mittheilungen. Zentralbl Chir 1881;8:776.
4. Amstutz HC, Hoy AS, Clarke IC. UCLA anatomic total shoulder arthroplasty. Clin Orthop 1981;155:7–20.
5. Averill RM, Sledge CB, Thomas WH. Neer total shoulder arthroplasty (abstract). Orthop Trans 1980;4:287.
6. Barr JS, Freiberg JA, Colonna PC, et al. A survey of end results on stabilization of the paralytic shoulder. J Bone Joint Surg 1942;24:699–707.
7. Barrett WP, Franklin JL, Jackins SE, et al. Total shoulder arthroplasty. J Bone Joint Surg 1987;69A:865–872.
8. Barton NJ. Arthrodesis of the shoulder for degenerative conditions. J Bone Joint Surg 1972;54A:1759–1764.
9. Beddow FH, Elloy MA. Clinical experience with the Liverpool shoulder replacement. In: Bayley I, Kessel L, eds. Shoulder surgery. New York: Springer-Verlag, 1982.
10. Beltran JE, Trilla JC, Barjau RR. A simplified compression arthrodesis of the shoulder. J Bone Joint Surg 1975;57A:538–541.
11. Bigliani LV, McCluskey III. Prosthetic replacement in acute fractures of the proximal humerus. In: Fenlin J Jr, ed. Seminars in arthroplasty. Philadelphia: WB Saunders, 1990;1:129–137.
12. Brett AL. A new method of arthrodesis of the shoulder joint, incorporating the control of the scapula. J Bone Joint Surg 1933;15:969–977.
13. Brittain HA. Architectural principles in arthrodesis. Edinburgh: Livingstone, 1942.
14. Brumfield RH Jr, Schilz J, Flinders BW. Total shoulder replacement arthroplasty: a clinical review of 21 cases (abstract). Orthop Trans 1981;5:398.
15. Buechel FF. Glenohumeral joint in the chimpanzee: comparative anatomical analysis for use in endoprosthetic replacement. J Med Primatol 1977;6:108–113.
16. Buechel FF, Pappas MJ, DePalma AF. Floating socket total shoulder replacement. Biomed Mater Res 1978;12:89–114.
17. Carroll RE. Wire loop in arthrodesis of the shoulder. Clin Orthop 1957;9:185–189.
18. Casuccio C. Internal prosthesis of the upper limbs. SICOT 10th Congress, Paris, France, September 4–9, 1966.
19. Charnley J. Compression arthrodesis of the ankle and shoulder. J Bone Joint Surg 1951;33B:180–191.
20. Charnley J, Houston JK. Compression arthrodesis of the shoulder. J Bone Joint Surg 1964;46B:614–620.
21. Clayton ML, Ferlic DC. Surgery of the shoulder in rheumatoid arthritis. Clin Orthop 1975;106:166–175.
22. Clayton ML, Ferlic DC, Jeffers PD. Prosthetic arthroplasties of the shoulder. Clin Orthop 1982;164:184–191.
23. Cofield RH. Status of total shoulder arthroplasty. Arch Surg 1977;112:1088–1091.
24. Cofield RH. Unconstrained total shoulder prostheses. Clin Orthop 1983;173:97–108.
25. Cofield RH. Total shoulder arthroplasty with the Neer prosthesis. J Bone Joint Surg 1984;66A:899–906.
26. Cofield RH. Subscapularis tendon transposition for large rotator cuff tears. Techniques Orthop 1989;3:58–64.
27. Cofield RH. Integral surgical maneuvers in prosthetic shoulder arthroplasty. Semin Arthroplasty 1990;1:112–123.
28. Cofield RH. Degenerative and arthritic problems of the glenohumeral joint. In: Rockwood CA Jr, Matsen FA III, eds. The shoulder. Philadelphia: WB Saunders, 1991;2:678–749.

29. Cofield RH, Briggs BT. Glenohumeral arthrodesis. J Bone Joint Surg 1979;61A: 668–677.

30. Cofield RH, Daly PJ. Total shoulder arthroplasty with a tissue-ingrowth glenoid component. J Shoulder Elbow Surg 1992;1:77–85.

31. Cofield RH, Edgerton BC. Total shoulder arthroplasty: complications and revision surgery. Instr Course Lect 1990;39:449–462.

32. Coughlin MJ, Morris JM, West WF. The semiconstrained total shoulder arthroplasty. J Bone Joint Surg 1979;61A:574–581.

33. Crossan JF, Vallance R. The shoulder joint in rheumatoid arthritis. In: Bayley I, Kessel L, eds. Shoulder surgery. New York: Springer-Verlag, 1982:131–143.

34. Cruess RL. Steroid-induced avascular necrosis of the head of the humerus. J Bone Joint Surg 1976;58B:313–317.

35. Cruess RL. Corticosteroid-induced osteonecrosis of the humeral head. Orthop Clin North Am 1985;16:789–796.

36. Cruess RL. Osteonecrosis of bone: current concepts as to etiology and pathogenesis. Clin Orthop 1986;208:30–39.

37. Curran JF, Ellman MH, Brown NL. Rheumatologic aspects of painful conditions affecting the shoulder. Clin Orthop 1983;173:27–37.

38. Davis JB, Cottrell GW. A technique for shoulder arthrodesis. J Bone Joint Surg 1962;44A:657–661.

39. Doody SG, Freedman L, Waterland JD. Shoulder movements during abduction in the scapular plane. Arch Phys Med Rehabil 1970;51:595.

40. Drvaric DM, Rooks MD, Bishop A, et al. Neuropathic arthropathy of the shoulder: a case report. Orthopedics 1988;11:301–304.

41. Ducci I. Sostituzione endoprotesica di estesa lesione omerale in granulomatosi eosinofila atipica. Arch Centr Traum Ortoped Inst Nzion Infort 1963;3:1.

42. Ellman MH, Curran JJ. Causes and management of shoulder arthritis. Compr Ther 1988;14:29–35.

43. Engelbrecht E, Heinert J. More than ten years' experience with unconstrained shoulder replacement. In: Kölbel R, Helbig B, Blauth W, eds. Shoulder replacement. Berlin: Springer-Verlag, 1987:85–91.

44. Engelbrecht E, Stellbrink G. Total schulterendoprosthese modell "St. Georg." Chirurg 1976;47:525–530.

45. Epps CH Jr. Painful hematologic conditions affecting the shoulder. Clin Orthop 1983;173:38–43.

46. Fenlin JM Jr. Total glenohumeral joint replacement. Orthop Clin North Am 1975; 6:565–583.

47. Fenlin JM Jr, Vaccaro A, Andreychik D, et al. Modular total shoulder: early experience and impressions. Semin Arthroplasty 1990;1:102–111.

48. Figgie HE III, Inglis AE, Goldberg VM, et al. An analysis of factors affecting the long-term results of total shoulder arthroplasty in inflammatory arthritis. J Arthroplasty 1988;3:123–130.

49. Franklin JL, Barrett WP, Jackins SE, et al. Glenoid loosening in total shoulder arthroplasty; association with rotator cuff deficiency. J Arthroplasty 1988;3: 39–46.

50. Friedman RJ. Glenohumeral translation after total shoulder arthroplasty. J Shoulder Elbow Surg 1992;1:312–316.

51. Friedman RJ, Ewald FC. Arthroplasty of the ipsilateral shoulder and elbow in patients who have rheumatoid arthritis. J Bone Joint Surg 1987;69A:661–666.

52. Friedman R, Thornhill ST, Thomas WH, et al. Non-constrained total shoulder replacement in patients who have rheumatoid arthritis and class-IV function. J Bone Joint Surg 1989;71A:494–498.

53. Fournie B, Railhac J-J, Monod P, et al. The enthesopathic shoulder. Rev Rhum Mal Osteoartic 1987;54:447–451.

54. Gill AB. A new operation for arthrodesis of the shoulder. J Bone Joint Surg 1931; 13:287–295.

55. Gristina AG, Romano RL, Kammire GC, et al. Total shoulder replacement. Orthop Clin North Am 1987;18:445–453.

56. Gristina AG, Webb LX. The trispherical total shoulder replacement. In: Bayley I, Kessel L, eds. Shoulder surgery. New York: Springer-Verlag, 1982:153–157.

57. Gristina AG, Webb LX, Carter RE. The monospherical total shoulder. Orthop Trans 1985;9:54–55.

58. Gschwend N, Kentsch A. Arthritic disorders: surgery of the rheumatoid shoulder. In: Bateman JE, Welsh RP, eds. Surgery of the shoulder. St. Louis: CV Mosby, 1984:269–280.

59. Halawa M, Lee AJ, Ling RS, et al. The shear strength of trabecular bone from the femur, and some factors affecting the shear strength of the cement-bone interface. Arch Orthop Trauma Surg 1978;92:19–20.

60. Halverson PB, Cheung HS, McCarty DJ, et al. "Milwaukee shoulder"—association of microspheroids containing hydroxyapatite crystals, active collagenase, and neutral protease with rotator cuff defects. II. Synovial fluid studies. Arthritis Rheum 1981;24:474–483.

61. Halverson PB, Cheung HS, McCarty DJ. Enzymatic release of microspheroids containing hydroxyapatite crystals from synovium and of calcium pyrophosphate dihydrate crystals from cartilage. Ann Rheum Dis 1982;41:527–531.

62. Halverson PB, Garancis JC, McCarty DJ. Histopathological and ultrastructural studies of synovium in Milwaukee shoulder syndrome—a basic calcium phosphate crystal arthropathy. Ann Rheum Dis 1984;43:734–741.

63. Halverson PB, McCarty DJ, Cheung HS, et al. Milwaukee shoulder syndrome: eleven additional cases with involvement of the knee in seven (basic calcium phosphate crystal deposition disease). Semin Arthritis Rheum 1984;14:36–44.

64. Hammond R. Transplantation of the fibula to replace bony defect in the shoulder joint. J Bone Joint Surg 1926;8:627–635.

65. Haraldsson S. Reconstruction of proximal humerus by muscle-sling prosthesis. Acta Orthop Scand 1969;40:225–233.

66. Hawkins RJ, Neer CS II. A functional analysis of shoulder fusions. Clin Orthop 1987;223:65–76.

67. Hawkins RJ, Neer CS II, Pianta RM, et al. Locked posterior dislocation of the shoulder. J Bone Joint Surg 1987;69A:9–18.

68. Hsu HC, Wu JJ, Chen TH, et al. The influence of abductor lever-arm changes after shoulder arthroplasty. J Shoulder Elbow Surg 1993;2:134–140.

69. Hughes M, Neer CS II. Glenohumeral joint replacement and postoperative rehabilitation. Phys Ther 1975;55:850–858.

70. Ianotti JP, Gabriel JP, Schneck SL, et al. The normal glenohumeral relationships. J Bone Joint Surg 1992;74A:491–500.

71. Imbriglia JE, Neer CS, Dick HM. Resection of proximal one-half of humerus in a child for chondrosarcoma. J Bone Joint Surg 1978;60A:262–264.

72. Inman VT, Saunders JB, Abbott LC. Observations on the function of the shoulder joint. J Bone Joint Surg 1944;26:1.

73. Jobbins B, Flowers M, Reeves BF. Fixation of orthopaedic implants under tensile loading. Biomed End 1973;7:380–383.

74. Jones L. The shoulder joint—observations on the anatomy and physiology: with an analysis of a reconstructive operation following extensive injury. Surg Gynecol Obstet 1942;75:433.

75. Kalamchi A. Arthrodesis for paralytic shoulder: review of ten patients. Orthopedics 1978;1:204–208.

76. Kelly IG, Foster RS, Fisher WD. Neer total shoulder replacement in rheumatoid arthritis. J Bone Joint Surg 1987;69B:723–726.

77. Kenmore PI, Maccartee C, Vitek B. A simple shoulder replacement. J Biomed Mater Res 1974;5(part 2):329–330.

78. Kessel L, Bayley I. Prosthetic replacement of shoulder joint: preliminary communication. J R Soc Med 1978;72:748–752.

79. Kessel L, Bayley I. The Kessel total shoulder replacement. In: Bayley I, Kessel L, eds. Shoulder surgery. New York: Springer-Verlag, 1982.
80. Kölbel R, Friedebold G. Schultergelenkersatz. Z. Orthop 1975;113:452–454.
81. Kölbel R, Rohlmann A, Bergmann G, et al. Shultergelenkersatz nach Kölbel-Friedebold. Aktuel Probl Chir Orthop 1977;1:50.
82. Kölbel R, Rohlmann A, Bergmann G. Biomechanical considerations in the design of a semi-constrained total shoulder replacement. In: Bayley I, Kessel L, eds. Shoulder surgery. New York: Springer-Verlag, 1982.
83. Kostuik JP, Schatzker J. Shoulder arthrodesis—A.O. technique. In: Bateman JE, Welsh, RP, eds. Surgery of the shoulder. Toronto: BC Decker, 1984:207–210.
84. Kraulis J, Hunter G. The results of prosthetic replacement in fracture-dislocations of the upper end of the humerus. Injury 1976;8:129–131.
85. Krueger FJ. A vitallium replica arthroplasty on shoulder: a case report of aseptic necrosis of the proximal end of the humerus. Surgery 1951;30:1005–1011.
86. Landon GC, Chao EY, Cofield RH. Three-dimensional analysis of angular motion of the shoulder complex. Trans Orthop Res Soc 1978;3:297.
87. Lettin AWF, Copeland SA, Scales JT. The Stanmore shoulder replacement. J Bone Joint Surg 1982;64B:47–51.
88. Lettin AWF, Scales JT. Total replacement of the shoulder joint. Proc R Soc Med 1972;65:373–374.
89. Lettin AWF, Scales JT. Total replacement arthroplasty of the shoulder in rheumatoid arthritis (abstract). J Bone Joint Surg 1973;55B:217.
90. Lucas DB. Biomechanics of the shoulder joint. Arch Surg 1973;107:425–435.
91. Lugli T. Artificial shoulder joint by Péan (1893): the facts of an exceptional intervention and the prosthetic method. Clin Orthop 1978;133:215–218.
92. Lynn TA, Alexakis PG, Bechtol CO. Stem prosthesis to replace lost proximal humerus. Clin Orthop 1965;13:245–247.
93. Macnab I, English E. Development of a glenohumeral arthroplasty for the severely destroyed shoulder joint (abstract). J Bone Joint Surg 1976;58B:137.
94. Makin M. Early arthrodesis for a flail shoulder in young children. J Bone Joint Surg 1977;59A:317–321.
95. Marmor L. Hemiarthroplasty for the rheumatoid shoulder joint. Clin Orthop 1977;122:201–203.
96. May VR Jr. Shoulder fusion: a review of fourteen cases. J Bone Joint Surg 1962;44A:65–76.
97. Mazas F, de la Caffiniere JY. Total arthroplasty of the shoulder: experience with 38 cases (abstract). Orthop Trans 1981;5:57.
98. McCarty D. Crystals, joints and consternation. Ann Rheum Dis 1983;42:243–253.
99. McCarty DJ, Halverson PB, Carrera GF, et al. "Milwaukee shoulder"—association of microspheroids containing hydroxyapatite crystals, active collagenase, and neutral protease with rotator cuff defects. I. Clinical aspects. Arthritis Rheum 1981;24:464–473.
100. Moseley HF. Arthrodesis of the shoulder in the adult. Clin Orthop 1961;20:156–162.
101. Neer CS. Articular replacement for humeral head. J Bone Joint Surg 1955;37A:215–228.
102. Neer CS. Prosthetic replacement of the humeral head: indications and operative technique. Surg Clin North Am 1963;43:1581–1597.
103. Neer CS II. The rheumatoid shoulder. In: Cruess RR, Mitchell NS, eds. Surgery of rheumatoid arthritis. Philadelphia: JB Lippincott, 1971:117–125.
104. Neer CS. Replacement arthroplasty for glenohumeral osteoarthritis. J Bone Joint Surg 1974;56A:1–13.
105. Neer CS, Brown TH, McLaughlin HL. Fracture of the neck of the humerus with dislocation of the head fragment. Am J Surg 1953;85:252–258.
106. Neer CS II, Craig EV, Fukuda H. Cuff-tear arthropathy. J Bone Joint Surg 1983;65A:1232–1244.

107. Neer CS II, Kirby RM. Revision of the humeral head and total shoulder arthroplasties. Clin Orthop 1982;170:189–195.
108. Neer CS II, McCann PD, Macfarlane EA, et al. Earlier passive motion following shoulder arthroplasty and rotator cuff repair: a prospective study. Orthop Trans 1987;2:231.
109. Neer CS, Morrison DC. Glenoid bone-grafting in total shoulder arthroplasty. J Bone Joint Surg 1988;70A:1154–1162.
110. Neer CS II, Watson KC, Stanton FJ. Recent experience in total shoulder replacement. J Bone Joint Surg 1982;64A:319–337.
111. Neviaser RJ, Neviaser TJ. Transfer of subscapularis and teres minor for massive defects of the rotator cuff. In: Bayley I, Kessel L, eds. Shoulder surgery. New York: Springer-Verlag, 1982:60–63.
112. Pahle JA, Kvarnes L. Shoulder synovectomy. Ann Chirurg Gynaecol 1985; 198(Suppl):37–39.
113. Péan JE. The classic: on prosthetic methods intended to repair bone fragments. Clin Orthop 1973;94:4.
114. Pollock RG, Deliz ED, McIlveen SJ, et al. Prosthetic replacement in rotator cuff-deficient shoulders. J Shoulder Elbow Surg 1992;1:173–186.
115. Poppen NK, Walker PS. Normal and abnormal motion of the shoulder. J Bone Joint Surg 1976;58A:195–201.
116. Poppen NK, Walker PS. Forces in the shoulder. In: Walker PS, ed. Human joints and their artificial replacements. Springfield, IL: Charles C. Thomas, 1977:87.
117. Post M. Constrained arthroplasty of the shoulder. In: Neviaser RJ, ed. Orthopedic clinics of North America. Philadelphia: WB Saunders, 1987:455–462.
118. Post M. Constrained arthroplasty (letter to the editor). Clin Orthop 1988;231:308–310.
119. Post M. Shoulder arthroplasty and total shoulder replacement. In: Post M, ed. The shoulder. Philadelphia: Lea & Febiger, 1988:221–278.
120. Post M. Constrained arthroplasty: its use and misuse. In: Fenlin J Jr, ed. Seminars on arthroplasty. Philadelphia: WB Saunders, 1990;1:151–159.
121. Post M. Unconstrained arthroplasty: long term results. Sixth International Congress on Shoulder Surgery, Helsinki, Finland, June 28, 1995.
122. Post M, Grinblat E. Complications of arthroplasty and total joint replacement in the shoulder. In: Epps CH Jr, ed. Complications in orthopaedic surgery. 3rd ed. Philadelphia: JB Lippincott, 1994.
123. Post M, Grinblat E. Preoperative clinical evaluation in arthroplasty of the shoulder. In: Friedman RJ, ed. Shoulder arthroplasty. New York: Thieme Medical Publishers, 1994:41–52.
124. Post M, Haskell S. Michael Reese total shoulder. Memphis, TN: Richards Manufacturing, 1978.
125. Post M, Haskell SS, Jablon M. Total shoulder replacement with a constrained prosthesis. J Bone Joint Surg 1980;62A:327–335.
126. Post M, Jablon M, Miller H, et al. Constrained total shoulder joint replacement: a critical review. Clin Orthop 1979;144:135–150.
127. Putti V. Arthrodesis for tuberculosis of the knee and of the shoulder. Chir Organi Mov 1933;18:217.
128. Rand JA, Sim FH. Total shoulder arthroplasty for the arthroplasty of hemochromatosis: a case report. Orthopedics 1981;4:658–660.
129. Reeves B, Jobbins B, Dowson D. The development of a total shoulder joint endoprosthesis. Conference on Human Locomotor Engineering, September 1971. London: Institution of Mechanical Engineers, 1971:108–122.
130. Reeves B, Jobbins B, Dowson D, et al. A total shoulder endo-prosthesis. Eng Med 1974;1:64–67.
131. Reeves B, Jobbins B, Flowers M. Biomechanical problems in the development of a total shoulder endoprosthesis. Proceedings of the British Orthopaedic Society. J Bone Joint Surg 1972;54B:193.

132. Richard A, Judet R, Rene L. Acrylic prosthetic construction of the upper end of the humerus for fracture-luxations. J Chir 1952;68:537–547.

133. Richards RR, Beaton D, Hudson AR. Shoulder arthrodesis with plate fixation: functional outcome analysis. J Bone Joint Surg 1993;2:225–239.

134. Richards RR, Waddell JP. Shoulder fusion's role in the treatment of brachial plexus palsy. Clin Orthop 1985;198:250–258.

135. Riggins RS. Shoulder fusion without external fixation—a preliminary report. J Bone Joint Surg 1976;58A:1007–1008.

136. Rossleigh MA, Smith J, Straus DJ, et al. Osteonecrosis in patients with malignant lymphoma. Cancer 1986;58:1112–1116.

137. Rovsing T. Et tilfaelde af fri knogletransplantation til erstatning of overarmens overste to trediedele ved hjaelp af patientens fibula. Hospitalstidende 1910;53:7.

138. Rowe CR. Re-evaluation of the position of the arm in arthrodesis of the shoulder in adult. J Bone Joint Surg 1974;56A:913–922.

139. Rydholm U, Sjögren J. Surface replacement of the humeral head in the rheumatoid shoulder. J Shoulder Elbow Surg 1993;2:286–295.

140. Saha AK. Surgery of the paralyzed and flail shoulder. Acta Orthop Scand 1967;97(Suppl):5–90.

141. Samilson RL, Prieto V. Dislocation arthropathy of the shoulder. J Bone Joint Surg 1983;65A:456–460.

142. Schroder HA, Frandsen PA. External compression arthrodesis of the shoulder joint. Acta Orthop Scand 1983;54:592–595.

143. Schulz OE. Arthrodesis acromio-humeralis osteoplastica. J Bone Joint Surg 1931; 13:722–724.

144. Sigholm G, Herberts P, Almstrom C, et al. Electromyographic analysis of shoulder muscle load. J Orthop Res 1984;1:379–386.

145. Steffee AD, Moore RW. Hemi-resurfacing arthroplasty of the shoulder. Contemp Orthop 1984;9:51–59.

146. Steindler A. Orthopedic operations: indications, technique, and end results. Springfield, IL: Charles C. Thomas, 1940:302.

147. Steindler A. Arthrodesis of the shoulder. American Academy of Orthopaedic Surgeons Instructional Course Lectures 1944;2:293.

148. Swanson AB. Bipolar implant shoulder arthroplasty in surgery of the shoulder. In: Bateman JE, Welsh RP, eds. Surgery of the shoulder. Toronto: BC Decker, 1984:211–223.

149. Tanner MW, Cofield RH. Prosthetic arthroplasty for fractures and fracture dislocations of the proximal humerus. Clin Orthop 1983;179:116–128.

150. Tully JG Jr, Latteri A. Paraplegia, syringomyelia tarda and neuropathic arthrosis of the shoulder: a triad. Clin Orthop 1978;134:244–248.

151. Vainio K. Orthopaedic surgery in the treatment of rheumatoid arthritis. Ann Clin Res 1975;7:216–224.

152. Watson-Jones R. Extra-articular arthrodesis of the shoulder. J Bone Joint Surg 1933;15:862–871.

153. Wolff R, Kölbel R. The history of shoulder joint replacement. In: Kölbel R, Helbig B, Blauth W, eds. Shoulder replacement. Berlin: Springer-Verlag, 1987:3–13.

154. Zippel J. Luxationssichere schulterendoprothese modell BME. Z Orthop 1975; 113:454–457.

155. Zuckerman JD, Cofield RH. Proximal humeral prosthetic replacement in glenohumeral arthritis. Orthop Trans 1986;10:231.

156. Zuckerman JD, Kummer FJ, Cuomo F, et al. The influence of coracoacromial arch anatomy on rotator cuff tears. J Shoulder Elbow Surg 1992;1:4–13.

157. Zuckerman JD, Matsen FA III. Complications about the glenohumeral joint related to the use of screws and staples. J Bone Joint Surg 1984;66A:175–180.

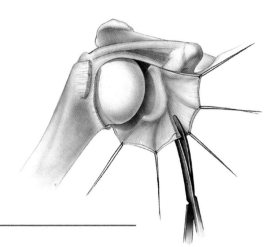

CHAPTER

4

Rotator Cuff Repair

LOUIS U. BIGLIANI

Introduction

Ernest A. Codman has been given the distinction as the first person who performed a rotator cuff repair. His initial report (20) on repair of the rotator cuff was in 1911 and was followed by his classic book (21) in 1934. In 1931, Wilson (83) introduced the concept of reinserting the torn rotator cuff tendon edge into a "bony trench" in the anatomic neck of the humerus. Over the next 30 years, McLaughlin (52–54) wrote on the pathogenesis and treatment of rotator cuff tears, including his report of 100 consecutive patients who underwent rotator cuff repair and whose progress was followed for an average of 3 years (54). Operative treatment of rotator cuff tears became a common surgical procedure, with many different techniques described (5, 16, 51–54, 80, 84). Initially, however, the outcome was not ideal; several series reported unsatisfactory results in as many as 26 to 46% of patients (16, 21, 22, 83).

The results of open rotator cuff repair improved significantly after Neer's report on anterior acromioplasty in combination with cuff mobilization and repair in 1972 (57). Recently, predictably satisfactory results have been reported in both pain relief and function with the use of this approach, which is the gold standard for operative treatment of rotator cuff tears (1, 24, 30, 34, 44, 60, 62, 65, 69). Over the past several years, however, shoulder arthroscopy has had a profound effect on the evaluation and treatment of rotator cuff disease (18, 31, 32). New information has resulted from the ability to visualize glenohumeral pathology during procedures previously performed through an open approach confined to the subacromial space. This information, as well as that available from improved imaging technology, has led to improved understanding in some areas and increased controversy in others. Treatment options have also been revolutionized as arthroscopically assisted ("mini-open") rotator cuff repair is now widely used, and arthroscopic repair is evolving. Not surprisingly, the arthroscope has worked most effectively in the hands of those surgeons who have treated it as one additional tool to be used according to principles established in the open treatment of rotator cuff disease.

133

Incidence/Etiology

Cadaver studies have shown an incidence of full-thickness tears of the rotator cuff to be quite high, with a range from 30 to 60%, which significantly increases with age. More recently, magnetic resonance imaging (MRI) studies (55, 72) have shown rotator cuff tears in up to 33% of asymptomatic shoulders, also increasing with age. Sher et al. (72) found that 54% of asymptomatic volunteers older than 60 years of age had a tear of the rotator cuff as diagnosed by MRI. The question of why some rotator cuff tears are well tolerated and others are associated with pain and functional disability is one of great debate, the answer to which is most certainly multifactorial.

The supraspinatus insertion on the greater tuberosity must repeatedly pass underneath the coracoacromial (CA) arch when the arm is used in overhead activity. Subacromial bursitis as well as rotator cuff tendinitis and tears are common disorders in the shoulder and can result in pain, weakness, and difficulties with activities of daily living (25, 58). Many factors have been implicated in the etiology of rotator cuff pathology, including extrinsic tendon injury due to compression from an abnormal CA arch (11, 13, 57, 63, 74, 85), abutment against the glenoid rim (77), tendon and bursal swelling in a confined space (39, 76), tensile overload (47), altered glenohumeral kinematics (e.g., instability) (47, 48), and intrinsic tendon injury from tendinitis (76), altered vascularity (70), or shear between different fiber bundles (36, 56).

Whether a primary factory or secondary effect, subacromial impingement is thought by many investigators to be an ongoing cause of tendon injury by the time surgical intervention is considered. Therefore, it is important to include subacromial decompression as part of the procedure in rotator cuff repair. Neer (57) proposed that variation in acromial slope and morphology were clinically relevant, and Bigliani et al. (11) demonstrated a relationship between acromial morphology and the incidence of rotator cuff tears in cadavers. Flatow et al. (35) performed contact studies on the subacromial space and found that contact was centered on the supraspinatus insertion, where cuff tears generally initiate. This contact involved the anteroinferior acromion, again supporting the removal of that region (anterior acromioplasty) in the treatment of rotator cuff impingement.

Classification

Due to different shapes of tendon defects as well as varying degrees of cuff elasticity and mobility, the development of a consistent and accurate classification for reporting rotator cuff tear size has been difficult. Partial-thickness rotator cuff tears are generally classified by their location (e.g., articular or bursal) and by the estimated percentage of the cuff thickness that the tear involves. The most commonly used system for the classification of full-thickness defects is that proposed by Post et al. (69), who defined small tears as those less than 1 cm at greatest diameter, medium tears as 1 to 3 cm, large tears as 3 to 5 cm, and massive tears as greater than 5 cm in diameter. In addition, Gerber et al. (41) described a classification of rotator cuff size based on the size of the defect after mobilization and the ability of the surgeon to approximate the tear to a bony trough near the greater tuberosity. Although some have advocated classifying tears by the number of tendons involved, this scheme is unreliable because the rotator cuff tendons become confluent near their insertion on the greater tuberosity (19), making anatomic differentiation difficult.

Evaluation

Despite the recent advances in imaging technology and arthroscopic techniques, history and physical examination continue to be the mainstay of evaluation of suspected rotator cuff pathology. The patient's chief complaint should direct the orthopaedic surgeon to an initial differential diagnosis. Symptoms referable to the rotator cuff are often shoulder pain, weakness, and an inability to perform certain activities of daily living, especially those involving use of the arm overhead. However, other primary shoulder disorders (e.g., adhesive capsulitis, instability, arthritis, and scapulothoracic disorders) and referred symptoms from the cervical spine, other areas of the upper extremity, and even visceral pathology must not be disregarded. The shoulder pain associated with rotator cuff pathology often extends down the lateral aspect of the upper arm (due to the extent of the subacromial/subdeltoid bursa) toward the deltoid insertion. This pain is frequently exacerbated by activities at or above the level of the shoulder and often occurs at night, interrupting sleep. Weakness is manifested either as an inability to raise or externally rotate the arm or as shoulder fatigue after repetitive activities. Daily activities that are often difficult to perform for the patient with rotator cuff pathology include fastening a bra, putting on a coat, placing dishes or clothes on shelves at or above the level of the shoulder, and lifting objects when the arm is abducted.

The physical examination should be thorough yet directed from the information gained in the history. For example, translation tests, apprehension signs, and relocation tests are usually not necessary in the 60-year-old patient who presents with shoulder pain of several months duration with an inability to lift his arm. The shoulder girdle should be inspected for signs of muscle atrophy or asymmetry, which may be present with long-standing rotator cuff tears. Discreet areas of tenderness to palpation (e.g., the acromioclavicular [AC] joint, greater tuberosity) should be noted. Both passive and active range of motion should be recorded in forward elevation in the scapular plane, external rotation both with the arm at the side and at 90° abduction, and internal rotation. The shoulder motion should then be compared with the contralateral shoulder. Patients with rotator cuff pathology often maintain the majority of shoulder motion, yet active external rotation and passive internal rotation can be limited. Strength testing in forward elevation, abduction, and external rotation is performed and again compared with the contralateral shoulder. Patients with partial-thickness or small full-thickness cuff tears rarely have clinically perceived weakness, whereas those with large and massive tears are unable to actively initiate shoulder abduction or sustain external rotation with the arm at the side. The impingement sign (57) reproduces shoulder pain with forward elevation of the internally rotated arm coincident with impingement of the supraspinatus tendon insertion on the undersurface of the CA arch. Selected lidocaine injections into the subacromial space and/or the AC joint can help differentiate true weakness from perceived weakness due to pain inhibition. Stability assessment is performed on those patients, especially throwing athletes, in whom the relative contributions of instability and rotator cuff pathology are uncertain. A thorough cervical spine and neurologic examination is necessary in all patients with suspected rotator cuff disease, and provocative tests (e.g., Yergason's test, Adson's maneuver) are used as clinically indicated.

Imaging

In the radiographic evaluation of rotator cuff disease, plain radiographs are useful to assess the bony aspects of impingement syndrome, to assess the position of the humeral head in relation to the glenoid fossa and acromion, and to rule out other potential causes of shoulder pain such as calcific tendonitis or early degenerative osteoarthritis. Anteroposterior (AP) views in neutral, internal, and external rotation; the supraspinatus outlet view (57–59); and an axillary view are obtained. The AP view may reveal excrescences on the greater tuberosity, AC arthritis, a subacromial spur, or a decrease in the acromiohumeral distance (Fig. 4.1A). However, other bony structures, such as the spine or body of the scapula, may prevent adequate visualization of subacromial pathology. The outlet view (Fig. 4.1B), a true lateral of the scapula with a 10° caudal tilt, reveals acromial morphology (11) and any spurs that may be present at the anteroinferior aspect of the acromion or in the substance of the CA ligament.

Magnetic resonance imaging may be used to assess the integrity of the rotator cuff when surgery is being considered. Clinical correlation of MRI findings is certainly important; studies have shown a significant incidence of rotator cuff abnormalities in the asymptomatic population (72). However, the

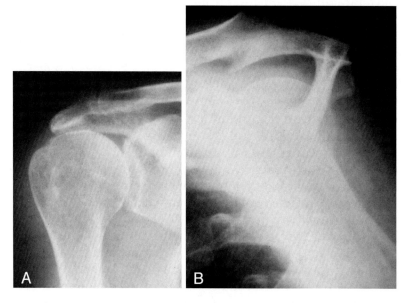

Figure 4.1. **(A)** Anteroposterior view of the shoulder showing superior humeral translation, excrescences on the greater tuberosity, and sclerosis on the undersurface of the acromion—all signs of rotator cuff disease. **(B)** Supraspinatus outlet view of the shoulder showing a large anteroinferior spur emanating from the coracoacromial ligament insertion.

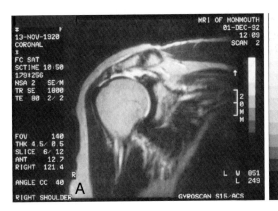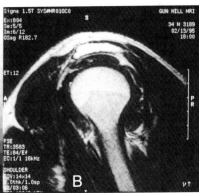

Figure 4.2. **(A)** Magnetic resonance imaging (coronal oblique) may be used preoperatively to determine the presence, size, and morphology of a rotator cuff tear. The information gained can help guide the surgical approach and also be used for appropriate preoperative patient counseling. This MRI image shows a large rotator cuff tear with retraction of the tendon edge nearly to the glenoid margin. **(B)** The sagittal oblique MRI view shows the morphology of the acromion and potential soft tissue components of the impingement syndrome (supraspinatus outlet, bursa, coracoacromial ligament).

MRI can be useful in the preoperative setting to determine the size and morphology of the rotator cuff tear and help guide the surgical approach (e.g., arthroscopic subacromial decompression with mini-open repair versus standard open decompression and repair) (Fig. 4.2A). In addition, the sagittal oblique view can show the lateral acromial morphology and potential soft tissue components of the impingement syndrome (e.g., supraspinatus outlet, bursa, CA ligament) (Fig. 4.2B).

Arthrography and ultrasonography may also be used for the evaluation of full-thickness rotator cuff tears. Neither, however, have the ability to reliably assess partial-thickness cuff tears or labral pathology. In addition, due to the invasive nature of arthrography and the technician-dependence of ultrasonography, MRI has become the modality of choice in most centers for evaluation of recalcitrant rotator cuff disease.

Surgical Indications

The mere presence of a rotator cuff tear is not necessarily an indication for operative repair. As mentioned previously, cadaver and MRI studies have shown that a significant number of rotator cuff tears occur in apparently asymptomatic individuals. Therefore, the indication for surgical intervention in rotator cuff disease is the presence of pain and/or functional deficits that interfere with activities and have not been successfully managed with nonoperative treatment.

The timing of surgical repair of rotator cuff tears is a factor that may potentially affect surgical outcome. Although some authors have recommended early repair after acute rotator cuff tears, many have reported that delaying repair does not adversely affect outcome. The question is whether an acute tear is the end-point of a degenerative process brought on by a trivial traumatic event or is an avulsion of a previously normal rotator cuff that occurred with forced contraction of an eccentrically loaded tendon. Many factors, such as age, previous symptoms, history of corticosteroid injections, and degree of traumatic injury, are incorporated into this decision-making process. The association of rotator cuff disruption occurring in the setting of concomitant acute anterior shoulder dislocation has been well described, and unrecognized and untreated disruption of the rotator cuff tear in this setting has a poor prognosis. Newer imaging technology, especially MRI, has helped in determining the size of the rotator cuff defect and amount of retraction of its tendons. Bassett and Cofield (6) have shown that in patients who have a significant acute injury and a full-thickness rotator cuff tear, repair done within 3 weeks of injury affords the best surgical results. They recommend early surgical repair of acute rotator cuff tears in active patients who place high demands on their shoulders. Thus, to establish a fixed requisite time period of conservative treatment before consideration of surgery for rotator cuff disease ignores the diversity of individual patient presentations and expectations.

The rationale of surgery includes decompressing impingement, debriding nonviable or inflamed tissue and thus presumably stimulating healing, repairing tendon defects, treating any associated pathology, and carefully staging and supervising a comprehensive rehabilitation program.

Techniques

The operative treatment of subacromial impingement and rotator cuff tears has evolved with improved understanding of subacromial pathology coincident with arthroscopic advancements. Our current algorithm for treatment of rotator cuff disease is summarized in Table 4.1. The majority of patients with

Table 4.1. Surgical treatment algorithm for subacromial impingement and rotator cuff tears

Continuum of Pathology	
Pathology	**Treatment**
Subacromial bursitis/tendonitis	Arthroscopic subacromial bursectomy
↓	↓
If prominent/worn coracoacromial ligament	Arthroscopic coracoacromial ligament excision
↓	↓
If prominent acromion, bone spur, < 50% thickness partial rotator cuff tear	Arthroscopic acromioplasty, cuff debridement
↓	↓
If > 50% thickness partial rotator cuff tear, small or medium full-thickness rotator cuff tear	Arthroscopically assisted (mini-open) rotator cuff repair
Large or massive rotator cuff tear	Open acromioplasty, rotator cuff repair, coracoacromial ligament preservation

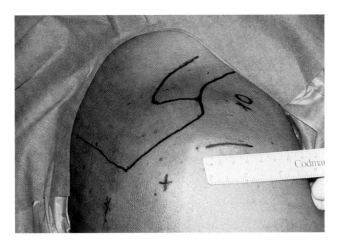

Figure 4.3. Before arthroscopy, bony landmarks are outlined and the portals are marked. The subacromial portals are approximately 4 cm lateral to the anterolateral and postero-lateral corners of the acromion. The mini-open approach is used if indicated.

chronic impingement syndrome with or without a partial rotator cuff tear can be managed arthroscopically. The advent of arthroscopically assisted (mini-open) rotator cuff repair has allowed the advantages of shoulder arthroscopy to be applied to patients with small and medium rotator cuff tears as well. However, patients with large or massive rotator cuff tears involving multiple tendons with retraction are preferably treated with the traditional open technique, as releases and tendon mobilization are facilitated, especially posteriorly. It must be emphasized that the rationale for arthroscopic intervention in rotator cuff disease should be based on sound principles established in the open treatment of the rotator cuff.

ARTHROSCOPY, SUBACROMIAL DECOMPRESSION, AND TREATMENT OF PARTIAL-THICKNESS ROTATOR CUFF TEARS

Preferably, arthroscopic procedures are performed using interscalene block anesthesia with intravenous sedation, thereby avoiding the associated morbidity and potential complications of general anesthesia (17). The patient is placed in a beach-chair position with the arm draped free so that it can be rotated throughout the procedure. It is important to have full access to the anterior, lateral, and posterior aspects of the shoulder. The bony superficial landmarks are outlined with a sterile marking pen (Fig. 4.3). This includes the coracoid; the anterior, lateral, and posterior aspects of the acromion; and the AC joint. Before the start of the procedure, 10 to 15 mL of 0.25% bupivacaine with epinephrine is injected into the subacromial space (Fig. 4.4). This distends the subacromial bursa, provides hemostasis, and helps provide anesthesia for an extended period. This injection should be done before arthroscopy of the joint so that there is time for the bupivacaine to bind to the soft tissues.

The initial part of the arthroscopy involves examination of the glenohumeral joint. A standard arthroscopy portal is made in the posterior aspect of the shoulder 2 cm inferior and medial to the posterolateral tip of the acromion. Gentle traction is placed on the arm, and ~20 mL of saline is injected through a spinal needle for joint distention. This facilitates entry of a blunt

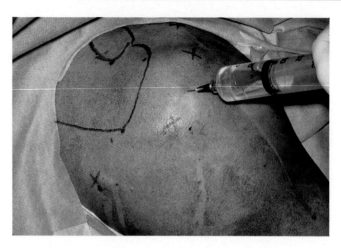

Figure 4.4. Before arthroscopic subacromial decompression, 10 to 15 mL of 0.25% bupivacaine with epinephrine is injected into the subacromial space to distend the bursa and provide hemostasis.

trocar into the glenohumeral joint. If pathology warrants, an anterior portal is made. This is performed by placing the spinal needle just lateral and a bit superior to the coracoid and arthroscopically visualizing the needle as it enters the joint in the triangle between the biceps and subscapularis tendons. The portal is then made with a plastic canula. Any inflamed synovium should be debrided and labral pathology addressed as indicated (27). Attention is then turned to the undersurface of the rotator cuff, which can be visualized with gentle external rotation and abduction of the arm.

In the era before arthroscopy, excision and repair of significant partial rotator cuff tears seemed logical and added little morbidity to the already open procedure (60). Currently, however, we generally treat patients with partial-thickness tears less than 50% the thickness of the tendon with arthroscopic debridement and subacromial decompression (2, 29, 40, 64) but warn them that their results may be less predictable, especially if a new trauma tears the weakened tendon. This debridement can be performed with a 5.5-mm full-radius resector. In the author's experience, reoperation has been so rarely required that routine open treatment seems unnecessary. However, if the rotator cuff is quite thin and the partial tear is greater than 50% of the tendon thickness, then mini-open repair is indicated following the arthroscopic decompression. The joint is then drained of saline, 10 mL of 0.25% bupivacaine is injected into the joint, and the arthroscope is removed.

For subacromial arthroscopy, two additional portals are made. A posterolateral portal, approximately 4 cm lateral to the posterolateral corner of the acromion, is made for the arthroscope; an anterolateral portal, approximately 4 cm lateral to the anterolateral tip of the acromion, is made as the working portal (Fig. 4.3). It is important to have these portals far enough from the bony acromion so that the rotator cuff and entire subacromial space can be visualized. One advantage of these portals is that visualization of the CA ligament in line with its fibers is possible (Fig. 4.5). This approach allows evaluation of the extent of overhang of the CA ligament. The 5.5-mm full-radius gator is placed through the anterolateral portal, and the thick bursa and undersurface of the CA ligament are debrided. This is done in a fanning-type fashion starting from the lateral aspect of the CA ligament and progressing to its medial aspect near the coracoid. In addition, the rotator cuff tendon can be inspected for a full-thickness tear and arthroscopically debrided before performing a mini-open repair.

The CA ligament is an important part of the CA arch and often extends inferior and lateral to the leading edge of the bony acromion. It has a broad insertion on the entire undersurface extending from the medial to the lateral side. Therefore, it may be the initial and primary source of subacromial impingement leading to disability, especially in overhead athletes. In patients who do not have a prominent acromion, it may be the only source of impingement. Adequate removal of the CA ligament is an important step in arthroscopic acromioplasty (7, 12). Removal enhances visualization of the acromion so that a more accurate determination can be made concerning the bony prominence of the anterior acromion and/or spur formation.

Technically, the CA ligament is sequentially removed using electro-cautery from the undersurface of the acromion starting laterally and extending medially (Fig. 4.6). An arthroscopic grasper is placed through the anterior portal and used to grasp the midsubstance of the anterolateral band of the CA ligament. The cautery is then used to resect this anterolateral band, which is then removed from the anterior portal (Fig. 4.7). The undersurface of the acromion is then exposed. The full-radius resector is then used to debride the soft tissue from the entire undersurface of the acromion so that the deltoid insertion into the acromion can be visualized. The AC joint can also be well visualized using the established portals and resected if it is symptomatic preoperatively. A 6.0-mm longitudinally tapered burr is preferred for the bony acromioplasty rather than a round burr. The thickness and morphology of the acromion (11) and the size of any bone spur will dictate the amount of bone removal in an individual case. On the average, however, only approximately 2 to 3 mm of bone is necessarily removed from the undersurface of the anteroinferior acromion. The amount of bone removed is not as important as the way in which it is removed. A smooth acromial undersurface should be achieved in establishing a smooth transition to the deltoid insertion (Fig. 4.8). No residual bone spurs or CA ligament attachment should be left at the anterolateral aspect of the acromion. The arthroscope may be

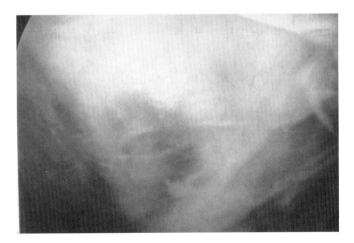

Figure 4.5. Direct visualization of the coracoacromial ligament in line with its fibers is possible through the posterolateral portal. Here, the ligament is seen with inflammation in its midsubstance.

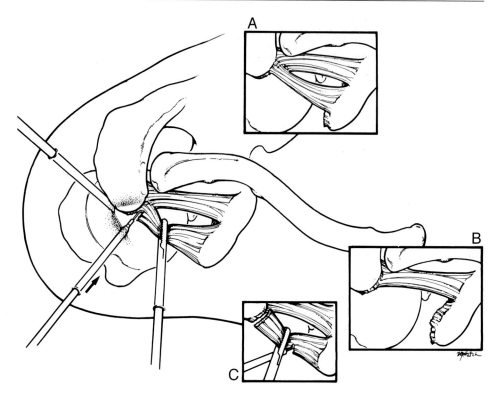

Figure 4.6. Arthroscopic excision of the coracoacromial ligament.

switched to the anterolateral portal or anterior portal to better assess this area for any residual bone. After decompression, the arthroscopic instruments are removed and portals are closed with absorbable suture and sterile bandage strips. The patient is then placed in a bulky dressing and sling. Postoperative exercises are generally started within the first 48 hours when the patient's pain has decreased.

MINI-OPEN ROTATOR CUFF REPAIR

The combination of arthroscopic subacromial decompression with an open tendon repair through a small deltoid split has become widely popular and increasingly accepted (4, 37, 49–51, 66, 68, 71, 79, 81). Arthroscopic localization of the tear allows precise incision placement, and newer suture-passing devices as well as implants have allowed the procedure to be performed through very small incisions. Small, easily mobilized tears are ideal for this approach, and tissue quality and elasticity are more important than exact tear size in determining repair potential (67). Reported results have been gratifying (4, 37, 49–51, 66, 68, 71, 79, 81). Perceived advantages over traditional open repair include deltoid preservation, quicker rehabilitation, shorter hospitalization, reduced early morbidity, a smaller scar, and the addition of glenohumeral inspection to elucidate other pathology. As mentioned previously, MRI can be extremely helpful in determining the size and morphology of the defect and whether a mini-open repair is appropriate.

After glenohumeral arthroscopy, identification and evaluation of the rotator cuff tear, and arthroscopic subacromial decompression, attention is turned to the mini-open aspect of the procedure. A portal-extension incision is made from the anterolateral subacromial arthroscopy portal and is only

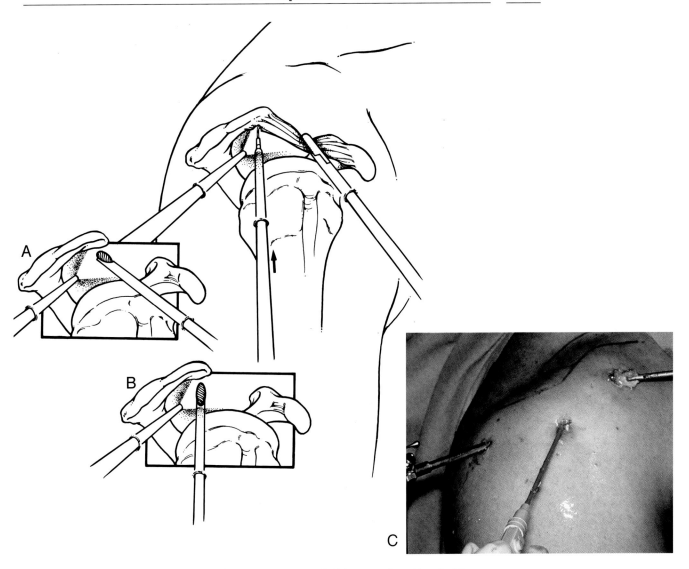

Figure 4.7. Removal of the anterolateral band of the coracoacromial ligament from the anterior portal.

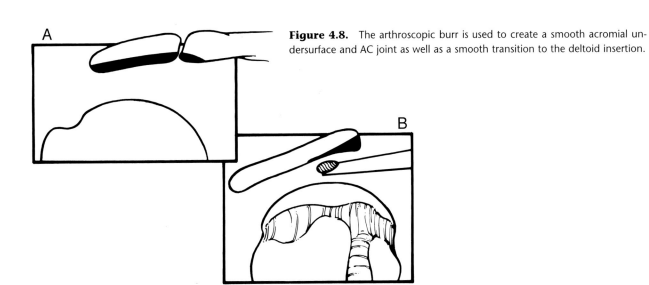

Figure 4.8. The arthroscopic burr is used to create a smooth acromial undersurface and AC joint as well as a smooth transition to the deltoid insertion.

approximately 3 to 4 cm in total length (Fig. 4.9). Subcutaneous flaps to the level of the deltoid fascia are raised. The deltoid muscle is then split in line with its fibers from the lateral aspect of the acromion for approximately 3 to 4 cm using needle-tip electrocautery. This deltoid split should incorporate the small defect caused by the introduction of arthroscopic instruments. Small retractors are used to retract the deltoid muscle anteriorly and posteriorly, and the rotator cuff tear is presented (Fig. 4.10). The entire extent of the tear can easily be identified by rotation of the arm (Fig. 4.11). In addition, abduction and rotation of the arm enables adequate exposure for bone tunnels through this small deltoid split. To facilitate the mobilization process, sutures may be placed in the tendon edge arthroscopically before performing the mini-open incision. The tear is then mobilized (Fig. 4.12) and repaired using standard open techniques (see below). After the tendon repair, the deltoid split is repaired with nonabsorbable zero or no. 1 sutures, and the skin is closed with a running subcuticular suture that provides a pleasing cosmetic result (Fig. 4.13).

Despite the already low morbidity of mini-open repair, efforts have continued to find methods for entirely arthroscopic tendon repair. Transfixing

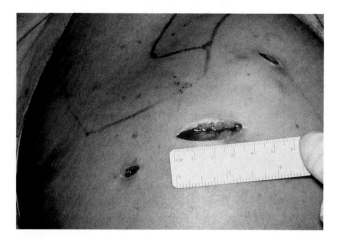

Figure 4.9. Mini-open tendon repair. A portal-extension incision is made in Langer's lines from the anterolateral subacromial arthroscopy portal and is only approximately 3 to 4 cm in length.

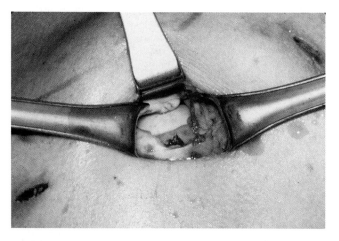

Figure 4.10. Mini-open tendon repair. After the deltoid muscle is split in line with its fibers from the lateral acromion, small retractors are used to present the rotator cuff tear.

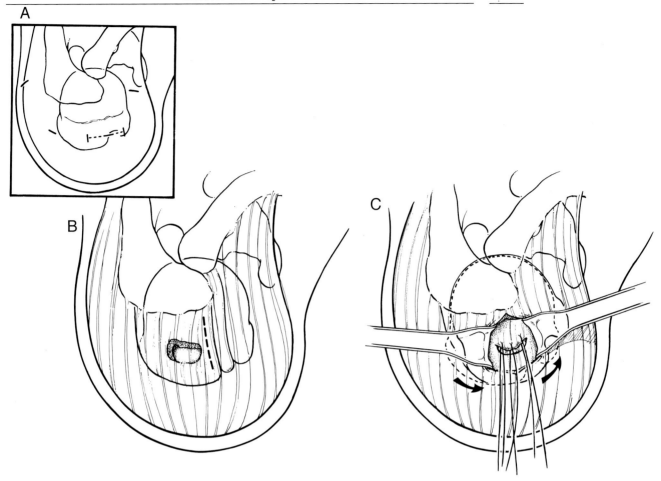

Figure 4.11. Mini-open tendon repair. Through rotation of the arm, the entire extent of the rotator cuff tear can be easily identified through the small deltoid split.

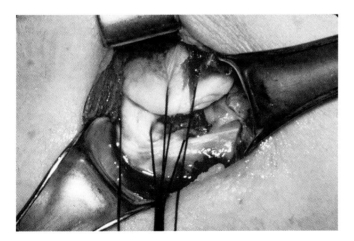

Figure 4.12. Mini-open tendon repair. Sutures are placed at the leading edge of the cuff tear; the tear is then mobilized and repaired using standard open techniques.

implants such as staples have been used (66), but problems with the metal staples have been worrisome (33, 38, 66). Biodegradable tacs have also been used (66). However, primate studies have shown that cuff repairs take up to 2 years to regain full strength (67) and are immediately stressed by early

Figure 4.13. Mini-open tendon repair. A running subcuticular closure provides a pleasing cosmetic result.

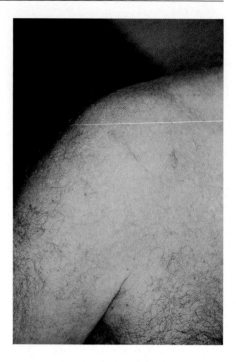

motion. Thus, most investigators have preferred permanent fixation. Snyder and Bachner (73) have developed a technique of repair using small screw suture-anchors in arthroscopic surgery, and early results are encouraging. However, the poor quality of greater tuberosity bone often seen in patients with cuff disease and osteoporosis has made this region less promising for implant technology than the glenoid neck. Currently, suture anchors are most helpful in the repair of subscapularis tears where the bone quality in the lesser tuberosity is better. Investigations into arthroscopic rotator cuff repair continue.

OPEN ROTATOR CUFF REPAIR

Patients with large and massive tears are best managed with standard open techniques. Open repair of a rotator cuff tear can be divided into four distinct phases: approach, decompression, repair of the cuff tear, and postoperative rehabilitation. Ideally, open procedures are also performed using interscalene block anesthesia with intravenous sedation. The analgesic effect of 0.5% bupivacaine will last for an extended period (8 to 10 hours), so that the patient does not have significant pain in the immediate postoperative period.

Approach

The patient is placed in a modified beach-chair position with the torso angled approximately 60° from the horizontal plane (Fig. 4.14). A head rest is used that allows access to the superior and posterior aspects of the shoulder. The arm is draped free allowing shoulder rotation, extension, and elevation, and two small towels are placed under the involved scapula to gently elevate the shoulder off the table. A first-generation cephalosporin is administered before the skin incision and is continued for 12 hours postoperatively.

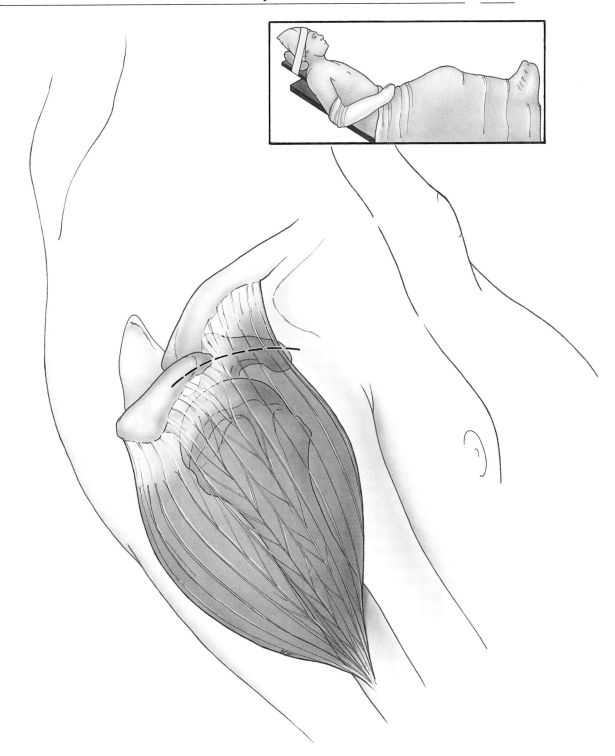

Figure 4.14. Open rotator cuff repair. The patient is positioned in a modified beach-chair position. The incision is made in the anterosuperior aspect of the shoulder in Langer's lines.

A 10- to 12-cm skin incision is made in the anterosuperior aspect of the shoulder in Langer's skin lines (Fig. 4.14), which provides a cosmetically pleasing scar and decreases the potential of scar spreading. The incision extends from just inside the lateral aspect of the anterior third of the acromion inferiorly to the lateral aspect of the coracoid. This places the incision perpendicular to the longitudinal orientation of the deltoid fibers. The incision is then deepened to the subcutaneous layer, and self-retaining Gelpi skin retractors are used to aid in exposure of the subcutaneous tissues. Mayo scissors or needle-tip electrocautery are used to expose the fascial layer of the deltoid. The needle-tip cautery is preferred because it significantly decreases bleeding. Subcutaneous flaps to the level of the deltoid fascia are then raised to allow access to the AC joint and 4 to 5 cm lateral to the lateral aspect of the acromion. At this point, it is important to identify the precise location of both the lateral tip of the acromion and the AC joint in preparation for the split in the deltoid.

The incision in the deltoid is started just anterior to the AC joint and extends laterally to the lateral edge of the acromion where it curves slightly posteriorly (Fig. 4.15). This will take the incision into the fibers of the middle deltoid, centering the split over the greater tuberosity. The deltoid origin is preserved as a 5- to 10-mm cuff of strong tissue is left on the anterior aspect of the acromion and the AC joint to facilitate closure of this split. The incision is usually extended 3 or 4 cm past the lateral tip of the acromion. A stay suture is then placed at the distal end of the split to avoid injury to the axillary nerve, which generally runs 5 to 6 cm from the tip of the lateral acromion. If more exposure is needed for a larger tear, the split can be carefully extended to 5 cm past the lateral tip of the acromion. The split is then deepened down to the area of the bursa using needle-tip cautery. At this stage, the superior aspect of the bursa is carefully opened and the lateral edge of the CA ligament is defined (Fig. 4.16). The entire CA ligament should then be identified. The superior part of the bursa lateral to the ligament should be removed. Before the ligament is subperiosteally dissected off the acromion, an attempt should be made to cauterize the artery that often bleeds in this portion of the approach, the acromial branch of the thoracoacromial trunk. A wide, flat retractor can then be placed underneath the acromion in the subacromial space and the humeral head can be levered inferiorly so that adequate exposure of the acromion and CA ligament can be achieved.

Using this approach, the split in the deltoid is centered more posteriorly over the greater tuberosity. This enables access to the entire rotator cuff through maneuvering the arm in flexion, extension, and internal and external rotation. Furthermore, the anterolateral aspect of the deltoid is anterior to the incision and does not block access to the posterior cuff.

Decompression

Subacromial impingement has been described by Neer et al. (57, 59, 60) as an important factor in the etiology of full-thickness rotator cuff tears. Impingement can occur at the CA ligament, the anterior acromion, and/or the AC joint. To perform an adequate decompression, the CA ligament is released and the anterior acromial "spur" is excised. The undersurface of the AC joint should also be examined for excrescences that may extend into the subacromial space. These can be easily removed with a rongeur or high-speed burr. The entire AC joint is only removed when there is preoperative tenderness, which occurs in only approximately 10 to 15% of cases. Currently, this is done from below with a rongeur and burr. The superior AC ligaments are preserved to maintain distal clavicle stability and cosmesis.

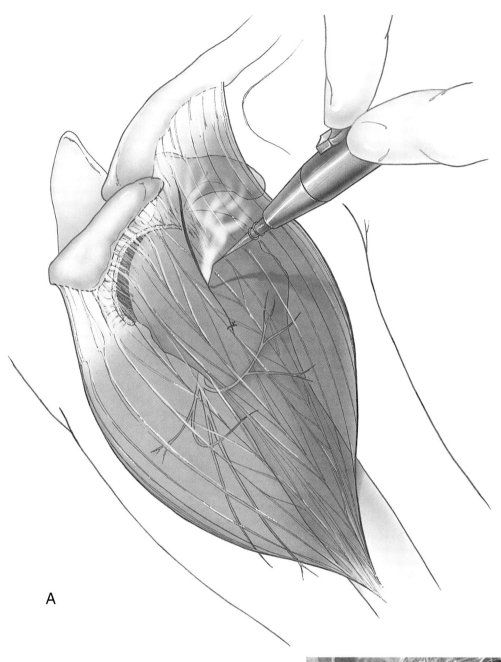

A

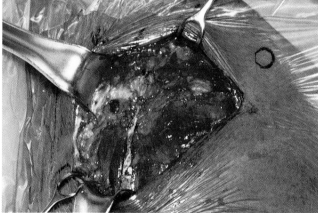

B

Figure 4.15. Open rotator cuff repair. The deltoid incision is made with needle-tip electrocautery. It is started just anterior to the AC joint and extends laterally to the lateral edge of the acromion. It then curves slightly posteriorly in line with fibers of the middle deltoid.

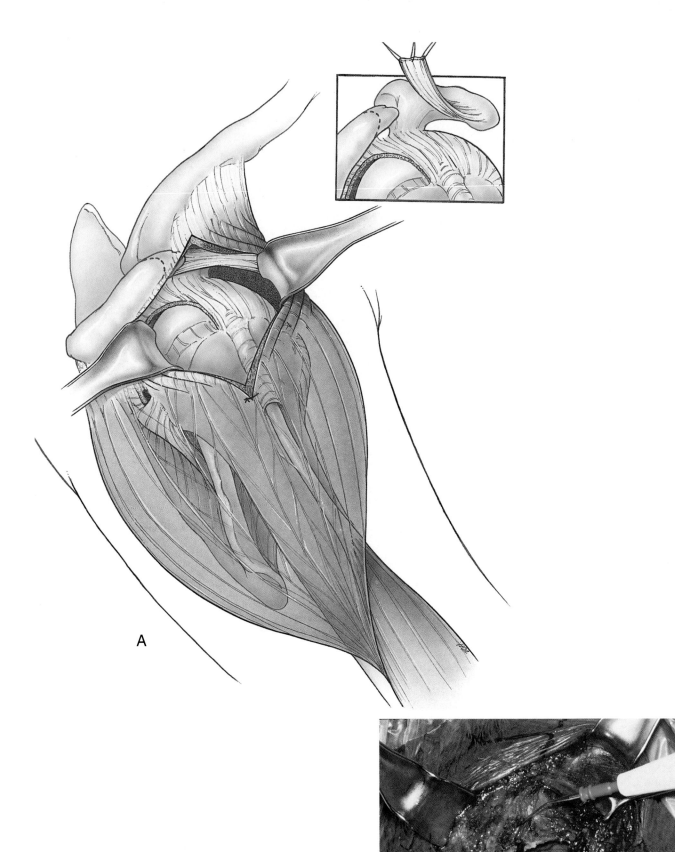

Figure 4.16. Open rotator cuff repair. The deltoid is retracted, and the coracoacromial ligament is identified. The ligament is subperiosteally dissected off the acromion, both from its anterior and inferior surface.

A

B

In preparation for the anterior acromioplasty, the lateral edge of the CA ligament is identified and subperiosteally removed from the undersurface of the acromion. It must be remembered that the ligament starts on the lateral aspect of the acromion and extends anteriorly and inferiorly to the coracoid. The author has recently modified his management of the CA ligament in patients with larger cuff tears (36). The CA arch has a passive, buffering function against superior humeral translation. If the dynamic head-depressing function of the cuff is lost and then the arch is overly resected, the head may translate superiorly to a subcutaneous position. Thus, in repairs of large and massive tears with associated superior migration of the humeral head, the author repairs the CA ligament back to the acromion in a more medial position after performing a conservative acromioplasty to preserve this soft tissue buffer (36). Following this, the remaining cuff of strong deltoid insertion tissue is meticulously elevated a few millimeters in a superior direction from the anterior part of the acromion and the AC joint.

The undersurface of the acromion is then cleared of bursal and/or rotator cuff tissue that is often adherent. It is important to check the thickness of the acromion with the thumb and index finger (Fig. 4.17A). The average acromion is only 8 mm thick in males and 6 mm thick in females. A thin, sharp, beveled osteotome is used to perform the anterior acromioplasty (Fig. 4.17B,C). The bevel is placed upward to protect from removing too much bone. Because the acromion may be very thin, especially in female patients, fracture of the acromion should be avoided. Traditionally, the amount of acromion removed has been approximately 7 to 8 mm in thickness and extended posteriorly approximately one-quarter to one-third the length of the acromion. Recent work in the author's laboratory, however, suggests that this may be too much bone and that only 3 to 4 mm of bone resection is necessary. The emphasis should be on contouring a smooth undersurface of the acromion for contact. However, the wedge of bone excised should consist of the full width of the acromion from the medial to the lateral border. A double-action laminectomy rongeur, rasp, or burr can be used to smooth the undersurface of the acromion and remove any remaining uneven ridges of bone (Fig. 4.17). In most cases, a properly performed acromioplasty removes a portion of the acromial aspect of the AC joint, often leaving the undersurface of the distal clavicle quite prominent; these rough edges should then be smoothed with a rongeur and rasp. This completes the modified AC arthroplasty that widens the subacromial space medially. If the entire distal clavicle needs to be removed, this can be done from beneath the superior AC ligaments with a burr or rongeur. Approaching the AC joint in this fashion prevents violation of the superior AC ligaments, helping to preserve AP stability of the joint.

Lateral or radical acromionectomy should be avoided (8, 28, 61). This procedure deforms the deltoid by removing its site of origin. Without this normal site of attachment, the deltoid is weakened and shoulder function is severely compromised. Transacromial approaches can also weaken the deltoid or result in nonunion and are not recommended. In addition, decompression is technically difficult to perform from this approach.

Rotator Cuff Repair

Attention is now turned toward mobilizing the torn rotator cuff tissue. The leading edge of the rotator cuff tear is identified, and sutures are placed into the leading edge of the tear using zero or no. 1 nonabsorbable sutures (Fig. 4.18).

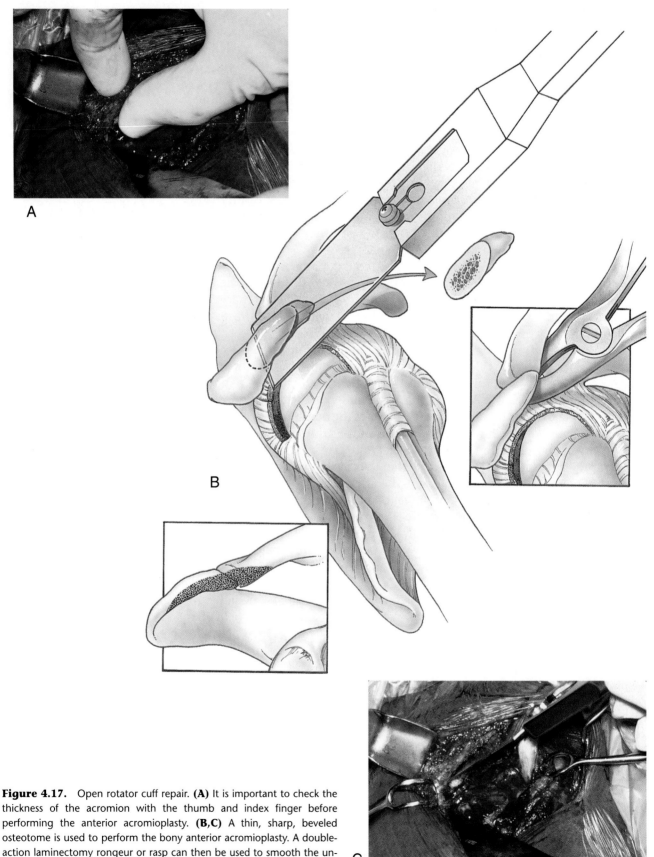

Figure 4.17. Open rotator cuff repair. **(A)** It is important to check the thickness of the acromion with the thumb and index finger before performing the anterior acromioplasty. **(B,C)** A thin, sharp, beveled osteotome is used to perform the bony anterior acromioplasty. A double-action laminectomy rongeur or rasp can then be used to smooth the undersurface of the acromion and/or distal clavicle.

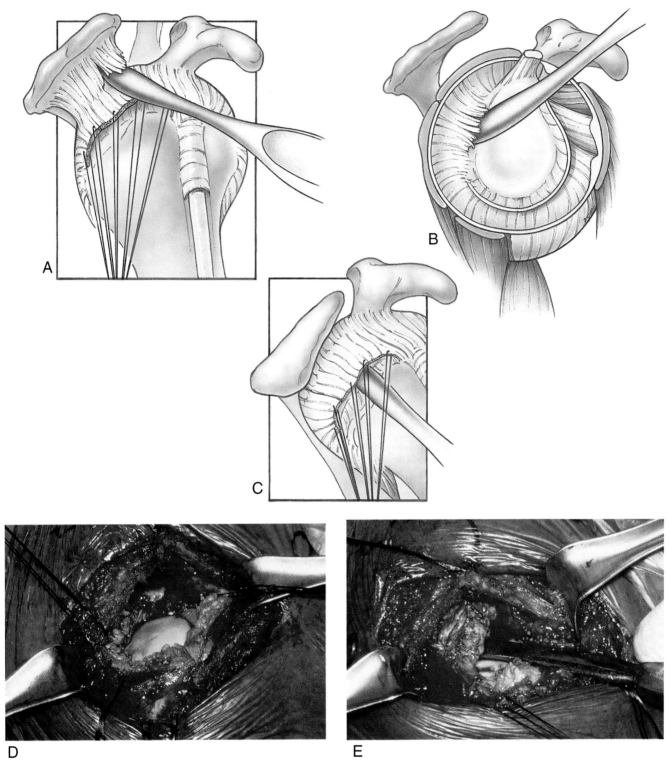

Figure 4.18. Open rotator cuff repair. Stay sutures are placed into the leading edge of the torn tendon, and the cuff is mobilized from anterior to posterior sequentially. **(A)** The cuff and bursal adhesions should be released from the undersurface of the acromion with an elevator. **(B)** The undersurface of the rotator cuff and glenohumeral capsule are often scarred to the glenoid rim. Undersurface release is carried out bluntly with an elevator. **(C)** The excursion of the torn tendons is assessed by pulling on the stay sutures; an elevator can be used to mobilize the tendon further. **(D)** A large rotator cuff tear before mobilization. **(E)** An elevator is used to mobilize the tendon.

An elevator is then used to sweep the superficial aspect of the bursa beneath the coracoid in the area of the subscapularis. It is important to remove only the superficial bursa, as the deep bursa may provide blood flow to the edges of the torn rotator cuff. Minimal tissue is debrided from the leading edge of the tear, as it has been shown that this tissue does have blood supply (75, 78).

The cuff is then mobilized from anterior to posterior in a sequential fashion (Fig. 4.18). Multiple stay sutures are placed at the visible edge of the torn tendons. Internal rotation and extension of the free arm helps to provide access to the posterior tissues. The posterior aspect of the cuff is also more accessible because of the "more posteriorly" placed deltoid split. Attention is initially turned toward the bursal surface of the cuff. A periosteal elevator or scissors can be used to mobilize the cuff and its associated bursa from the undersurface of the acromion. It is important to re-emphasize that the undersurface of the acromion is a common location for cuff and bursal adhesions and that this area should be released before the acromioplasty to prevent inadvertent extension of the tear (Fig. 4.18A). These rotator cuff adhesions are often underneath the posterolateral aspect of the acromion and the deltoid muscle and become readily apparent after the acromioplasty is performed. The previously placed stay sutures are used to advance the torn edge of the rotator cuff anteriorly. To gain additional posterior exposure, the humeral head can be depressed with a blunt retractor while in a position of internal rotation and extension. Also, a Gerber retractor may be helpful to depress the humeral head. This device is a laminar spreader that has been modified with a ring to depress the humeral head (Fig. 4.19). After complete bursal surface release and exposure, the posterior tissues are assessed to determine the full extent of the tear. Usually a portion of the infraspinatus and/or the teres minor remain attached to the humeral head. The surgeon should be careful not to remove these tendon insertions during attempts at mobilization and release of surrounding adhesions.

Attention is then turned toward mobilization and release of the undersurface of the rotator cuff. The undersurface is commonly scarred to the glenoid rim and base of the coracoid. Undersurface release is generally carried out bluntly with an elevator (Fig. 4.18B). Sharp dissection may be done with scissors, but this should be done with caution. Sharp release of this portion of the

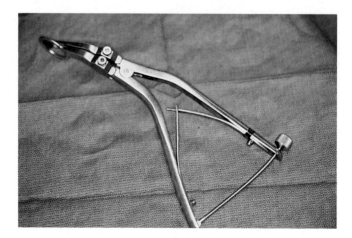

Figure 4.19.   Open rotator cuff repair. The Gerber retractor, a modified laminar spreader, enables excellent posterior exposure of difficult large and massive rotator cuff tears.

capsule not only places the suprascapular nerve at risk at the base of the scapular spine, but also risks cutting the posterior rotator cuff muscle as it is closely adherent to this posterior capsule. If scissors are used, spreading is more advisable than cutting. After a complete and systematic release of the undersurface of the cuff, the excursion of the torn tendons are assessed by pulling on the stay sutures (Fig. 4.18C). To ensure a successful repair, the edges of the torn tendon should reach the anatomic neck of the humerus with the arm in a functional position of 10° to 15° of forward elevation and 10° of abduction.

There are several maneuvers that can be performed if sufficient tendon cannot be mobilized to bring the leading edge of the cuff to the anatomic neck (Fig. 4.20A). The rotator interval and coracohumeral ligament should be released to the base of the coracoid (Fig. 4.20C). The coracohumeral ligament is often contracted, thus inhibiting the lateral and distal advancement of the supraspinatus tendon. This complete release of the rotator interval and coracohumeral ligament to the base of the coracoid is termed "the interval slide" and will allow the supraspinatus to be mobilized up to 1.0 to 1.5 cm. The author has avoided the need to transfer the upper portion of the subscapularis by using this maneuver. However, if the subscapularis transfer is performed (23), it is important not to transfer the underlying capsule because this may lead to instability. The posterior aspect of the rotator cuff, between the portion of the tendon still attached to bone and the free tendon edge, may have to be released from scarring at the posterior glenoid. This is best done by slowly using scissors in a spreading motion so that posterior cuff tissue is not damaged by cutting (Fig. 4.20B). Thus, it is important to release the apex of the posterior tear so that it can be properly tensioned and later sutured. In the majority of cases, these maneuvers will provide sufficient mobilization to allow the torn rotator cuff tendons to reach the anatomic neck with the shoulder in the desired position. The author has found the use of synthetic material or allografts to be helpful in repairs. With mobilization complete, the next step becomes the actual repair of the rotator cuff to bone.

The greater tuberosity is prepared for tendon repair by "scarifying" the anatomic neck area with a large curette. A deep trough is not used because it increases the amount of tendon mobilization required and has not been found necessary to promote tendon-to-bone healing. Multiple drill holes (four or five) are then placed into the greater tuberosity starting medially in the anatomic neck. Corresponding lateral tuberosity holes are made, leaving a 1.0- to 1.5-cm bridge of tuberosity bone between the holes and thereby creating a bony tunnel for suture repair to bone. Zero or no. 1 braided nylon sutures are then passed through the tunnels with a curved needle (Fig. 4.21). Although suture anchors can be used in the greater tuberosity (3), the bone may be osteoporotic, allowing for potential pull-out of the anchors.

During the repair, the arm is held in approximately 10 to 15° of flexion and 10° of abduction as well as a slight amount of internal rotation. The sutures are tied over the bony bridges. This allows excellent apposition of the bone and rotator cuff edge (Fig. 4.21). If an interval slide has been performed, the rotator interval should be closed in such a way as to realign the mobilized supraspinatus edge further laterally than the corresponding subscapularis edge of the interval (Fig. 4.22). If there is a split between the infraspinatus and teres minor (generally the "apex" of the tear), this should also be closed. The side-to-side "apex stitch" should be sutured before reapproximation of the distal edges of the tear to allow proper restoration of the intratendinous relationships of the posterior cuff (Fig. 4.21B,D).

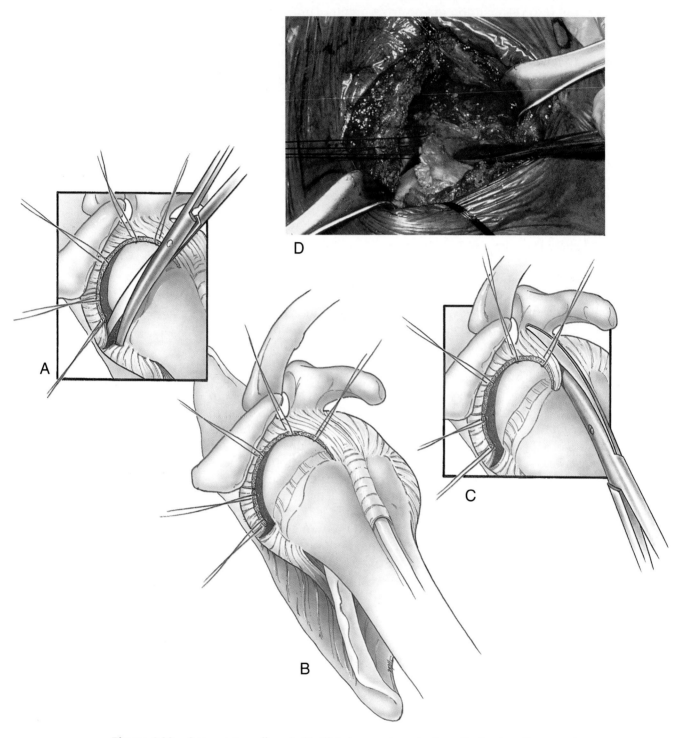

Figure 4.20. Open rotator cuff repair. **(A, B)** In large and massive tears, the tendon often cannot initially be mobilized to the anatomic neck. The apex of the tear posteriorly can be scarred down to the posterior glenoid. Blunt mobilization using scissors and an elevator is used to mobilize the posterior cuff. **(C)** The rotator interval and coracohumeral ligaments are released with scissors to the base of the coracoid. This complete release is termed the interval slide. **(D)** An elevator is showing where the interval slide should occur. The scissors are placed from the edge of the tear and directed toward the base of the coracoid.

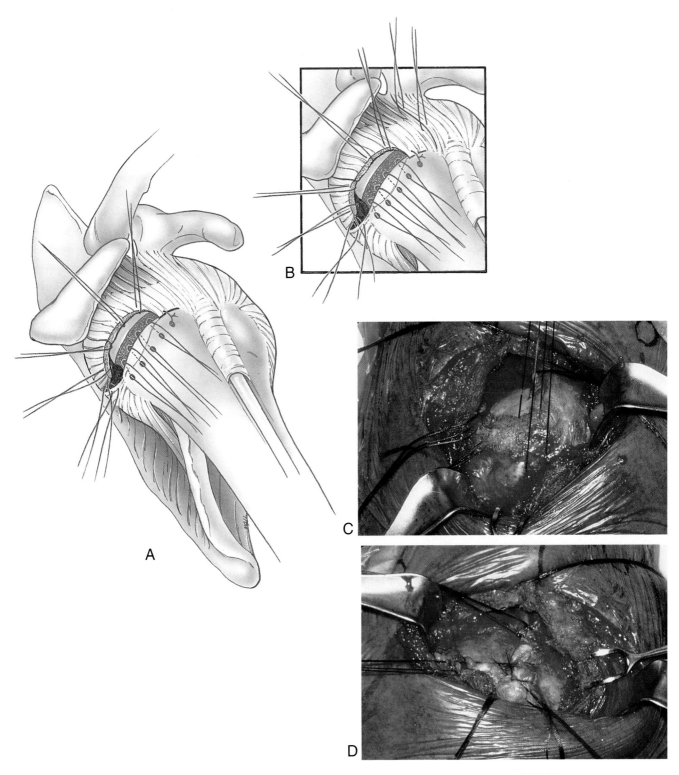

Figure 4.21. Open rotator cuff repair. **(A)** Multiple drill holes are used for zero or no. 1 braided nylon sutures. **(B)** The anterior and posterior aspects of the repair are tied down first, thus reestablishing the intratendinous relationships of the rotator cuff. **(C)** Placing sutures through a strong bony bridge helps prevent failure at the bone-suture interface. **(D)** The rotator cuff tear is reapproximated after mobilization techniques. Tendon-to-tendon repair of the anterior and posterior aspects of the tear are tied first, as is the apex of the tear.

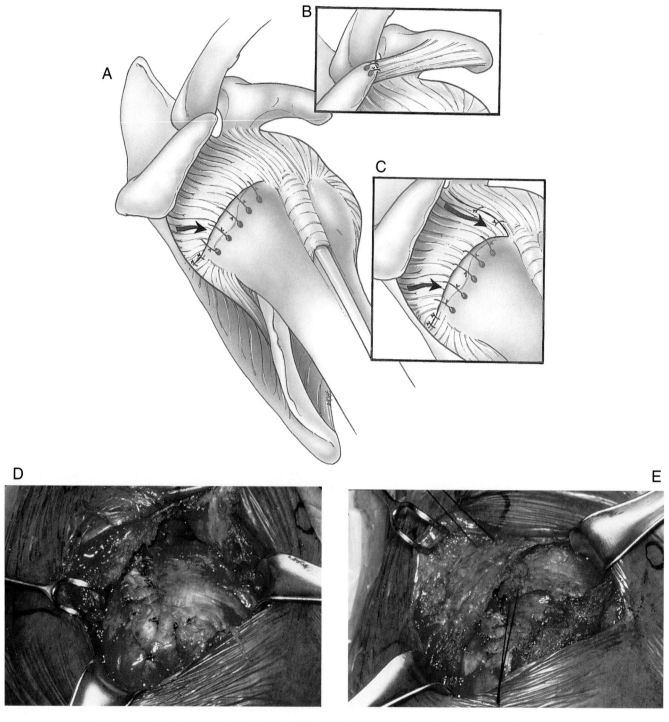

Figure 4.22. Open rotator cuff repair. **(A)** The tendon edge is brought to the anatomic neck and sutured with the arm in approximately 10–15° of flexion and 10° of abduction. **(B)** After the rotator cuff repair, the coracoacromial ligament is reattached to the acromion in a slightly more medial position. **(C)** The rotator interval and posterior cuff have been mobilized and repaired in a realigned position, thus decreasing stress across the repair at the anatomic neck. **(D)** Rotator cuff repair with complete reestablishment of tendinous continuity. **(E)** In large and massive rotator cuff repairs, the coracoacromial ligament is reattached.

If there is a large or massive cuff tear with deficiency of the superomedial aspect of the CA arch, the preserved CA ligament is now reattached medially (Fig. 4.22B,E). As mentioned previously, this provides a superomedial buttress that may provide restraint from superior migration of the humeral head (36, 82). The deltoid is then meticulously repaired to the cuff of strong deltoid origin that was preserved, and the stay suture in the distal deltoid split is removed (Fig. 4.23). If the cuff of the deltoid origin tissue is of poor quality, drill

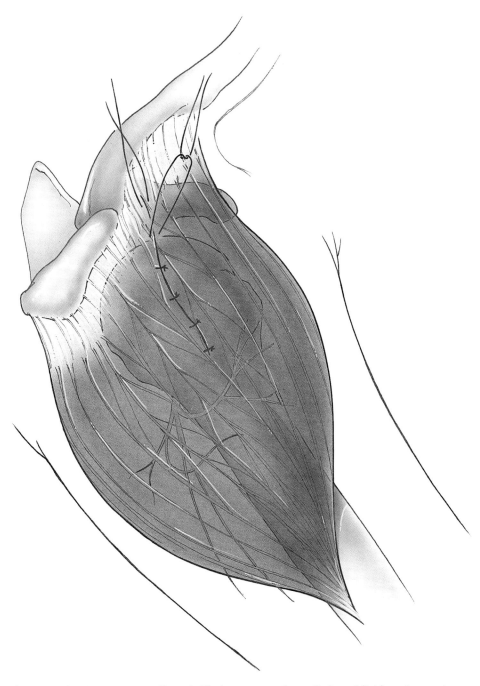

Figure 4.23. Open rotator cuff repair. The importance of a meticulous deltoid repair cannot be overemphasized. Zero or no. 1 nonabsorbable sutures are used to repair the deltoid back to the cuff of strong deltoid origin that was preserved in the approach.

holes are placed in the acromion and the deltoid is repaired directly to bone. A few subcutaneous absorbable sutures are placed, followed by a subcuticular skin closure with an absorbable suture. The arm is immobilized in a sling and swathe for approximately 24 hours. If an abduction pillow is believed to be necessary, it is important to avoid placing the arm in extension, which increases tension across the repair. In addition, it is unwise to abduct the arm in more than 60° of abduction in the pillow. The swathe is removed at 24 hours, and precise range of motion exercises are initiated.

Rehabilitation

In large and massive tears, the normal Neer Phase I Rehabilitation Program (59) is altered. In the first 6 weeks, only three exercises are performed. These include pendulum exercises, supine external rotation using a stick to 30°, and assisted passive forward elevation to 140°. Extension and pulley exercises are avoided in the first 4 to 6 weeks, because this puts stress across the rotator cuff repair. Isometric and active assistive exercises are usually started at 6 to 8 weeks. These generally begin with active supine external rotation, elastic band exercises, and active supine forward elevation. Once these exercises are performed, erect forward elevation with the help of a stick is started. This is done initially with a stick alone and is then followed with weights from 1 to 5 lb. A hand weight can then be used in the supine position to raise the arm. Weights can be increased to 3 lb but should not be increased over this weight to avoid placing undue stress on the cuff repair. Once these exercises can be performed without difficulty, more active strengthening exercises can be added.

Results

Since Neer's 1972 report on the routine use of anterior acromioplasty in combination with rotator cuff mobilization and repair (57), rotator cuff repair has been associated with improved results. In a review on rotator cuff repairs, Cofield (24) found that an average of 85% of patients could be expected to achieve satisfactory results, with a range from 65 to 100% reported in the literature. Black et al. (15) have reported results of rotator cuff repair on 481 patients and found that 92% of patients had a satisfactory result, with pain relief reliably achieved in 96%. The fact that pain relief is predictable and nearly universally achieved reinforces the premise that pain remains the primary indication for rotator cuff repair.

Functional results after rotator cuff repair, however, are more difficult to quantify and have been a topic of controversy. Walker et al. (78) showed by isometric strength testing of 33 postoperative shoulders that external rotation strength reached 90% of normal by 1 year after surgery, which was an improvement over that measured at 6 months. They also showed no difference in external rotation strength when comparing small and large tears. On the other hand, Heikel (45) demonstrated that 55% of patients had moderate or considerable weakness in shoulder abduction and flexion at an average of 35 months after rotator cuff repair. Gore et al. (42) objectively measured postoperative isokinetic strength in 63 shoulders at an average of 5.5 years after cuff repair and found abduction strength 78% of normal and flexion strength 90% of normal; abduction strength, however, significantly decreased as the size of the tear increased. They also found a positive correlation between the objective results of isometric shoulder strength and range of motion with their patient's subjective results postoperatively. Although the degree of functional improvement reported in studies is difficult to compare, most reports indicate that approximately 75 to 95% of patients have significant improvement in shoulder function after rotator cuff repair.

Separating and categorizing potential clinical factors that may affect the result after rotator cuff surgery is extremely difficult, as these factors are frequently highly interdependent (14, 46). The most commonly cited factor that affects surgical outcome is rotator cuff size. Although McLaughlin and Asherman (54) and others have stated that the overall results of rotator cuff surgery were not significantly affected by cuff tear size, Cofield et al. (26) found that tear size is the single most important factor influencing long-term results. Also, several studies have found that results after rotator cuff repair are better and more predictable with smaller tears (8–10, 28, 30, 43, 60, 61). When results are unsatisfactory after rotator cuff repair, the majority are due to decreased strength and function that is attributable to the poor quality of existing rotator cuff tissue in patients with larger tears, rather than unsatisfactory pain relief. Bigliani et al. (8) reported 92% satisfactory pain relief after repair of massive rotator cuff tears, which is in agreement with the observation of Hawkins et al. (44) and others that the achievement of satisfactory pain relief after rotator cuff repair is independent of cuff tear size. Although it is now generally agreed that the best overall results are seen with repair of smaller rotator cuff tears, surgical repair of massive tears is worthwhile due to the high level of pain relief achievable in this difficult patient population. Although repair of a massive rotator cuff tear is a tedious, demanding procedure, the results are rewarding if technical principles are strictly followed.

Summary

Symptomatic full-thickness tears of the rotator cuff can be successfully managed with operative repair. Performing an adequate subacromial decompression, maintaining the integrity of the deltoid, mobilizing and preserving the remaining rotator cuff tissue, and carefully staging and supervising the rehabilitation program are factors that will lead to favorable results. Patient satisfaction and pain relief are reliably achieved in the majority of patients. By following the techniques of repair as presented, the presence of a large or massive tear does not preclude a satisfactory result and/or adequate pain relief.

Arthroscopy has improved our diagnostic assessment of rotator cuff disease, especially in understanding patterns of articular and bursal surface partial-thickness tears. Despite continued controversy, most partial-thickness rotator cuff tears may be satisfactorily treated by arthroscopic debridement and decompression. The role for debridement and decompression without repair for full-thickness rotator cuff tears seems less than initially suggested, as several recent independent studies have documented results inferior to open repair. Arthroscopically assisted mini-open repair of small and medium full-thickness rotator cuff tears is a reliable procedure. Arthroscopic repair appears promising, but it is not yet well enough documented to be considered a standard of treatment.

REFERENCES

1. Adamson GJ, Tibone JE. Ten-year assessment of primary rotator cuff repairs. J Shoulder Elbow Surg 1993;2:57–63.
2. Andrews JR, Broussard TS, Carson WG. Arthoscopy of the shoulder in the management of partial tears of the rotator cuff: a preliminary report. Arthroscopy 1985;1:117–122.
3. Armstrong JH. Rotator cuff repair using anchor sutures. Orthop Trans 1994;18:312–313.
4. Baker CL, Liu SH. Comparison of open and arthroscopically assisted rotator cuff repairs. Am J Sports Med 1995;23:99–104.
5. Bartolozzi A, Andreychik D, Ahmad S. Determinants of outcome in the treatment of rotator cuff disease. Clin Orthop 1994;308:90–97.
6. Bassett RW, Cofield RH. Acute tears of the rotator cuff: the timing of surgical repairs. Clin Orthop 1983;175:18–24.
7. Bigliani LU, Codd TP, Flatow EL. Arthroscopic coracoacromial ligament resection. Tech Orthop 1994;9:95–97.
8. Bigliani LU, Cordasco FA, McIlveen SJ, et al. Operative treatment of massive rotator cuff tears: long-term results. J Shoulder Elbow Surg 1992;1:120–130.
9. Bigliani LU, Cordasco FA, McIlveen SJ, et al. Operative treatment of failed repairs of the rotator cuff. J Bone Joint Surg 1992;74A:1505–1515.
10. Bigliani LU, Kimmel J, McCann PD, et al. Repair of rotator cuff tears in tennis players. Am J Sports Med 1992;20:2;112–117.
11. Bigliani LU, Morrison DS, April EW. The morphology of the acromion and its relationship to rotator cuff tears. Orthop Trans 1986;10:228.
12. Bigliani LU, Rodosky MW, Newton PD, et al. Arthroscopic coracoacromial ligament resection for impingement in the overhead athlete. American Shoulder and Elbow Surgeons, Tenth Open Meeting, New Orleans, Louisiana, February 1994.
13. Bigliani LU, Ticker JB, Flatow EL, et al. The relationship of acromial architecture to rotator cuff disease. Clin Sports Med 1991;10:823–838.
14. Björkenheim J, Paavolainen P, Ahovuo J, et al. Surgical repair of the rotator cuff and surrounding tissues: factors influencing the results. Clin Orthop 1988;236:148–153.
15. Black AD, Codd TD, Rodosky MW, et al. Surgical management of rotator cuff disease. Presented at the American Academy of Orthopaedic Surgeons 62nd Annual Meeting, Orlando, Florida, February 16–21, 1995.
16. Bosworth DM. An analysis of twenty-eight consecutive cases of incapacitating shoulder lesions, radically explored and repaired. J Bone Joint Surg 1940;22:369–392.
17. Brown AR, Weiss R, Greenberg C, et al. Interscalene block for shoulder arthroscopy: comparison with general anesthesia. Arthroscopy 1993;9:295–300.
18. Burns TP, Turba JE. Arthroscopic treatment of shoulder impingement in athletes. Am J Sports Med 1992;20:13–16.
19. Clark JM, Harryman DT II. Tendons, ligaments, and capsule of the rotator cuff: gross and microscopic anatomy. J Bone Joint Surg 1992;74:713–725.
20. Codman EA. Complete rupture of the supraspinatus tendon: operative treatment with report of two successful cases. Boston Med Surg J 1911;164:708–710.
21. Codman EA. The shoulder, rupture of the supraspinatus tendon and other lesions in or about the subacromial bursa. Boston: Thomas Todd, 1934.
22. Codman EA. Rupture of the supraspinatus. J Bone Joint Surg 1937;19:643–652.
23. Cofield RH. Subscapular muscle transposition for repair of chronic rotator cuff tears. Surg Gynecol Obstet 1982;154:667–672.
24. Cofield RH. Tears of the rotator. Instructional Course Lectures 1981;30:258–273.
25. Cofield RH. Rotator cuff disease of the shoulder. J Bone Joint Surg 1985;67A:974–979.

26. Cofield RH, Hoffmeyer P, Lanzar WH. Surgical repair of chronic rotator cuff tears. Orthop Trans 1990;14:251–252.

27. Cordasco FA, Steinmann S, Flatow EL, et al. Arthroscopic treatment of glenoid labral tears. Am J Sports Med 1993;21:425–431.

28. DeOrio JK, Cofield RH. Results of a second attempt at surgical repair of a failed initial rotator cuff repair. J Bone Joint Surg 1984;66A:563–567.

29. Ellman H. Diagnosis and treatment of incomplete rotator cuff tears. Clin Orthop 1990;254:64–74.

30. Ellman H, Hanker G, Baer M. Repair of the rotator cuff: end-result study of factors influencing reconstruction. J Bone Joint Surg 1986;68A:1136–1144.

31. Ellman H, Kay SP. Arthroscopic subacromial decompression for chronic impingement: two- to five-year results. J Bone Joint Surg 1991;73B:395–398.

32. Esch JC, Ozerkis LR, Helgager JA, et al. Arthroscopic subacromial decompression: results according to the degree of rotator cuff tear. Athroscopy 1988;4:241–249.

33. Flatow EL, Bigliani LU. Complications of rotator cuff repair. Complications Orthop 1992;8:298–303.

34. Flatow EL, Fischer RA, Bigliani LU. Results of surgery. In: Ianotti JP, ed. Rotator cuff disorders: evaluation and treatment. Park Ridge, IL: American Academy of Orthopaedic Surgeons, 1991:53–63.

35. Flatow EL, Soslowsky LJ, Ticker JB, et al. Excursion of the rotator cuff under the acromion: patterns of subacromial contact. Am J Sports Med 1994;22:779–788.

36. Flatow EL, Weinstein DM, Duralde XA, et al. Coracoacromial ligament preservation in rotator cuff surgery. J Shoulder Elbow Surg 1994;3(Suppl):73.

37. Flynn LM, Flood SJ, Clifford S, et al. Arthroscopically assisted rotator cuff repair with the Mitek anchor. Am J Arthoscopy 1991;1:15–18.

38. France EP, Paulos LE, Harner CD, et al. Biomechanical evaluation of rotator cuff fixation methods. Am J Sports Med 1989;17:176–181.

39. Fukuda H, Hamada K, Nakajima T, et al. Pathology and pathogenesis of the intratendinous tearing of the rotator cuff viewed from en bloc histologic sections. Clin Orthop 1994;304:60–67.

40. Gartsman GM. Arthroscopic acromioplasty for lesions of the rotator cuff. J Bone Joint Surg 1990;72A:169–180.

41. Gerber C, Schneeberger AG, Beck M, et al. Mechanical strength of repairs of the rotator cuff. J Bone Joint Surg 1994;76B:371–380.

42. Gore DR, Murray MP, Sepic SB, et al. Shoulder muscle strength and range of motion following surgical repair of full-thickness rotator cuff tears. J Bone Joint Surg 1986;68A:266–272.

43. Harryman DT, Mack LA, Wang KY, et al. Repairs of the rotator cuff: correlation of functional results with integrity of the cuff. J Bone Joint Surg 1991;73A:982–989.

44. Hawkins RJ, Missnore GW, Hobecka PE. Surgery for full-thickness rotator cuff tears. J Bone Joint Surg 1985;67A:1349–1355.

45. Heikel HVA. Rupture of the rotator cuff of the shoulder: experiences of surgical treatment. Acta Orthop Scand 1968;39:499–502.

46. Iannotti JP. Full-thickness rotator cuff tears: factors affecting surgical outcome. J Am Acad Orthop Surg 1994;2:87–95.

47. Jobe FW, Bradley JP. Rotator cuff injuries in baseball: prevention and rehabilitation. Sports Med 1988;6:378–387.

48. Jobe FW, Kvitne RS. Shoulder pain in the overhand or throwing athlete: the relationship of anterior instability and rotator cuff impingement. Orthop Rev 1989;18:963–975.

49. Levy HJ, Uribe JW, Delaney LG. Arthroscopic assisted rotator cuff repair: preliminary results. Arthroscopy 1990;6:55–60.

50. Liu SH. Arthroscopically-assisted rotator-cuff repair. J Bone Joint Surg 1994;76B:592–595.

51. Liu SH, Baker CL. Arthroscopically assisted rotator cuff repair: correlation of functional results with integrity of the cuff. Arthroscopy 1994;10:54–60.

52. McLaughlin HL. Lesions of the musculotendinous cuff of the shoulder: 1. the exposure and treatment of tears with retraction. J Bone Joint Surg 1944;26:31–51.

53. McLaughlin HL. Repair of major cuff ruptures. Surg Clin North Am 1963;43:1535–1540.

54. McLaughlin HL, Asherman EG. Lesions of the musculotendinous cuff of the shoulder: IV. some observations based upon the results of surgical repair. J Bone Joint Surg 1951;33A:76–86.

55. Miniaci A, Dowdy PA, Willits KR, et al. Magnetic resonance imaging evaluation of the rotator cuff tendons in the asymptomatic shoulder. Am J Sports Med 1995;23(2):142–145.

56. Nakajima T, Rokuuma N, Hamada K, et al. Histologic and biomechanical characteristics of the supraspinatus tendon: reference to rotator cuff tearing. J Shoulder Elbow Surg 1994;3:79–87.

57. Neer CS II. Anterior acromioplasty for the chronic impingement syndrome in the shoulder: a preliminary report. J Bone Joint Surg 1972;54:41–50.

58. Neer CS II. Impingement lesions. Clin Orthop 1983;173:70–77.

59. Neer CS II. Shoulder reconstruction. Philadelphia: WB Saunders, 1990:41–142.

60. Neer CS II, Flatow EL, Lech O. Tears of the rotator cuff: long term results of anterior acromioplasty and repair. Orthop Trans 1988;12:735.

61. Neer CS II, Marberry TA. On the disadvantages of radical acromionectomy. J Bone Joint Surg 1981;63A:416–419.

62. Neviaser TJ, Neviaser RJ, Neviaser JS, et al. The four-in-one arthroplasty for the painful arc syndrome. Clin Orthop 1982;163:107–112.

63. Nicholson GP, Goodman DA, Flatow EL, et al. The acromion: morphologic condition and age-related changes: a study of 420 scapulae. J Shoulder Elbow Surg 1996;5(1):1–11.

64. Olsewski JM, Depew AD. Arthroscopic subacromial decompression and rotator cuff debridement for stage II and stage III impingement. Arthroscopy 1994;10:61–68.

65. Packer NP, Calvert PT, Bayley JIL, et al. Operative treatment of chronic ruptures of the rotator cuff of the shoulder. J Bone Joint Surg 1983;65B:171–175.

66. Paletta GA Jr, Warner JJP, Altchek DW, et al. Arthroscopic-assisted rotator cuff repair: evaluation of results and a comparison of techniques. Orthop Trans 1993;17:139.

67. Paulos LE, France EP, Boam GW, et al. Augmentation of rotator cuff repair: in vivo evaluation in primates. Orthop Trans 1990;14:404.

68. Paulos LE, Kody MH. Arthroscopically enhanced miniapproach to rotator cuff repair. Am J Sports Med 1994;22:19–25.

69. Post M, Silver R, Singh M. Rotator cuff tear: diagnosis and treatment. Clin Orthop 1983;173:78–92.

70. Rathbun JB, Macnab I. The microvascular pattern of the rotator cuff. J Bone Joint Surg 1970;52B:540–553.

71. Seltzer DG, Zvijac J. The technique of arthroscopy-assisted rotator cuff repair. Tech Orthop 1994;8:212–224.

72. Sher JS, Uribe JW, Posada A, et al. Abnormal findings on magnetic resonance images of asymptomatic shoulders. J Bone Joint Surg 1995;77(1):10–15.

73. Snyder SJ, Bachner EJ. Arthroscopic fixation of rotator cuff tears: a preliminary report. Arthroscopy 1993;9:342.

74. Soslowsky LJ, An CH, Johnston SP, et al. Geometric and mechanical properties of the coracoacromial ligament and their relationship to rotator cuff disease. Clin Orthop 1994;304:10–17.

75. Swointkowsky MF, Iannotti JP, Boulas HJ, et al. Intraoperative assessment of rotator cuff vascularity using laser doppler flowmetry. In: Post M, Morrey BF, Hawkins RI, eds. Surgery of the shoulder. St. Louis: Mosby-Year Book, 1990:202–212.

76. Uhthoff HK, Hammond DI, Sarkar K, et al. The role of the coracoacromial ligament in the impingement syndrome: a clinical, radiological and histological study. Int Orthop 1988;12:97–104.

77. Walch G, Boileau P, Noel E, et al. Impingement of the deep surface of the supraspinatus tendon on the posterosuperior glenoid rim: an arthroscopic study. J Shoulder Elbow Surg 1992;1:238–245.
78. Walker SW, Couch WH, Boester GA, et al. Isokinetic strength of the shoulder after repair of a torn rotator cuff. J Bone Joint Surg 1987;69:1041–1044.
79. Warner JJP, Altchek DW, Warren RF. Arthroscopic management of rotator cuff tears with emphasis on the throwing athlete. Operative Tech Orthop 1991;1: 235–239.
80. Watson M. Major ruptures of the rotator cuff: the results of surgical repair in 89 patients. J Bone Joint Surg 1985;67B:618–624.
81. Weber SC, Schaefer R. "Mini-open" versus traditional open repair in the management of small and moderate size tears of the rotator cuff. Arthroscopy 1993;9:365–366.
82. Wiley AM. Superior humeral dislocation: a complication following decompression and debridement for rotator cuff tears. Clin Orthop 1991;263:135–141.
83. Wilson PD. Complete rupture of the supraspinatus tendon. JAMA 1931;96: 433–438.
84. Wolfgang GL. Surgical repair of tears of the rotator cuff of the shoulder: factors influencing the result. J Bone Joint Surg 1974;56A:14–26.
85. Zuckerman JD, Klummer FJ, Cuomo F, et al. The influence of the coraco-acromial arch anatomy on rotator cuff tears. J Shoulder Elbow Surg 1992;1:4–14.

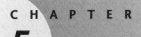

CHAPTER

5

Glenohumeral Instability

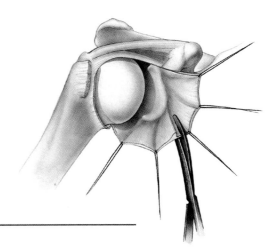

EVAN L. FLATOW

Introduction

Glenohumeral instability has been recognized to be a disabling problem since antiquity, and a wide variety of treatments have been recommended over the years (1–3, 15, 16, 20, 22, 33, 34, 47, 49, 63, 65–67, 72, 94, 96, 100–102, 114, 116, 122, 123, 126, 128, 129, 131, 132, 134–137, 145, 148–150, 156, 158, 170, 171, 176, 177, 183, 186, 188, 190, 193, 195, 197, 200, 201, 203, 209, 217, 218, 221, 229, 233–235, 238). Until quite recently, surgical repairs were generally undertaken only for recurrent, locked, anterior glenohumeral dislocations, and success was measured by the rate of recurrent postoperative dislocations. By this standard, many different procedures were effective, and most orthopaedic surgeons were happy with whichever repair they had learned during training. Several recent trends in shoulder surgery have combined to transform this relatively straightforward situation into the complex and controversial subject that glenohumeral instability is today. First, the recognition that subluxations may be a source of clinical symptoms (29, 77, 84, 198) expanded the indications for surgery beyond recurrent dislocations, thus shifting from a fairly "clean" diagnosis (e.g., the old rule in many residency programs that a patient could not be scheduled for surgery unless a radiograph documenting an anterior dislocation could be produced) to a more subtle one, with frequent clinical overlap (e.g., between glenohumeral subluxation and rotator cuff impingement in young, athletic patients). Furthermore, a growing disenchantment with repairs that achieve stability by restricting motion has prompted the search for more anatomic procedures, so that the criteria for success has expanded beyond a low recurrence rate to concerns for motion, strength, and function, especially for athletic use (46, 110, 159). Also, clinical and basic science studies of the role of inferior, posterior, and multidirectional instability have suggested the need for procedures tailored to the specific pattern of instability encountered rather than the use of a standard repair in all cases (21, 24, 27, 32, 48, 54, 57, 64, 69, 75, 83, 88, 95, 124, 139, 140, 144, 146, 151, 152, 154, 155, 157, 166, 191, 205, 208, 222, 224, 225, 228, 231). In addition, the growing use of arthroscopy has uncovered a bewildering variety of ligament variations, labral lesions, and associated rotator cuff and articular abnormalities, the significance of which are still controversial (5, 13, 23, 39, 40, 43, 50, 103, 118, 120, 138, 142, 144, 147, 165, 167, 172, 174, 210). Finally, the growing awareness that overly tight or improperly balanced repairs can lead to glenohumeral arthritis has further emphasized the need for precise balancing of the soft tissues (78, 89, 130, 154, 155, 164, 167, 202, 215, 237).

For all these reasons, the clinical challenge in modern instability surgery is to accurately assess and correct the specific pathology present in each case, restoring normal anatomy and function as best possible.

Incidence

The glenohumeral joint is the most frequently dislocated major joint in the body; in some series, glenohumeral dislocations are more common than all other joint dislocations combined (220). In a series of 1600 shoulder injuries, Cave (42) reported that 394 were dislocations, of which 84% were anterior glenohumeral dislocations, 12% were acromioclavicular, 2.5% were sternoclavicular, and 1.5% were posterior glenohumeral. Traumatic dislocations account for the majority of dislocations, with an incidence of 96 to 98% in various studies. The male to female ratio ranges from 2:1 to 5.5:1 (61, 62, 141, 180, 190, 216). There is no statistical difference in right versus left shoulder injuries.

Classification

The literature on shoulder instability can be confusing because of inconsistent use of nomenclature and varying classification schemes.

DEGREE

Episodes of instability may range from dislocations, in which the humeral articular surface is completely out of contact with the glenoid, to subluxations, in which the humeral head is partially translated out of concentric reduction but is still in contact with a portion of the glenoid. It is important to realize that not all transient episodes represent subluxations; patients may have full dislocations that spontaneously reduce and do not lock out.

DURATION

A dislocation may be acute or chronic. Although chronic unreduced posterior dislocations are far more common (4, 68, 206), chronic unreduced anterior dislocations do occur, especially in debilitated patients or those with altered mental status (19, 35, 44, 52, 55, 59, 60, 71, 87, 90, 93, 98, 104, 160, 161, 163, 181, 182, 194, 199, 204, 207, 211). Such a patient may present with new pain after an injury, and if the chronicity of the dislocation is not recognized, an attempt at closed reduction may produce a fracture (71). Recurrent instability consists of repeated episodes of dislocations, subluxations, or both.

DIRECTION

Dislocation or subluxation in one direction, anterior or posterior, is termed unidirectional instability. The patient with multidirectional instability has symptomatic glenohumeral instability in more than one direction: anterior, inferior, and posterior (21, 27, 69, 154, 157, 232). Patients with instability in all three directions have been thought of as having classic multidirectional instability. However, it has been recognized that many patients, especially athletes, present with intermediate degrees of instability. (6, 24). The term bidirectional has been used for patients with two major directions, usually either anterior and inferior or posterior and inferior (178).

ETIOLOGY (TRAUMA)

Hippocrates classified recurrent instabilities as traumatic versus atraumatic (2). Neer added acquired instability to this classification (154, 157). An initial traumatic dislocation results from a single, forceful trauma (58, 153) and frequently produces a Bankart lesion. The atraumatic dislocation frequently occurs in a patient with multiple joint laxities who has often experienced subluxations before suffering a minor injury to the shoulder joint that results in the dislocation (38, 41, 76). Capsular laxity is common, and frank Bankart lesions are infrequently found if surgery becomes necessary.

The patient with acquired instability (repetitive microtrauma) develops an enlarged shoulder joint capsule secondary to repeated stress and minor injuries from sports such as swimming (back stroke and butterfly), weightlifting, gymnastics, and baseball pitching (14, 76). Because the injuries occur in many different arm positions, varying regions of the glenohumeral capsule are attenuated with each episode, resulting in global enlargement over time. These patients may have loose shoulders but no laxity in other joints (76). A traumatic episode may put them "over the edge," so that they present with a first locked dislocation. However, the traumatic component is now only a part of the pathology.

VOLUNTARY VERSUS INVOLUNTARY

Neer used the term involuntary in 1980 in reference to the patients who "were so unstable they dislocated against their will" (157). Voluntary refers to the patient who purposely dislocates his or her shoulder due to psychiatric problems or for secondary gain (196) (Fig. 5.1). Not all voluntary dislocators have

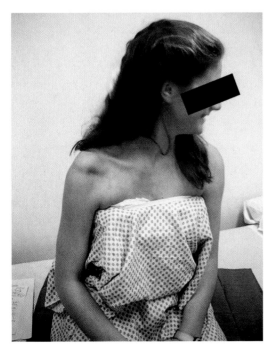

Figure 5.1. Voluntary instability. This adolescent patient is subluxing her humerus inferiorly through asymmetric muscle concentration. Although she says this is disabling, she is smiling and watching her mother's horrified reaction.

Figure 5.2. This motivated patient is plagued with unwanted posterior instability during daily activities. When asked by the examiner, she can demonstrate the instability by placing her arm in the at-risk position—flexion, adduction, and internal rotation.

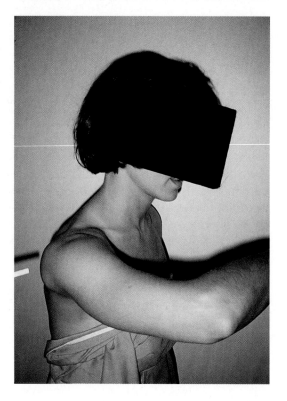

psychiatric disturbance, however. Some patients may put their shoulder out with asymmetric muscle contractions as an unconscious behavioral tic (219). Surgical intervention in voluntary dislocation is discouraged (17, 86, 196). Another group of patients can demonstrate their instability, if asked, by placing their arm in a susceptible position (e.g., flexion and internal rotation to cause posterior subluxation) (Fig. 5.2). These positional dislocators generally complain of unwanted episodes of instability during everyday activities which bring their arm into such positions and are reasonable candidates for surgical repair.

Evaluation

Careful and meticulous evaluation of a patient with suspected shoulder instability is essential before treatment may be initiated (187, 239).

HISTORY

The patient's chief complaint should be elucidated. Is it pain, a sensation of instability, or frank dislocations? The circumstances of the first episode of symptoms should be determined (99). Was there hard trauma (113, 117, 133) (e.g., a fall skiing), a minor injury (e.g., spiking the ball during volleyball), or no trauma (e.g., putting an arm up on a sofa)?

It is important to know if a locked dislocation occurred, if a reduction performed by a physician was required, and if there were any associated injuries (56) (especially nerve injuries). The frequency and character of subsequent episodes should be clarified, especially if dislocations are occurring more easily or more frequently.

The pattern of pain may be complex and nonspecific, especially because patients with recurrent subluxation can have diffuse ache from synovitis, posterior shoulder pain from rotator cuff traction injury, or snapping and pain from an associated labral injury. However, the association of symptoms with certain provocative activities may suggest the direction(s) of instability involved. Pain on carrying suitcases, especially when accompanied by traction (brachial plexus) paresthesias, may implicate inferior instability. Symptoms with the arm externally rotated and abducted are common in anterior instability, whereas pain and slipping with the arm internally rotated and flexed (especially when pushing open doors) is suggestive of posterior instability. Patients may complain of dislocations only (and be fine between episodes), subluxation only, or both. Some patients may have little pain and only rare dislocations but be quite disabled because they avoid all at-risk activities. Thus, it is important to understand the patient's functional demands and current limitations.

Associated symptoms such as a painful clicking or popping may suggest a labral tear but can be nonspecific. A family history of loose joints or shoulder instability may be an important clue that the instability may be multidirectional, especially if the patient's first episode was atraumatic.

Physical Examination

Visual inspection usually fails to discern deformity or atrophy unless there has been a nerve injury (106) or associated fracture. Axillary nerve injury is not rare after traumatic dislocations (30, 36, 51, 143, 223, 226), and spinati atrophy may indicate a rotator cuff tear that can accompany a dislocation in an older patient. Evidence of generalized ligamentous laxity (which would raise the suspicion of multidirectional instability) is sought and includes the ability to press the thumbs back to the forearms, to hyperextend the elbows, and to hyperextend the index metacarpophalangeal joint beyond 90°. Examination of the uninvolved shoulder may demonstrate anterior, inferior, and/or posterior laxity, which may be an important clue that the involved shoulder (which may be hard to examine due to pain and muscle guarding) is multidirectional.

Palpation for acromioclavicular tenderness is important; otherwise, pain from this joint may be incorrectly attributed to a loose but asymptomatic glenohumeral joint. Tenderness over the anterior or posterior glenohumeral joint line is a nonspecific finding.

Range of motion is usually full unless there is muscle guarding or a history of surgery. The essential part of the examination is the reproduction of the patient's symptoms with provocative maneuvers. In the classic anterior apprehension test, the seated patient's arm is placed in 90° of abduction and maximal extension and external rotation while applying an anterior force to the back of the proximal humerus (23). Classically, patients with anterior instability would report a sense of dread and a fear that subluxation or dislocation is imminent. More commonly, especially in patients who sublux but do not dislocate, pain alone is produced. This is less specific and may be found in rotator cuff disease. Jobe et al. (110) have proposed that performing the apprehension test supine is more specific if pain is produced by anterior pressure on the humerus and then eliminated by posterior pressure (relocation test). However, this test may also be unable to consistently differentiate instability from impingement unless true apprehension (rather than just pain) is elicited (and then relieved by posterior pressure on the humeral head) (213). Anesthetic infection of the subacromial space may also be helpful. If a significant portion of the pain produced by overhead maneuvers is eliminated, then some degree of subacromial inflammation is likely involved, although again this may not be due to a primary rotator cuff problem if there is secondary impingement from underlying instability.

A posterior stress test is performed by placing the arm in adduction, internal rotation, and 90° of flexion and applying a posterior force (by grasping the elbow) (178). True apprehension is rarely produced; pain and a reproduction of the discomfort associated with symptomatic episodes are the usual results in patients with posterior instability (92).

Inferior instability can be assessed by performing the sulcus test, by pulling down on the affected arm in adduction, and by pressing down on the humerus in 90° abduction (157). A variety of other maneuvers can be helpful, such as anterior and posterior load and shift tests, Fukuda test, and others (91). The aim is to produce humeral translations anteriorly, inferiorly, or posteriorly and to be sure that these translations are reliably accompanied by the patient's usual pain and symptoms.

Imaging Studies

Radiographs should be taken in three orthogonal planes (155, 175, 185). We usually obtain an anteroposterior view in the plane of the scapula (true glenohumeral joint anteroposterior) in internal and external rotation, a lateral of the scapular ("Y" view), and an axillary view (192). If there is recent trauma with pain and spasm, a Velpeau axillary view may be used instead of an abducted supine axillary (31).

Radiographic images are often normal, especially in patients with subluxation alone. Reactive bone wear at the glenoid rim may be demonstrated in patients with a history of dislocation, Hill-Sachs lesions (169) (Fig. 5.3), loose hardware from prior operations (11), and/or fractures (10, 45, 70, 82, 127). Computed tomography (CT) scans are rarely needed but can be helpful in assessing the size of glenoid fractures (Fig. 5.4) and Hill-Sachs lesions (97) and in assessing the rare case of abnormal glenoid version (e.g., due to glenoid hypoplasia). CT arthrography can document excessive capsular volume and labral tears (144) and detachments (73, 184) (Fig. 5.5). Magnetic resonance imaging is less reliable for these lesions but helpful if an associated rotator cuff injury is suspected (74, 81, 162).

Nonoperative Management

After a diagnosis of instability has been established, a prolonged course of rehabilitation is instituted with emphasis on strengthening the deltoid, rotator cuff, and parascapular muscles (9, 37, 173, 236). This is begun gently, below the horizontal, and avoiding pain. If secondary impingement and rotator cuff tendinitis is present, a subacromial steroid injection may reduce inflammation enough to facilitate rehabilitation. A brief course of nonsteroidal, antiinflammatory medication may be helpful, especially when a baseline joint ache results form secondary inflammation. Activities are modified to avoid those that cause pain or apprehension.

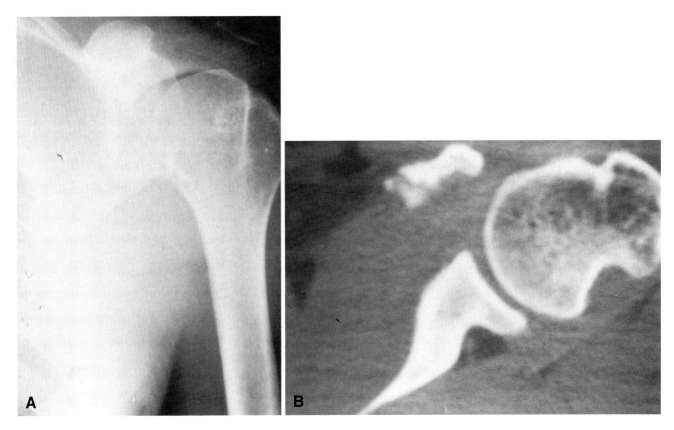

Figure 5.3. **(A)** Hill-Sachs defect seen as a dense line (the edge of the compression fracture) on an internally rotated anteroposterior radiograph. **(B)** The same Hill-Sachs lesion seen on CT scan (note coracoid fracture). (Reproduced with permission from Raven Press, Sports Medicine and Arthroscopy Review, 1:190–201, 1993).

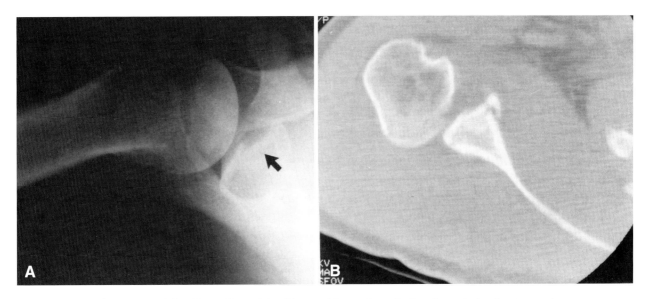

Figure 5.4. **(A)** Axillary radiograph in a 30-year-old man after reduction of an anterior glenohumeral dislocation. A depressed glenoid fracture is noted (arrow). **(B)** CT scan. (Reproduced with permission from Raven Press, Sports Medicine and Arthroscopy Review, 1:190–201, 1993).

Figure 5.5. (A) Bankart lesion (detachment of anterior labrum and attached glenohumeral ligaments) demonstrated on CT arthrography. **(B)** Same lesion seen at surgery.

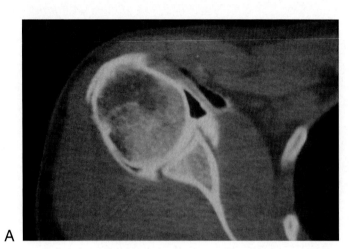

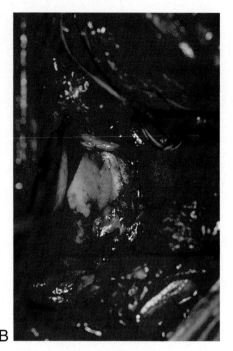

A   B

Imbalance in muscle coordination has been noted in studies of patients with generalized laxity (121). Deficiency in shoulder joint proprioception, possibly important in controlling the dynamic stabilizers in response to capsular or ligamentous stretch, has been noted in unstable shoulders (125). Therapy is aimed at improving muscle tone and coordination and generally increasing the patient's functional adaptation.

Indications for Surgery

Surgical repair is considered if the patient has prolonged symptoms of pain and disability due to recurrent subluxation or dislocation despite extensive nonoperative treatment. It is important to carefully assess patient motivation, both to be sure that the patient will cooperate with postoperative rehabilitation and to screen out voluntary cases (189).

Arthroscopy and examination under anesthesia can define the extent of instability and characterize intraarticular pathology such as labral lesions, early arthritic changes, partial-thickness and full-thickness rotator cuff tears, ligaments avulsions, and capsular redundancy (5, 13, 23, 40, 43, 50, 103, 110, 119, 138, 147, 210). Although many surgeons prefer to perform diagnostic arthroscopy at the time of open or arthroscopic stabilization, isolated diagnostic arthroscopy is rarely needed. This is because most patients can be evaluated and treatment planned after a history, physical examination, and routine radiographs.

However, arthroscopy without stabilization can be helpful in certain situations. In overlap cases, especially in young athletes, there can be rotator cuff tendinitis and bursal scarring secondary to underlying instability and overuse. Some of these patients will not improve with rehabilitation, because the bursal pain prevents muscle strengthening. Arthroscopic evaluation can define the extent of bursal and rotator cuff involvement, and soft tissue debridement of the subacromial space (e.g., debriding a thickened coracoacromial ligament or bursal scarring) can relieve pain and facilitate renewed rehabilitation (28). It may seem illogical to not address the instability surgically. However, most instability can be managed nonoperatively (37), and in these patients nonoperative treatment may be successful once secondary bursal lesions are treated.

The value of arthroscopic debridement of glenoid labral tears (as opposed to repair of labral avulsions [Bankart lesions] as part of an instability repair) is controversial. Although early reports suggested that labral tears might be symptomatic (142, 172), others have suggested that there is usually an underlying mechanical disorder (120). In addition, the results of labral debridement have been disappointing (7, 50). Nevertheless, in a patient with pain and clicking rather than giving way or dislocation as a chief complaint, arthroscopic evaluation and debridement of any labral tears discovered can be helpful, even if subtle underlying instability is suspected.

The choice of arthroscopic or open stabilization is controversial (18, 53, 79, 80, 85, 111, 112, 115, 168, 227). Arthroscopic repair has been associated with a higher recurrence rate than open repair, perhaps because arthroscopic techniques (although effective in repairing Bankart lesions) are less reliable in reducing capsular stretch (107). Arthroscopic repair may be especially effective after a first traumatic dislocation in an athlete in whom the Bankart lesion is the most significant component of the injury and the associated capsular stretching may heal and contract with postoperative immobilization (8). In the setting of recurrent instability, the author and colleagues have preferred open repair because it has been a versatile method of correcting pathology with a high percentage of satisfactory results. Reported relative contraindications to arthroscopic repair include a large Hill-Sachs lesion, glenoid fracture, return to contact sports, poor quality capsular tissue, and inferior capsular laxity. Contraindications to open or arthroscopic repair include voluntary instability, active infection, and paralysis.

Technique

RATIONALE

The inferior capsular shift was introduced for multidirectional instability (157). It is designed to reduce capsular volume on all sides by both thickening and overlapping the capsule on the side of greatest instability (anterior or posterior) and by tensioning the capsule on the inferior and opposite sides. For unidirectional anterior instability, a variety of anterior capsular procedures have been effective. We prefer to use a modified inferior capsular shift procedure, essentially a laterally based "T" capsulorrhaphy, without the complete mobilization of the capsule around the humeral neck to the posterior capsule, as would be done in a full inferior capsular shift procedure (24, 147, 179). The advantages of such a unified surgical approach for shoulder instability include the following.

1. Shoulder instability constitutes a spectrum from unidirectional to bidirectional to multidirectional (24, 178). The inferior capsular shift approach allows titration of the degree of capsular mobilization, so that intermediate degrees of capsular redundancy may be dealt with precisely. Furthermore, the surgeon is not committed to one or the other procedure from the beginning and may adjust the degree of capsular takedown around the humeral neck as the full extent of the inferior pouch is appreciated.

2. The capsule is shaped like a funnel, with a larger circumference laterally. A laterally based capsular incision allows shifting tissue a larger distance and provides more capsular overlap.

3. Detachment of the capsule laterally is less close to the axillary nerve as it passes along the undersurface of the midcapsule.

4. Use of a "T" capsulorrhaphy allows independent adjustment of tension medial-lateral and superior-inferior. Superior-inferior tensioning is usually more important than medial-lateral, which if overdone can result in loss of external rotation.

5. Although rare, capsular avulsions from the humerus do occur (12), and a lateral incision best detects and treats these lesions.

Bankart lesions can be easily repaired "inside-out" during a laterally based capsulorrhaphy. However, one advantage of a medial or transverse capsulorrhaphy is that in cases of unidirectional anterior subluxation, it allows a subscapularis splitting approach and fashioning of a capsular buttress at the glenoid margin (108–110).

The aim of repair is to restore normal anatomy. If a Bankart lesion is present, it is repaired. However, there is usually some degree of capsular laxity, and a concomitant capsulorrhaphy is performed. The translations that result from an isolated Bankart lesion induced experimentally are quite small (212). Furthermore, tensile tests have shown that the inferior glenohumeral ligament stretches in midsubstance before it fails, even when failure ultimately occurs at the insertion (e.g., Bankart lesions) (27). Indeed, Jobe (107) has pointed out that the capsule and labrum must deform and stretch from superior to inferior if the labrum is to pull away from the glenoid, much as a turtleneck collar must stretch to be pulled over one's head (Fig. 5.6). This may account for the higher failure rate seen after many arthroscopic Bankart re-

Figure 5.6. For the labrum and capsule to pull off the glenoid rim, they must deform circumferentially (redrawn after Jobe C. Symposium on Anterior Shoulder Instability, Fourth Congress of the European Society for Surgery of the Shoulder and the Elbow, Milan, Italy, October 1990).

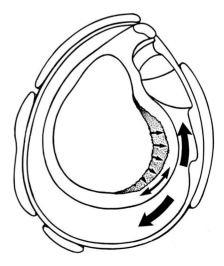

pairs; these minimally invasive procedures do not cause scarring of the lax capsule, whereas open approaches either include an explicit capsulorrhaphy or at least reduce capsular stretch through scarring from the open approach.

CHOICE OF APPROACH

The approach is performed on the side of greatest instability. Although all sides of the capsule may be tensioned from either an anterior or a posterior approach, the side of the approach can be best reinforced and strengthened by the overlap of flaps and the scar of the approach. Multidirectional shoulders that dislocate both anteriorly and posteriorly are approached from the anterior side.

Examination under anesthesia can be helpful in confirming the components of instability, especially in the occasional patient whose examination is clouded by pain and muscle spasm. Usually, however, the direction of greatest instability has been determined preoperatively, after assessment of the history, multiple examinations, plain radiographs, and any additional imaging studies. It is rare to charge the approach intraoperatively on the basis of the examination under anesthesia.

ANTERIOR REPAIR

The patient is placed in the beach-chair position but not as tilted up as for rotator cuff repair. Interscalene block regional anesthesia is used routinely because it provides excellent muscle relaxation and avoids many of the complications of general anesthesia. A concealed anterior axillary skin incision measuring 7 to 8 cm is used (Fig. 5.7). A few milliliters of local anesthetic are infiltrated around the lower part of the axillary wound, because there is thoracic cross-innervation not covered by the block in this region. Subcutaneous flaps are elevated until the inferior aspect of the clavicle is palpated. The deltopectoral interval is developed, and the cephalic vein is taken laterally with the deltoid. Occasionally, the upper 1 to 2 cm of the insertion of the pectoralis major is incised for exposure, if needed. The clavipectoral fascia is incised lateral to the coracoid muscles (Fig. 5.8), which are gently retracted medially. Coracoid osteotomy is unnecessary for exposure and may lead to injury to the medial neuromuscular structures (230). A small wedge of the anterior fascicle of the coracoacromial ligament may be excised to allow better visualization of the rotator interval and upper part of the subscapularis muscle (Fig. 5.9).

The upper and lower borders of the subscapularis are identified, and the circumflex vessels are ligated and divided (Fig. 5.10). Although the inferior muscular fibers of the subscapularis may be preserved in some unidirectional cases, this can compromise the inferior capsular dissection required if there is a significant inferior component requiring correction. The tendon is detached, leaving a stump for repair (Fig. 5.11). Bluntly elevating the muscle belly medially may allow early identification of the plane between the tendon and capsule. A portion of the deep surface of the tendon may be left with the capsule to reinforce a thin or laterally avulsed capsule but is not usually necessary.

The axillary nerve should be gently palpated and protected during the procedure (Fig. 5.12). The capsule is incised laterally near its insertion, leaving a 1-cm cuff of tissue for repair. Keeping the arm adducted and externally

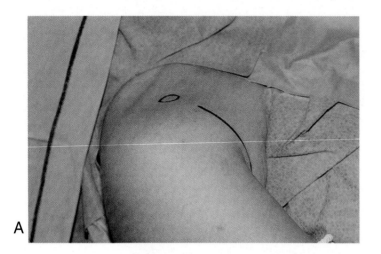

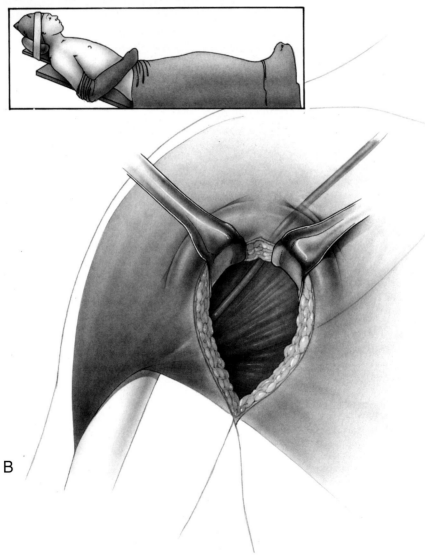

Figure 5.7. **(A)** A concealed axillary incision begins approximately 3 cm below
the coracoid and extends inferiorly for 8 cm into the axillary crease.
(B) Skin flaps are elevated to expose the deltopectoral interval.

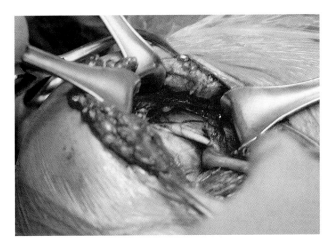

Figure 5.8. After the deltopectoral interval has been developed, the clavipectoral fascia is incised and the strap muscles are bluntly elevated from the underlying subscapularis.

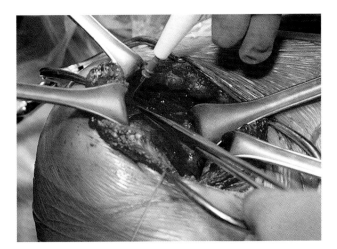

Figure 5.9. A wedge-shaped portion of the coracoacromial ligament is excised for improved exposure on the rotator interval and upper border of the subscapularis.

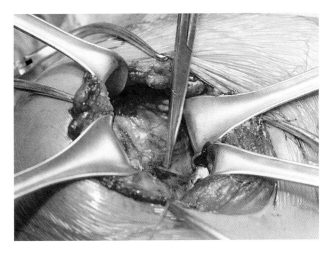

Figure 5.10. The anterior circumflex vessels (shown by clamp) are ligated or coagulated and divided.

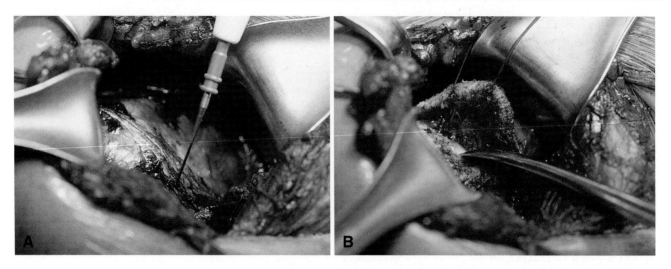

Figure 5.11. **(A)** The subscapularis tendon is sharply separated from the capsule with the needle-tip cautery. **(B)** More medially, the plane between muscle and capsule may be bluntly developed.

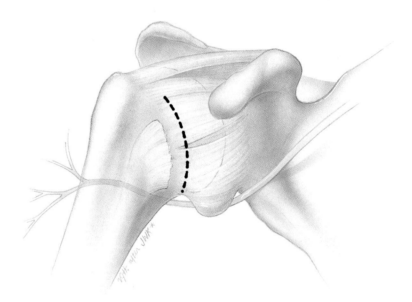

Figure 5.12. The axillary nerve is close to the inferior capsule at the midcapsule or slightly medial.

rotated will maximize the distance to the axillary nerve (Fig. 5.13). The incision progresses from superior to inferior, and traction sutures are placed in the free edge. As the humerus is externally rotated and flexed, the capsule is incised around the neck of the humerus with a blade or an elevator while protecting the axillary nerve (Fig. 5.14). A finger may be placed in the inferior pouch to assess how large it is and how much redundant capsule needs to be released before shifting. If pulling up on the sutures pushes the finger out and obliterates this pouch, then enough mobilization has been accomplished for an effective shift (Fig. 5.15).

The degree of capsular takedown and shifting will vary in each case. In a unidirectional anterior case, only the anterior capsule is mobilized. If there is both anterior instability and inferior instability in abduction and a large pouch, then the inferior capsular is mobilized and the pouch obliterated. If there is frank multidirectional instability with anterior, inferior, and posterior instability, the capsule is taken down all the way around the neck to the posterior capsule, which can then be tensioned as the detached inferior capsule is shifted anteriorly.

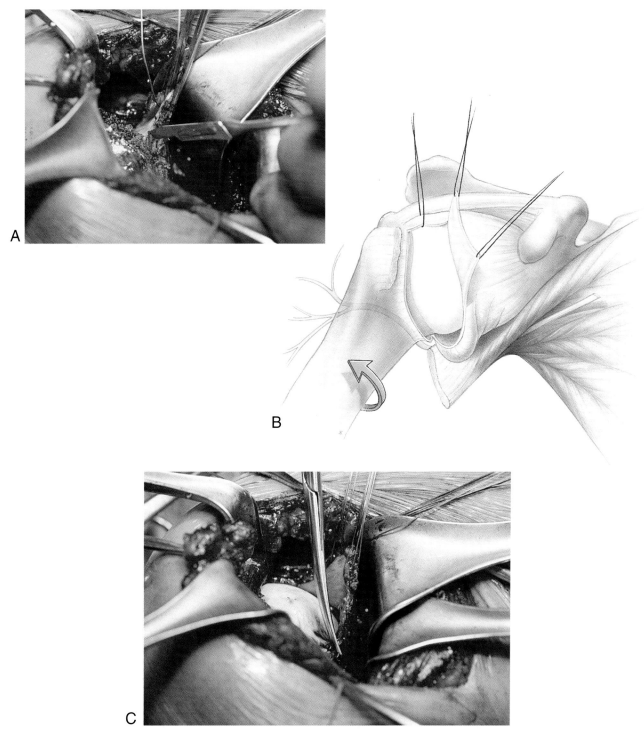

Figure 5.13. **(A)** After the subscapularis takedown, the capsule is incised. **(B)** The arm is kept adducted and externally rotated. **(C)** Scissors or an elevator may be used to take the capsule down around the humeral neck.

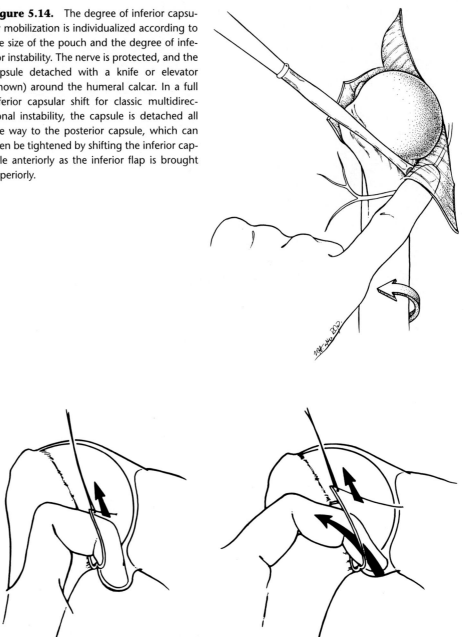

Figure 5.14. The degree of inferior capsular mobilization is individualized according to the size of the pouch and the degree of inferior instability. The nerve is protected, and the capsule detached with a knife or elevator (shown) around the humeral calcar. In a full inferior capsular shift for classic multidirectional instability, the capsule is detached all the way to the posterior capsule, which can then be tightened by shifting the inferior capsule anteriorly as the inferior flap is brought superiorly.

Figure 5.15. **(Left)** A finger may be used to assess the size of the inferior pouch. **(Right)** If the inferior flap has been adequately mobilized, pulling up on it will force the finger out of the pouch.

Neer and Forster (157) referred to the gap between the supraspinatus and subscapularis tendons as the rotator interval, while calling the deeper capsular interval at the same location the cleft between the superior and middle glenohumeral ligaments. They believed that this cleft was generally enlarged in patients with multidirectional instability and described closing it as part of an inferior capsular shift. We repair it when it is widened, especially if there is a preoperative sulcus sign with symptomatic inferior instability. However, the interval should not be overly tightened because this may restrict motion, especially external rotation.

The horizontal limb of the "T" is made between the inferior and middle glenohumeral ligaments (Fig. 5.16). A Fukuda or other head retractor is then placed and the glenoid is inspected (Fig. 5.17). If the capsule is thin and redundant medially, a "barrel" stitch may be used to tension it. This can also serve to bunch up tissue at the glenoid rim to reconstruct a bumper to compensate for a deficient labrum (Fig. 5.18). When the glenohumeral ligaments and labrum are found to be avulsed medially from the bone, they are reattached to the glenoid rim. This is done inside-out before the capsulorrhaphy, because the capsulorrhaphy must be anchored medially to the glenoid for a shift to be effective. The anterior glenoid neck is freshened to bleeding bone.

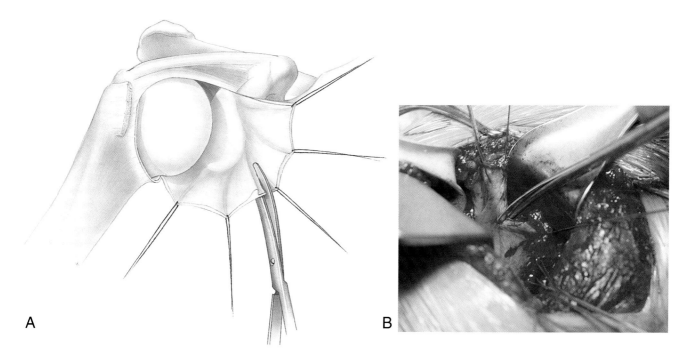

A   B

Figure 5.16. **(A)** The horizontal limb of the "T" is made between the inferior and middle glenohumeral ligaments. **(B)** The incision comes to but not through the labrum.

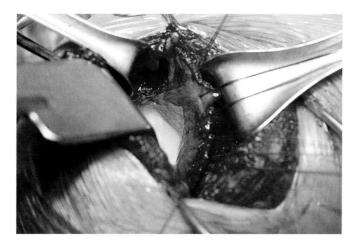

Figure 5.17. A Fukuda retractor is placed, and the glenoid is inspected.

Two to three sets of drill holes placed through the glenoid rim are used (Fig. 5.19). Small curved awls, small angled curettes, and heavy towel clip-like tools are helpful in making the tunnel. Zero nonabsorbable braided sutures are passed through the bone tunnels. Both ends of each suture are passed through the labrum and tied on the outside capsule (Fig. 5.19). Alternatively, suture anchors may be used. These should be placed adjacent to the articular cartilage and not medially to avoid a step-off and to bring the labrum and capsule right to the rim as a buttress.

The glenoid margin may be compromised either by a glenoid rim fracture or wear from repeated dislocations (10). Defects representing less than 25% of the surface area of the glenoid may be rendered extraarticular by repairing the detached labrum and capsule back to the edge of the remaining intact glenoid articular cartilage (214). If a chip of bone has been avulsed with the capsule and ligaments attached, then it is repaired back with sutures as in a standard repair. If the fragment is large enough and can be mobilized, a cannulated screw may be used, burying the head in the substance of the fragment. If the defect is larger than 25% and there is no fragment to be repaired, then the coracoid tip with attached muscle is transferred into the defect

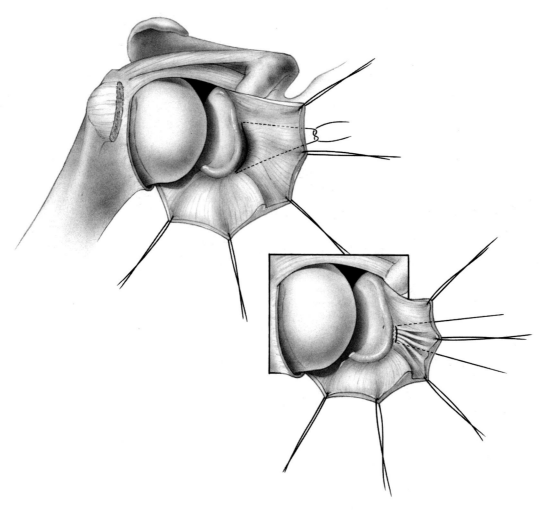

Figure 5.18.   If the capsule is thin and redundant medially, a "barrel" stitch may be used to tension it. This can also serve to bunch up tissue at the glenoid rim to reconstruct a bumper to compensate for a deficient labrum.

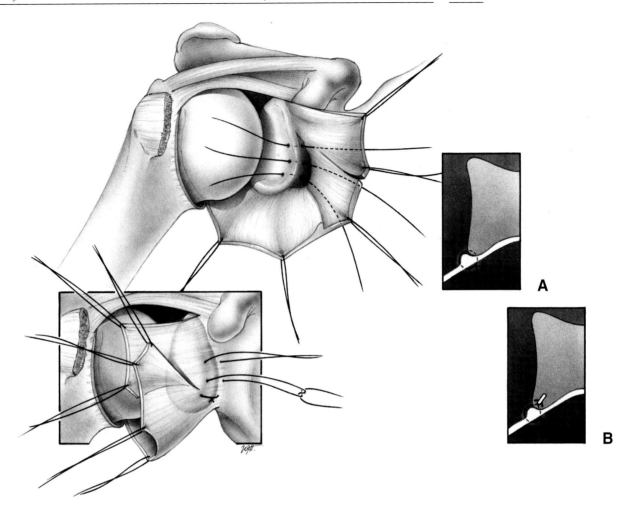

Figure 5.19. A capsulolabral avulsion from the glenoid rim should be repaired inside-out before the capsulorrhaphy. Sutures are passed through the glenoid rim **(top)**. Both ends are passed through the medial capsule-labrum and tied on the outside **(bottom)**. Bone sutures **(A)** or suture anchors **(B)** may be used.

behind the repaired capsule (extraarticular). A screw and washer are generally used. The aim is to deepen the socket, not to act as a bone block.

The arm is positioned in at least 20° of external rotation and 30° of abduction during the capsular shift. For overhead athletes with anterior subluxation, more abduction and external rotation are used. For multidirectional patients with generalized laxity, the capsule is repaired in a more neutral position (but still slight abduction) to allow balanced tension in the anterior and posterior capsule. The inferior flap is shifted superiorly, and then the superior flap is brought inferiorly (Fig. 5.20). It is initially important that the inferior flap be free and untethered if is to be shifted, and any adherent muscle or other tissue must be gently freed. A stitch may be added between the two flaps more medially (Fig. 5.18). The subscapularis is then repaired (Fig. 5.21), and a layered closure effected with a cosmetic, subcuticular stitch.

Patients who undergo a modified shift for unidirectional or bidirectional instability are protected in a sling for 6 weeks but begin exercises with a protected range after 10 days. From 10 days to 2 weeks, they perform isometric exercises and external rotation to 10° and elevation to 90°. From 2 to 4 weeks,

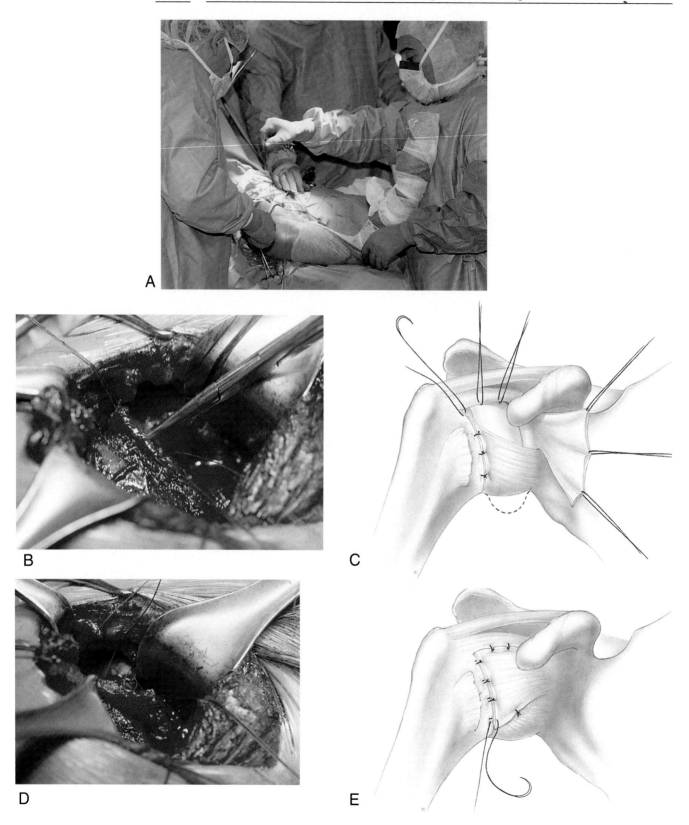

Figure 5.20. **(A)** The inferior flap is brought superiorly with the arm in approximately 20° external rotation and 30° abduction. **(B)** The flap is held in place. **(C)** The flap is repaired to its lateral stump. **(D)** The superior flap is then shifted inferiorly over the inferior flap. **(E)** The rotator interval has been precisely closed.

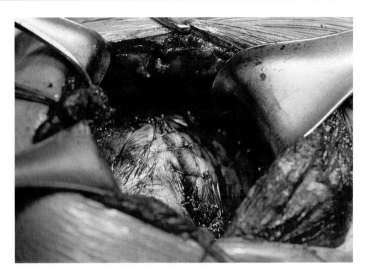

Figure 5.21.   The subscapularis is anatomically repaired.

external rotation is allowed to 30° and elevation to 140°. From 4 to 6 weeks, external rotation is increased to 40° and elevation to 160°, and resistive exercises are begun. After 6 weeks, external rotation is increased to 50° and terminal elevation stretching allowed. After 3 months, terminal external rotation stretching is added. These are general protocols and are modified on an individual basis as indicated. The aim is gain motion over several months. Progression that is too rapid may lead to recurrent instability. This is especially true in patients with generalized joint laxity. Careful and frequent follow-up care is needed. Patients who are not progressing quickly enough may need an accelerated program, and those who are regaining motion too quickly may need to be slowed. Return to contact sports is generally restricted until 9 to 12 months have elapsed.

Patients with classic multidirectional instability undergoing a full inferior capsular shift are immobilized for 6 weeks in a brace, with the arm in slight abduction and neutral rotation, allowing only gentle isometric exercises and supervised elbow range of motion. At 6 weeks, the brace is discontinued, and range of motion exercises are very gradually introduced. At 12 weeks, progressive strengthening is instituted.

POSTERIOR REPAIR

The patient is placed in the lateral decubitus position. General anesthesia is administered. An oblique 10- to 12-cm skin incision is used, angled 40 to 60° from the scapular spine and extending 2 to 3 cm beyond the posterolateral corner of the acromion (Fig. 5.22). The deltoid is split along the direction of it fibers for no more than 5 cm from the posterolateral corner of the acromion. A stay suture is placed at the distal aspect of the split to prevent its propagation with retraction that might injure the axillary nerve. The deltoid is then detached from the scapular spine for 3 to 4 cm medially and from the lateral acromion for 1 to 2 cm anteriorly.

The infraspinatus is then differentiated from the supraspinatus superiorly and the teres minor inferiorly. The latter distinction is aided by two considerations. First, the infraspinatus is bipennate, and so three "groups" of muscle fibers are usually seen—the upper two are the infraspinatus, and the lower

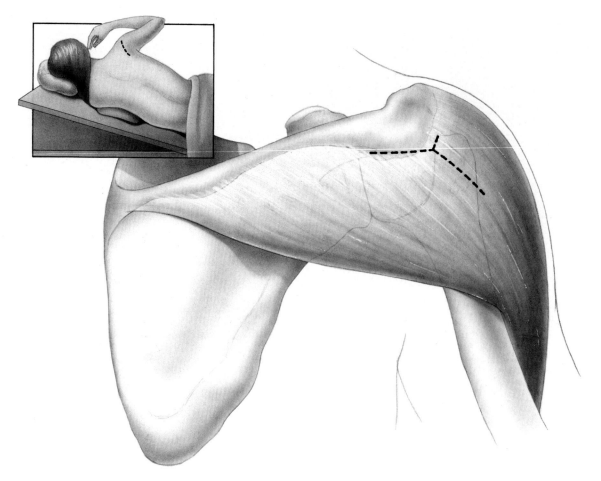

Figure 5.22. An oblique skin incision is used with the patient in the lateral decubitus position. The deltoid is taken down from the spine of the scapula for 3 to 4 cm and from the posterior lateral acromion for 1 to 2 cm, and a 4- to 5-cm split is made from the posterolateral corner of the acromion.

one is the teres minor. Second, there is a broad facet on the greater tuberosity for the infraspinatus tendon and a distinct smaller one, which is palpable, for the teres minor. After defining the infraspinatus, it is separated from the underlying capsule. This can be tedious but becomes easier with experience. It is often helpful to bluntly elevate it more medially where the muscle belly separates easily, and then add sharp dissection proceeding laterally where the tendon is fused to the capsule. Passing a Penrose drain around the muscle belly can aid in controlling the muscle. The tendon is then incised 1 cm medial to the greater tuberosity (Fig. 5.23). Occasionally, a flap to be used later to reinforce the capsule is created by incising the tendon obliquely, starting medial and superficial and proceeding laterally and deeply; however, this is not usually necessary.

The posterior capsule is then incised 1 cm medial to its humeral insertion, starting superiorly and proceeding inferiorly around the humeral neck. The degree of capsular takedown is determined in a manner similar to that previously described for anterior repairs, so that the more inferior capsule is mobilized when there is a large pouch and more than simple unidirectional posterior instability. The rare posterior labral detachment is repaired inside-out in a fashion similar to that described for anterior repairs. Posterior bone grafts are occasionally used in the (rare) case of glenoid hypoplasia or in revision cases in which the soft tissues posteriorly are deficient.

The horizontal limb of the "T" is then created so that the medial junction of the two flaps is at the middle of the glenoid. The superior flap is then mobilized as necessary from the overlying supraspinatus tendon and brought inferiorly and repaired to the lateral cuff of the capsule (Fig. 5.24). The inferior

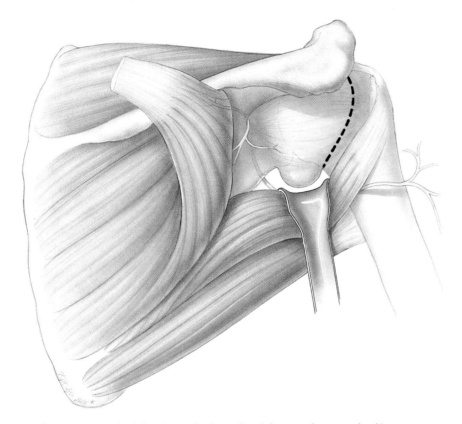

Figure 5.23.   The infraspinatus is elevated and the capsule exposed, taking care to avoid the axillary nerve inferiorly and the suprascapular nerve medially.

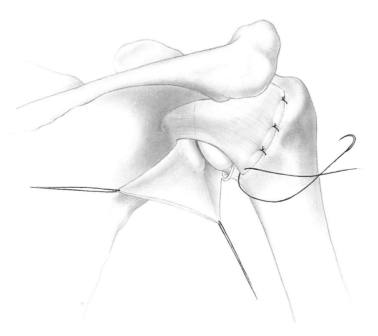

Figure 5.24.   The superior flap is brought inferiorly.

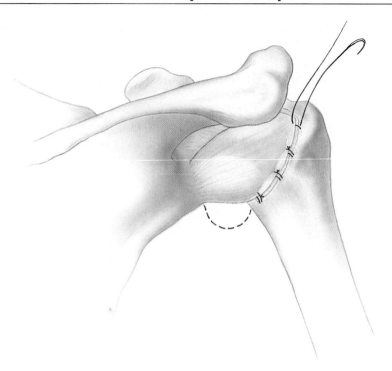

Figure 5.25. The inferior flap is brought up across the superior flap to obliterate the inferior pouch and thicken the posterior capsule.

flap is then shifted superiorly to obliterate the inferior pouch and to reinforce the posterior capsule (Fig. 5.25). The flaps are repaired with the arm in slight abduction and neutral rotation. The infraspinatus is then repaired. If a superficial reinforcement flap was created, it is sutured over the capsular repair before repairing the infraspinatus. The deltoid is then repaired anatomically, and a layered closure effected.

The patient is then immobilized in a custom plastic brace (measured preoperatively) for 6 weeks in slight abduction and neutral rotation. Mobilization after this is individualized, being quicker in unidirectional posterior instability after trauma and very gradual in multidirectional cases with generalized laxity (delaying internal rotation and horizontal adduction especially).

Results

The results of instability repairs have been gratifying. Pollock et al. (179) reported 90% successful results in 151 shoulders having had an anterior inferior capsular shift procedure, with a recurrence rate (instability) of 5%. In another series of 63 athletes having a similar procedure for anterior and inferior instability (24), 94% of patients had satisfactory results. Fifty-eight of 63 patients (92%) returned to their major sports; 47 patients (75%) returned at the same competitive level.

Bigliani et al. (25) reported results with posterior repair in a series of 36 shoulders with an average follow-up of 5 years. The posterior inferior capsular shift was found to yield overall satisfactory results in 80%. Recurrent instability was noted in 11% of cases. Five of six failures were reoperations, so that 96% of the primary repairs achieved satisfactory results. Results with the inferior capsular shift for classic multidirectional instability have also been recently reported (26). Fifty-two repairs were performed (36 from an anterior approach and 16 from posterior). All were completely immobilized in a brace for 6 weeks postoperatively. Forty-nine shoulders were followed for 2 to 11 years (average, 5 years). Satisfactory results were achieved in 94% of cases.

Conclusions

The inferior capsular shift allows precise correction of pathology with a high percentage of successful results. Future directions include better definition of optimum arm positioning for tensioning, greater understanding of the role of discreet repairs (e.g., tension of the rotator interval alone), and improved arthroscopic techniques.

REFERENCES

1. Aamoth GM, O'Phelan EH. Recurrent anterior dislocation of the shoulder: a review of 40 athletes treated by a subscapularis transfer (modified Magnuson-Stack procedure). Am J Sports Med 1977;5:188–190.
2. Adams FL. The genuine works of Hippocrates, volumes 1 and 2. William Wood: New York, 1891.
3. Adams JC. Recurrent dislocation of the shoulder. J Bone Joint Surg 1948;30B: 26–38.
4. Ahlgren O, Lorentzon R, Larsson SE. Posterior dislocation of the shoulder associated with general seizures (abstract). Acta Orthop Scand 1981;52:694–695.
5. Altchek DW, Skyhar MJ, Warren RF. Shoulder arthroscopy for shoulder instability. American Academy of Orthopaedic Surgeons Instructional Course Lectures 1989;38:187–198.
6. Altchek DW, Warren RF, Skyhar MJ, et al. T-Plasty modification of the Bankart procedure for multidirectional instability of the anterior and inferior types. J Bone Joint Surg 1991;73A:105–112.
7. Altchek DW, Warren RF, Wickiewicz TL, et al. Arthroscopic labral debridement: a three-year follow-up. Am J Sports Med 1992;20:702–706.
8. Arciero RA, Wheeler JH III, Ryan JB, et al. Arthroscopic Bankart repair versus nonoperative treatment for acute, initial anterior shoulder dislocations. Am J Sports Med 1994;22:589–594.
9. Aronen JG, Regan K. Decreasing the incidence of recurrence of first time anterior shoulder dislocations with rehabilitation. Am J Sports Med 1984;12:283–291.
10. Aston JW Jr, Gregory CF. Dislocation of the shoulder with significant fracture of the glenoid. J Bone Joint Surg 1973;55A:1531–1533.
11. Bach BR Jr. Arthroscopic removal of painful Bristow hardware. Arthroscopy 1990;6:324–326.
12. Bach BR, Warren RF, Fronek J. Disruption of the lateral capsule of the shoulder: a cause of recurrent dislocation. J Bone Joint Surg 1988;70B:274–276.
13. Baker CL, Uribe JW, Whitman C. Arthroscopic evaluation of acute initial anterior shoulder dislocations. Am J Sports Med 1990;18:25–28.
14. Bankart ASB. The pathology and treatment of recurrent dislocation of the shoulder joint. Br J Surg 1939;26:23–29.
15. Barry TP, Lombardo SJ, Kerlan RK, et al. The coracoid transfer for recurrent anterior instability of the shoulder in adolescents. J Bone Joint Surg 1985;67A: 383–387.

16. Bassey L. Alte und vernachlassigte schulterluxationen als indikation fur die Bankart'sche operation. Unfallchir 1988;91:85–90.
17. Beall MS Jr, Diefenbach G, Allen A. Electromyographic biofeedback in the treatment of voluntary posterior instability of the shoulder. Am J Sports Med 1987;15: 175–178.
18. Benedetto KP, Glotzer W. Arthroscopic Bankart procedure by suture technique: indications, technique, and results. Arthroscopy 1992;8:111–115.
19. Bennett GE. Old dislocations of the shoulder. J Bone Joint Surg 1936;18:594–606.
20. Berg EE, Ellison AE. The inside-out Bankart procedure. Am J Sports Med 1990;18: 129–133.
21. Bigliani LU. Anterior and posterior capsular shift for multidirectional instability. Tech Orthop 1989;3:36–45.
22. Bigliani LU, Endrizzi DP, McIlveen SJ, et al. Operative management of posterior shoulder instability. Orthop Trans 1989;13:232.
23. Bigliani LU, Flatow EL. History, physical examination, and diagnostic modalities. In: McGinty JB, Caspari RB, Jackson RW, et al., eds. Operative arthroscopy. New York: Raven, 1991:453–464.
24. Bigliani LU, Kurzweil PR, Schwartzbach CC, et al. Inferior capsular shift procedure for anterior inferior shoulder instability in athletes. Am J Sports Med 1994; 22:578–584.
25. Bigliani LU, Pollock RG, McIlveen SJ, et al. Shift of the posteroinferior aspect of the capsule for recurrent posterior glenohumeral instability. J Bone Joint Surg 1995;77A:1011–1020.
26. Bigliani LU, Pollock RG, Owens JM, et al. The inferior capsular shift procedure for multidirectional instability of the shoulder. Orthop Trans 1993;17:576.
27. Bigliani LU, Pollock RG, Soslowsky LJ, et al. The tensile properties of the inferior glenohumeral ligament. J Orthop Res 1992;10:187–197.
28. Bigliani LU, Rodosky MW, Newton PD, et al. Arthroscopic coracoacromial ligament resection for impingement in the overhead athlete. J Shoulder Elbow Surg 1994;4(Suppl):54.
29. Blazina ME, Satzman JS. Recurrent anterior subluxation of the shoulder in athletics: a distinct entity. J Bone Joint Surg 1969;51A:1037–1038.
30. Blom S, Dahlback LO. Nerve injuries in dislocations of the shoulder joint and fractures of the neck of the humerus. Acta Chir Scand 1970;136:461–466.
31. Bloom MH, Obata WG. Diagnosis of posterior dislocation of the shoulder with use of Velpeau axillary and angle-up roentgenographic views. J Bone Joint Surg 1967;49A:943–949.
32. Bost FC, Inman VT. The pathological changes in recurrent dislocation of the shoulder. J Bone Joint Surg 1942;24A:595–613.
33. Braly WG, Tullos HS. A modification of the Bristow procedure for recurrent anterior shoulder dislocation and subluxation. Am J Sports Med 1985;13:81–86.
34. Breasted JH. The Edwin Smith surgical papyrus. University of Chicago Press, 1930. Reprinted by The Classics of Surgery Library, Gryphon Editions Ltd., Birmingham, AL, 1984:354–357.
35. Bridle SH, Ferris BD. Irreducible acute anterior dislocation of the shoulder: interposed subscapularis. J Bone Joint Surg 1990;72B:1078–1079.
36. Brown JT. Nerve injuries complicating dislocation of the shoulder (abstract). J Bone Joint Surg 1952;34B:526.
37. Burkhead WZ Jr, Rockwood CA Jr. Treatment of instability of the shoulder with an exercise program. J Bone Joint Surg 1992;74A:890–896.
38. Calandra JJ, Baker CL, Uribe J. The incidence of Hill-Sachs lesions in initial anterior shoulder dislocations. Arthroscopy 1989;5:254.
39. Callaghan JJ, McNiesh LM, DeHaven JP, et al. A prospective comparison study of double contrast computed tomography (CT) arthrography and arthroscopy of the shoulder. Am J Sports Med 1988;16:13–20.
40. Caspari RB, Meyers JF, Savoie FH, et al. Arthroscopic management of shoulder instability. In: Post M, Morrey BF, Hawkins RJ, eds. Surgery of the shoulder. St. Louis: Mosby Year Book, 1989:117–120.

41. Cautilli RA, Joyce MF, Mackell JV Jr. Posterior dislocations of the shoulder: a method of post reduction management. Am J Sports Med 1978;6:397–399.
42. Cave EM, ed. Fractures and other injuries. Chicago: Year Book Medical Publishers, 1961.
43. Cerulli G, Caraffa A, Buompadre V, et al. Arthroscopic findings in acute shoulder dislocations. Presented at the 4th Congress of the European Society for Surgery of the Shoulder and the Elbow. Milan, Italy, October, 1990.
44. Chen W. Modified Bristow-Helfet procedure in treatment of chronic unreduced anterior dislocation of the shoulder joint. In: Post M, Morrey BF, Hawkins RJ, eds. Surgery of the shoulder. St. Louis: Mosby Year Book, 1990:73–76.
45. Christophe K. A functioning false shoulder joint following an old dislocation. J Bone Joint Surg 1939;21:916–917.
46. Collins HR, Wilde AH. Shoulder instability in athletics. Orthop Clin North Am 1973;4:759–774.
47. Cooper A. Treatise on dislocations and fractures of the joints. 2nd American ed. Boston: Lilly & Wait and Carter & Hendee, 1832.
48. Cooper DE, Arnoczky SP, O'Brien SJ, et al. Anatomy, histology and vascularity of the glenoid labrum: an anatomic study. Presented at The American Shoulder and Elbow Surgeons, Seventh Open Meeting, Anaheim, California, March 1991.
49. Cooper RA, Brems JJ. The inferior capsular-shift procedure for multidirectional instability of the shoulder. J Bone Joint Surg 1992;74A:1516–1521.
50. Cordasco FA, Steinmann S, Flatow EL, et al. Arthroscopic treatment of glenoid labral tears. Am J Sports Med 1993;21:425–430.
51. Corner NB, Milner SM, MacDonald R, et al. Isolated musculocutaneous nerve lesion after shoulder dislocation. J R Army Med Corps 1990;136:107–108.
52. Costigan PS, Binns MS, Wallace WA. Undiagnosed bilateral anterior dislocation of the shoulder. Injury 1990;21:409.
53. Coughlin L, Rubinovich M, Johansson J, et al. Arthroscopic staple capsulorrhaphy for anterior shoulder instability. Am J Sports Med 1992;20:253–256.
54. Craig EV. The posterior mechanism of acute anterior shoulder dislocations. Clin Orthop 1984;190:212–216.
55. Cubbins WR, Callahan JJ, Scuderi CS. The reduction of old or irreducible dislocations of the shoulder joint. Surg Gynecol Obstet 1934;58:129–135.
56. Curr JF. Rupture of the axillary artery complicating dislocation of the shoulder: report of a case. J Bone Joint Surg 1970;52B:313–317.
57. Danzig LA, Greenway G, Resnick D. The Hill-Sachs lesion: an experimental study. Am J Sports Med 1980;8:328–332.
58. Davids JR, Talbott RD. Luxatio erecta humeri: a case report. Clin Orthop 1990;252:144–149.
59. Delbet P. Des luxations anciennes et irreductibles delepaule. Arch Gen Med 1893;31:19–39.
60. Deliz E, Flatow EL. Chronic unreduced shoulder dislocations. In: Bigliani LU, ed. Complications of shoulder surgery. Baltimore: Williams & Wilkins, 1993:127–138.
61. DePalma AF. Factors influencing the choice of a modified Magnuson procedure for recurrent anterior dislocation of the shoulder with a note on technique. Surg Clin North Am 1963;43:1647–1649.
62. DePalma AF. Surgery of the shoulder. 3rd ed. Philadelphia: JB Lippincott, 1983.
63. Dickson JW, Devas MB. Bankart's operation for recurrent dislocation of the shoulder. J Bone Joint Surg 1957;39B:114–119.
64. Endo H, Takigawa T, Takata K, et al. A method of diagnosis and treatment for loose shoulder (in Japanese). Cent Jpn J Orthop Surg Trauma 1971;14:630–632.
65. Epps CH. Complications in orthopaedic surgery. 1st ed. Philadelphia: JB Lippincott, 1978:198–203.
66. Ferlic DC, DiGiovine NM. A long-term retrospective study of the modified Bristow procedure. Am J Sports Med 1988;16:469–474.
67. Finckh J. Ueber die reponibilitat der veralteten schultergelenks-luxationen. Beitr Z Klin Chir 1897;17:751–774.

68. Fipp GJ. Simultaneous posterior dislocation of both shoulders: report of a case. Clin Orthop 1966;44:191–195.
69. Flatow EL. Multidirectional instability. In: Kohn D, Wirth CJ, eds: Die schulter: aktuelle operative therapie. Stuttgart: Thieme, 1992:180–187.
70. Flatow EL, Cuomo FC, Miller SR, et al. Open reduction and internal fixation of 2-part displaced greater tuberosity fractures of the proximal humerus. J Bone Joint Surg 1991;73:1213–1218.
71. Flatow EL, Miller SR, Neer CS II. Chronic anterior dislocation of the shoulder. J Shoulder Elbow Surg 1993;2:2–10.
72. Flower WH. On the pathological changes produced in the shoulder-joint by traumatic dislocation, as derived from an examination of all the specimens illustrating this injury in the museums of London. Trans Pathol Soc Lond 1861;12:179–200.
73. Freeland AE, Higgins RW. Anterior shoulder dislocations with posterior displacement of the long head of the biceps tendon: arthrographic findings. Orthopedics 1985;8:468–469.
74. Friedman RJ, Bonutti PM, Genez B, et al. Cine magnetic resonance imaging of the glenohumeral joint. Orthop Trans 1993;17:1018–1019.
75. Fronek J, Warren RF, Bowen M. Posterior subluxation of the glenohumeral joint. J Bone Joint Surg 1989;71A:205–216.
76. Ganel A, Horoszowski H, Heim M, et al. Persistent dislocation of the shoulder in elderly patients. J Am Geriatr Soc 1980;28:282–284.
77. Garth WP Jr, Allman FL, Armstrong WS. Occult anterior subluxations of the shoulder in noncontact sports. Am J Sports Med 1987;15:579–585.
78. Glasgow MT, Weinstein DM, Flatow EL, et al. Glenohumeral arthroplasty for arthritis after instability surgery. Presented at American Academy of Orthopaedic Surgeons, Sixtieth Annual Meeting, San Francisco, California, February 1993.
79. Grana WA, Buckley PD, Yates CK. Arthroscopic Bankart suture repair. Am J Sports Med 1993;21:348–353.
80. Gross RM. Arthroscopic shoulder capsulorrhaphy: Does it work? Am J Sports Med 1989;17:495–500.
81. Gross ML, Seeger LL, Smith JB, et al. Magnetic resonance imaging of the glenoid labrum. Am J Sports Med 1990;18:229–234.
82. Hall RH, Isaac F, Booth CR. Dislocations of the shoulder with special reference to accompanying small fractures. J Bone Joint Surg 1959;41A:489–494.
83. Harryman DT, Sidles JA, Harris SL, et al. Laxity of the normal glenohumeral joint: a quantitative in vivo assessment. J Shoulder Elbow Surg 1992;1:66–76.
84. Hastings DE, Coughlin LP. Recurrent subluxation of the glenohumeral joint. Am J Sports Med 1981;9:352–355.
85. Hawkins RB. Arthroscopic stapling repair for shoulder instability: a retrospective study of 50 cases. Arthroscopy 1989;5:122.
86. Hawkins RH, Hawkins RJ. Failed anterior reconstruction for shoulder instability. J Bone Joint Surg 1985;67B:709–714.
87. Hawkins RJ. Unrecognized dislocations of the shoulder. American Academy of Orthopaedic Surgeons Instructional Course Lectures 1985;34:258–263.
88. Hawkins RJ, Abrams JS, Schutte J. Multidirectional instability of the shoulder: an approach to diagnosis. Orthop Trans 1987;11:246.
89. Hawkins RJ, Angelo RL. Glenohumeral osteoarthrosis. J Bone Joint Surg 1990;72A:1193–1197.
90. Hawkins RJ, Bell RH, Hawkins RH, et al. Anterior dislocation of the shoulder in the older patient. Clin Orthop 1986;206:192–195.
91. Hawkins RJ, Bokor DJ. Clinical evaluation of shoulder problems. In: Rockwood CA, Matsen FA, eds. The shoulder. 1st ed. Philadelphia: WB Saunders, 1990:167–171.
92. Hawkins RJ, Koppert G, Johnston G. Recurrent posterior instability (subluxation) of the shoulder. J Bone Joint Surg 1984;66A:169–174.

93. Hejna WF, Fossier CH, Goldstein TB, et al. Ancient anterior dislocation of the shoulder. J Bone Joint Surg 1969;51A:1030–1031.

94. Helfet AJ. Coracoid transplantation for recurring dislocation of the shoulder. J Bone Joint Surg 1958;40B:198–202.

95. Hertz H. Die bedeutung des limbus glenoidalis fur die stabilitat des schulterge- lenks. Wien Klin Wochenschr 1984;152(Suppl):1–23.

96. Hill JA, Lombardo SJ, Kerlan RK, et al. The modified Bristow-Helfet procedure for recurrent anterior shoulder subluxations and dislocations. Am J Sports Med 1981;9:283–287.

97. Hill HA, Sachs MD. The grooved defect of the humeral head: a frequently un- recognized complication of dislocations of the shoulder joint. Radiology 1940; 35:690–700.

98. Hejna WE, Fossier CH, Goldstein TB, et al. Ancient anterior dislocations of the shoulder. J Bone Joint Surg 1969;54A:1030–1031.

99. Henry JH, Genung JA. Natural history of glenohumeral dislocation revisited. Am J Sports Med 1982;10:135–137.

100. Hovelius L. Anterior dislocation of the shoulder in teen-agers and young adults: five-year prognosis. J Bone Joint Surg 1987;69A:393–399.

101. Hovelius L, Akermark C, Albrektsson B, et al. Bristow-Latarjet procedure for recurrent anterior dislocation of the shoulder: a 2-5 year follow-up study on the results of 112 cases. Acta Orthop Scand 1983;54:284–290.

102. Hovelius L, Eriksson K, Fredin H, et al. Recurrences after initial dislocation of the shoulder. J Bone Joint Surg 1983;65:343–349.

103. Hurley JA, Anderson TE. Shoulder arthroscopy: its role in evaluating shoulder disorders in the athlete. Am J Sports Med 1990;18:480–483.

104. Inao S, Hirayama T, Takemitsu Y. Irreducible acute anterior dislocation of the shoulder: interposed bicipital tendon. J Bone Joint Surg 1990;72B:1079–1080.

105. Jardon OM, Hood LT, Lynch RD. Complete avulsion of the axillary artery as a complication of shoulder dislocation. J Bone Joint Surg 1973;55A:189–192.

106. Jerosch J, Castro WHM, Geske B. Damage of the long thoracic and dorsal scapu- lar nerve after traumatic shoulder dislocation: case report and review of the lit- erature. Acta Orthop Belg 1990;56:625–627.

107. Jobe C. Symposium on Anterior Shoulder Instability, Fourth Congress of the Eu- ropean Society for Surgery of the Shoulder and the Elbow, Milan, Italy, October 1990.

108. Jobe FW, Giangarra CE, Kvitne RS, et al. Anterior capsulolabral reconstruction of the shoulder in athletes in overhead sports. Am J Sports Med 1991;19:428–434.

109. Jobe FW, Glousman RE. Anterior capsulolabral reconstruction. Tech Orthop 1989;3:29–35.

110. Jobe FW, Tibone JE, Jobe CM, et al. The shoulder in sports. In: Rockwood CA Jr, Matsen FA III, eds: The shoulder. Philadelphia: WB Saunders, 1990:961–990.

111. Johnson LL. Symposium on shoulder arthroscopy. Arthroscopy Assoc North Am 1986.

112. Johnson LL. Arthroscopic stapling capsulorrhaphy. Presented at the Fourth In- ternational Conference on Surgery of the Shoulder, New York, New York, Octo- ber 1989.

113. Johnston GW, Lowry JH. Rupture of the axillary artery complicating anterior dis- location of the shoulder. J Bone Joint Surg 1962;44B:116–118.

114. Karadimas J, Rentis G, Varouchas G. Repair of recurrent anterior dislocation of the shoulder using transfer of the subscapularis tendon. J Bone Joint Surg 1980; 62A:1147–1149.

115. Kaveney MF, Wilson FD. Arthroscopic staple capsulorrhaphy for recurrent shoul- der instability. Orthop Trans 1988;12:728.

116. Kazar B, Relovszky E. Prognosis of primary dislocation of the shoulder. Acta Or- thop Scand 1969;40:216–224.

117. Kirker JR. Dislocation of the shoulder complicated by rupture of the axillary ves- sels: report of a case. J Bone Joint Surg 1952;34B:72–73.

118. Kirtland S, Resnick D, Sartoris DJ, et al. Chronic unreduced dislocations of the glenohumeral joint: imaging strategy and pathologic correlation. J Trauma 1988;28:1622–1631.
119. Kneisl JS, Sweeney HJ, Paige ML. Correlation of pathology observed in double contrast arthrotomography and arthroscopy of the shoulder. Arthroscopy 1988;4:21–24.
120. Kohn D. The clinical relevance of glenoid labrum lesions. Arthroscopy 1987;3:223–230.
121. Kronberg M, Brostrom L-A, Nemeth G. Differences in shoulder muscle activity between patients with generalized joint laxity and normal controls. Clin Orthop 1991;269:181–192.
122. Kummel BM. Fractures of the glenoid causing chronic dislocation of the shoulder. Clin Orthop 1970;69:189–191.
123. Latarjet M. A propos du traitement des luxations récidivantes l'épaule. Lyon Chir 1954;49:994–997.
124. Lebar RD, Alexander AH. Multidirectional shoulder instability: clinical results of inferior capsular shift in an active-duty population. Am J Sports Med 1992;20:193–198.
125. Lephart SM, Warner JJP, Borsa PA, et al. Proprioceptions of the shoulder in healthy unstable and surgically repaired shoulders. J Shoulder Elbow Surg 1994;3:371–380.
126. Leslie JT Jr, Ryan TJ. The anterior axillary incision to approach the shoulder joint. J Bone Joint Surg 1962;44A:1193–1196.
127. Lindholm TS, Elmstedt E. Bilateral posterior dislocation of the shoulder combined with fracture of the proximal humerus: a case report. Acta Orthop Scand 1980;51:485–488.
128. Lombardo SJ, Kerlan RK, Jobe FW, et al. The modified Bristow procedure for recurrent dislocation of the shoulder. J Bone Joint Surg 1976;58A:256–261.
129. Loomer R, Fraser J. A modified Bankart procedure for recurrent anterior/inferior shoulder instability. Am J Sports Med 1989;17:374–379.
130. MacDonald PB, Hawkins RJ, Fowler PJ, et al. Release of the subscapularis for internal rotation contracture and pain after anterior repair for recurrent anterior dislocations of the shoulder. J Bone Joint Surg 1992;74A:734–737.
131. Magnuson PB, Stack JK. Recurrent dislocation of the shoulder. J Am Med Assoc 1943;123:889–892.
132. Maki NJ. Arthroscopic stabilization for recurrent shoulder instability. In: Post M, Morrey BF, Hawkins RJ, eds. Surgery of the shoulder. St. Louis: Mosby Year Book, 1989:121–123.
133. Mallon WJ, Bassett FH, Goldman RD. Luxatio erecta: the inferior glenohumeral dislocation. J Orthop Trauma 1990;4:19–24.
134. Marans HJ, Angel KR, Schemitsch EH, et al. The fate of traumatic anterior dislocation of the shoulder in children. J Bone Joint Surg 1992;74A:1242–1244.
135. Matsen FA III, Thomas SC, Rockwood CA Jr. Anterior glenohumeral instability. In: Rockwood CA Jr, Matsen FA III, eds. The shoulder. Philadelphia: WB Saunders, 1990.
136. Matthews LS, Vetter WL, Oweida SJ, et al. Arthroscopic staple capsulorrhaphy for recurrent anterior shoulder instability. Arthroscopy 1988;4:106–111.
137. May VR. A modified Bristow operation for anterior recurrent dislocation of the shoulder. J Bone Joint Surg 1970;52A:1010–1016.
138. McGlynn FJ, Caspari RB. Arthroscopic findings in the subluxating shoulder. Clin Orthop 1984;183:173–178.
139. McLaughlin HL. Dislocation of the shoulder with tuberosity fracture. Surg Clin North Am 1963;43:1615–1620.
140. McLaughlin HL, Cavallaro WU. Primary anterior dislocation of the shoulder. Am J Surg 1950;80:615–621.
141. McLaughlin HL, MacLellan DI. Recurrent anterior dislocation of the shoulder. J Trauma 1967;7:191–201.

142. McMaster WC. Anterior glenoid labrum damage: a painful lesion in swimmers. Am J Sports Med 1986;14:383–387.

143. Merle D'Aubigne R. Nerve injuries in fractures and dislocations of the shoulder. Surg Clin North Am 1963;43:1685–1689.

144. Mendoza F, Nicholas JA, Reilly JP. Anatomic patterns of anterior glenoid labrum tears. Orthop Trans 1987;11:264.

145. Miller LS, Donahue JR, Good RP, et al. The Magnuson-Stack procedure for treatment of recurrent glenohumeral dislocation. Am J Sports Med 1984;12:133–137.

146. Mitzuno K, Itakura Y, Muratso H. Inferior capsular shift for inferior and multidirectional instability of the shoulder in young children: report of two cases. J Shoulder Elbow Surg 1992;1:200–206.

147. Mok DWH, Fogg AJB, Hokan R, et al. The diagnostic value of arthroscopy in glenohumeral instability. J Bone Joint Surg 1990;72B:698–700.

148. Morgan CD. Arthroscopic Bankhart suture repair: 2–5 year results. Orthop Trans 1989;13:231.

149. Morgan CD. Arthroscopic transglenoid Bankart suture repair. Operative Tech Orthop 1991;1:171–179.

150. Morgan CD, Bodenstab AB. Arthroscopic Bankart suture repair: technique and early results. Arthroscopy 1987;3:111–122.

151. Mosley JB, Jobe FW, Perry J, et al. EMG analysis of the scapular rotator muscles during a baseball rehabilitation program. Orthop Trans 1990;14:252.

152. Moseley HF, Overgaard B. The anterior capsular mechanism in recurrent anterior dislocation of the shoulder. J Bone Joint Surg 1962;44B:913–927.

153. Mustonen PK, Kouri KJ, Oksala IE. Axillary artery rupture complicating anterior dislocation of the shoulder. Acta Chir Scand 1990;156:643–645.

154. Neer CS II. Involuntary inferior and multidirectional instability of the shoulder: etiology, recognition, and treatment. American Academy of Orthopaedic Surgeons Instructional Course Lectures 1985;34:232–238.

155. Neer CS II. Shoulder reconstruction. Philadelphia: WB Saunders, 1990:273–341.

156. Neer CS II, Fithian TF, Hansen PE, et al. Reinforced cruciate repair for anterior dislocations of the shoulder. Orthop Trans 1985;9:44.

157. Neer CS II, Foster CR. Inferior capsular shift for involuntary inferior and multidirectional instability of the shoulder. J Bone Joint Surg 1980;62A:897–908.

158. Neer CS II, Perez-Sanz JR, Ogawa K. Causes of failure in repairs for recurrent anterior dislocations. Presented at New York Orthopaedic Hospital Alumni Annual Meeting, 1983. As cited in Neer CS II. Shoulder reconstruction. Philadelphia: WB Saunders, 1990:279.

159. Neer CS II, Welsh RP. The shoulder in sports. Orthop Clin North Am 1977;8: 583–591.

160. Neviaser JS. An operation for old dislocation of the shoulder. J Bone Joint Surg 1948;30A:997–1000.

161. Neviaser JS. The treatment of old unreduced dislocations of the shoulder. Surg Clin North Am 1963;43:1671–1678.

162. Nevaiser RJ, Nevaiser TJ, Nevaiser JS. Concurrent rupture of the rotator cuff and anterior dislocation of the shoulder in the older patient. J Bone Joint Surg 1988; 70A:1308–1311.

163. Noack W, Strohmeier M. Die behandlung der veralteten vorderen schulterluxation. Unfallchir 1988;14:184–190.

164. Norris TR, Bigliani LU. Analysis of failed repair for shoulder instability: a preliminary report. In: Bateman JE, Welsh RP, eds. Surgery of the shoulder. Decker: Philadelphia, 1984:111–116.

165. Nottage WM, Duge WD, Fields WA. Computed arthro-tomography of the glenohumeral joint to evaluate anterior instability: correlation with arthroscopic findings. Arthroscopy 1987;3:273–276.

166. O'Brien SJ, Neves MC, Arnockzky SP, et al. The anatomy and histology of the inferior glenohumeral ligament complex of the shoulder. Am J Sports Med 1990; 18:449–456.

167. O'Driscoll SW, Evans DC. Long-term results of staple capsulorrhaphy for anterior instability of the shoulder. J Bone Joint Surg 1993;75A:249–258.
168. Ogilvie-Harris DJ, Wiley AM. Arthroscopic surgery of the shoulder. J Bone Joint Surg 1986;68B:201–207.
169. Oppenheim WL, Dawson EG, Quinlan C, et al. The cephaloscapular projection: a special diagnostic aid. Clin Orthop 1985;195:191–193.
170. Osmond-Clarke H. Habitual dislocation of the shoulder: the Putti-Platt operation. J Bone Joint Surg 1948;30B:19–25.
171. Palmer I, Widen A. The bone block method for recurrent dislocation of the shoulder joint. J Bone Joint Surg 1948;30B:53–58.
172. Pappas AM, Goss TP, Kleinman PK. Symptomatic shoulder instability due to lesions of the glenoid labrum. Am J Sports Med 1983;11:279–288.
173. Pasila M, Kiviluoto O, Jaroma H, et al. Recovery from primary shoulder dislocation and its complications. Acta Orthop Scand 1980;51:257–262.
174. Paulos LE, Grauer JD, Smutz WP. Traumatic lesions of the biceps tendon, rotator cuff interval and superior labrum. Arthroscopy 1990;6:159.
175. Pavlov H, Warren RF, Weiss CB Jr, et al. The roentgenographic evaluation of anterior shoulder instability. Clin Orthop 1985;194:153–158.
176. Pemiceni T, Augereau B, Apoil A. Traitement des luxations antero-internes anciennes de l'epaule par reduction sanglante et butee armee costale: a propos de trois cas. Ann Chir 1982;36:235–239.
177. Perthes G. Uber operationen bei habitueller schulterluxation. Deutsche Zeitschr F Chir 1906;85:199–227.
178. Pollock RG, Bigliani LU. Recurrent posterior shoulder instability. Clin Orthop 1993;291:85–96.
179. Pollock RG, Owens JM, Nicholson GP, et al. Anterior inferior capsular shift procedure for anterior glenohumeral instability: long term results. Orthop Trans 1993;17:974
180. Post M. The shoulder: Surgical and non-surgical management. Philadelphia: Lea & Febiger, 1978:429–456.
181. Postacchini F, Facchini M. The treatment of unreduced dislocation of the shoulder: a review of twelve cases. Ital J Orthop Traumatol 1987;13:15–26.
182. Pritchett JW, Clark JM. Prosthetic replacement for chronic unreduced dislocations of the shoulder. Clin Orthop 1987;216:89–93.
183. Protzman RR. Anterior instability of the shoulder. J Bone Joint Surg 1980;62A:909–918.
184. Rafii M, Minkoff J, Bonamo J, et al. Computed tomography (CT) arthrography of shoulder instabilities in athletes. Am J Sports Med 1988;16:352–361.
185. Richardson JB, Ramsey A, Davidson JK, et al. Radiographs in shoulder trauma. J Bone Joint Surg 1988;7OB:457–460.
186. Richmond JC, Donaldson WR, Fu F, et al. Modification of the Bankart reconstruction with a suture anchor: report of a new technique. Am J Sports Med 1991;19:343–346.
187. Rockwood CA Jr. Subluxation of the shoulder: the classification, diagnosis and treatment. Orthop Trans 1979;4:306.
188. Rockwood CA Jr. Dislocations about the shoulder. In: Rockwood CA Jr, Green DP, eds. Fractures. 2nd ed. Philadelphia: JB Lippincott, 1984;1:722–985.
189. Rockwood CA, Gerber C. Analysis of failed surgical procedures for anterior shoulder instability. Orthop Trans 1985;9:48.
190. Rockwood CA Jr, Thomas SC, Matsen FA III. Subluxations and dislocations about the glenohumeral joint. In: Rockwood CA Jr, Green DP, eds. Fractures in adults. Philadelphia: JB Lippincott, 1991.
191. Rodosky MW, Harner CD, Fu FH, et al. The role of the long head of the biceps muscle and the superior glenoid labrum in anterior stability of the shoulder. Am J Sports Med 1994;22:121–130.
192. Rokous JR, Feagin JA, Abbott HG. Modified axillary roentgenogram: a useful adjunct in the diagnosis of recurrent instability of the shoulder. Clin Orthop 1972;82:84–86.

193. Rowe CR. Prognosis in dislocations of the shoulder. J Bone Joint Surg 1956;38A: 957–977.
194. Rowe CR. Chronic unreduced dislocations. In: Rowe CR, ed. The shoulder. New York: Churchill Livingstone, 1988:244–254.
195. Rowe CR, Patel D, Southmayd WW. The Bankart procedure: a long-term end-result study. J Bone Joint Surg 1978;60A:1–16.
196. Rowe CR, Pierce DS, Clark JG. Voluntary dislocation of the shoulder: a preliminary report on a clinical, electromyographic, and psychiatric study of twenty-six patients. J Bone Joint Surg 1973;55A:445–460.
197. Rowe CR, Sakellarides HT. Factors related to recurrences of anterior dislocations of the shoulder. Clin Orthop 1961;20:40–47.
198. Rowe CR, Zarins B. Recurrent transient subluxation of the shoulder. J Bone Joint Surg 1981;63A:863–872.
199. Rowe CR, Zarins B. Chronic unreduced dislocations of the shoulder. J Bone Joint Surg 1982;64A:494–505.
200. Rowe CR, Zarins B, Ciullo JV. Recurrent anterior dislocation of the shoulder after surgical repair: apparent causes of failure and treatment. J Bone Joint Surg 1984; 66A:159–168.
201. Rubenstein DL, Jobe FW, Glousman RE, et al. Anterior capsulolabral reconstruction of the shoulder in athletes. J Shoulder Elbow Surg 1992;1:229–237.
202. Samilson RL, Prieto V. Dislocation arthropathy of the shoulder. J Bone Joint Surg 1983;65A:456–460.
203. Schlaepfer K. Uncomplicated dislocations of the shoulder: their rational treatment and late results. Am J Med Sci 1924;167:244–255.
204. Schulz TJ, Jacobs B, Patterson RL. Unrecognized dislocations of the shoulder. J Trauma 1969;9:1009–1023.
205. Schwartz RE, O'Brien SJ, Warren RF, et al. Capsular restraints to anterior-posterior motion of the shoulder. Orthop Trans 1988;12:727.
206. Scougall S. Posterior dislocation of the shoulder. J Bone Joint Surg 1957;39B: 726–732.
207. Seradge H, Orme G. Acute irreducible anterior dislocation of the shoulder. J Trauma 1982;22:330–332.
208. Shea K, O'Keefe R, Fulkerson JP. Initial failure strength of arthroscopic Bankhart suture and staple repairs. Arthroscopy 1990;6:158.
209. Simonet NW, Cofield RH. Prognosis in anterior shoulder dislocation. Am J Sports Med 1984;12:19–24.
210. Snyder SJ, Karzel RP, Del Pizzo W, et al. S.L.A.P. lesions of the shoulder. Arthroscopy 1990;6:274–279.
211. Souchon E. Operative treatment of irreducible dislocations of the shoulder joint, recent or old, simple or complicated. Trans Am Surg Assoc 1897;15:311–451.
212. Speer KP, Deng X, Borrero S, et al. Biomechanical evaluation of the Bankart lesion. J Bone Joint Surg 1994;76A:1819–1826.
213. Speer KP, Hannafin JA, Altchek DW, et al. An evaluation of the shoulder relocation test. Am J Sports Med 1994;22:177–183.
214. Steinman S, Bigliani LU, McIlveen SJ. Glenoid fractures associated with recurrent anterior dislocations of the shoulder. Presented at the American Academy of Orthopaedic Surgeons, Fifty-Seventh Annual Meeting, February, 1990.
215. Steinmann SR, Flatow EL, Pollock RG, et al. Evaluation and surgical treatment of failed shoulder instability repairs. Orthop Trans 1992;16:727.
216. Symeonides PP. The significance of the subscapularis muscle in the pathogenesis of recurrent anterior dislocation of the shoulder. J Bone Joint Surg 1972;54B:476–483.
217. Symeonides PP. Reconsideration of the Putti-Platt procedure and its mode of action in recurrent traumatic anterior dislocation of the shoulder. Clin Orthop 1989;246:8–15.
218. Thomas SC, Matsen FA III. An approach to the repair of avulsion of the glenohumeral ligaments in the management of traumatic anterior glenohumeral instability. J Bone Joint Surg 1989;71A:506–512.

219. Thompson FR, Moga JJ, Fielding JW. Unusual habitual shoulder dislocations combined operative repair. Audio-visual Presentation at the Annual Meeting of the American Academy of Orthopaedic Surgeons, New York, New York, 1965.
220. Thorndike A. Athletic injuries. Philadelphia: Lea & Febiger, 1956:152.
221. Torg JS, Balduini FC, Bonci C, et al. A modified Bristow-Helfet-May procedure for recurrent dislocation and subluxation of the shoulder. J Bone Joint Surg 1987; 69A:904–913.
222. Townley CO. The capsular mechanism in recurrent dislocations of the shoulder. J Bone Joint Surg 1950;32A:370–380.
223. Travlos J, Goldberg I, Boome RS. Brachial plexus lesions associated with dislocated shoulders. J Bone Joint Surg 1990;72B:68–71.
224. Tsutsui H, Yamamoto R, Kuroki Y, et al. Biochemical study on collagen from the loose shoulder joint capsules. In: Post M, Morrey BF, Hawkins RJ, eds. Surgery of the Shoulder. St. Louis: Mosby, 1990.
225. Turkel SJ, Panio MW, Marshall JL, et al. Stabilizing mechanisms preventing anterior dislocation of the glenohumeral joint. J Bone Joint Surg 1981;63A: 1208–1217.
226. Volpin G, Langer R, Stein H. Complete infraclavicular brachial plexus palsy with occlusion of axillary vessels following anterior dislocation of the shoulder joint. J Orthop Trauma 1990;4:121–123.
227. Ward WG, Bassett FH III, Garrett WE Jr. Anterior staple capsulorrhaphy for recurrent dislocation of the shoulder: a clinical and biomechanical study. South Med J 1990;83:510–518.
228. Warner JP, Deng XH, Warren RF, et al. Static capsuloligamentous restraints to superior-inferior translation of the glenohumeral joint. Am J Sports Med 1992; 20:675–685.
229. Warner JP, Pagnani M, Warren RF, et al. Arthroscopic Bankhart repair utilizing an absorbable cannulated fixation device. Presented at the American Academy of Orthopaedic Surgeons, Fifty-Eighth Annual Meeting, Anaheim, California, March 1991.
230. Warren JC. History of a case of ligature of the left subclavian artery between the scaleni muscles, attended with some peculiar circumstances. Am J Med Sci 1846; 11:539–541.
231. Weber SC, Caspari RB. A biomechanical evaluation of the restraint to posterior shoulder dislocation. Arthroscopy 1989;5:115.
232. Welsh RP, Trimmings N. Multidirectional instability of the shoulder. Orthop Trans 1987;11:231.
233. Wheeler JH, Ryan JB, Arciero RA, et al. Arthroscopic versus nonoperative treatment of acute shoulder dislocations in young athletes. Arthroscopy 1989;5: 213–217.
234. Wiley AM. Arthroscopy for shoulder instability and a technique for arthroscopic repair. Arthroscopy 1988;4:25–30.
235. Wredmark T, Tornkvist H, Johansson C, et al. Long-term functional results of the modified Bristow procedure for recurrent dislocations of the shoulder. Am J Sports Med 1992;20:157–161.
236. Yoneda B, Welsh RP, MacIntosh DL. Conservative treatment of shoulder dislocation in young males (abstract). J Bone Joint Surg 1982;64B:254–255.
237. Young DC, Rockwood CA Jr. Complications of a failed Bristow procedure and their management. J Bone Joint Surg 1991;73A:969–981.
238. Zarins B. Bankart repair for anterior shoulder instability. Tech Orthop 1989;3: 23–28.
239. Zuckerman JD, Matsen FA III. Complications about the glenohumeral joint related to the use of screws and staples. J Bone Joint Surg 1984;66A:175–180.

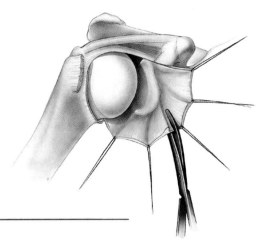

CHAPTER

6

Orthopaedic Management of
Neuromuscular Disorders

M E L V I N   P O S T

Introduction

A variety of neuromuscular disorders affecting the shoulder girdle and causing severe and often painful disability are amenable to surgical treatment
(42, 43, 52, 59). The surgeon must accurately assess functional neuromuscular deficits and choose the best methods for restoring function around the
shoulder girdle after an irreparable muscle loss. A decision must be made
whether to perform an arthrodesis, for example, which has a greater chance
for success and produces strength and power but diminished motion and
placement of the hand, or a muscle transfer, which can produce a greater
range of shoulder motion. Moreover, release of an entrapped nerve, especially before severe muscle atrophy ensues, may dramatically relieve a
chronic disability. This chapter reviews the principles, indications, and operative techniques for the restoration of shoulder function in treating some of
the more common neurologic lesions that affect the shoulder.

The surgeon must rely on a thorough history and physical examination,
including complete clinical neurologic evaluation as well as imaging studies
and electromyography (EMG), to achieve an accurate diagnosis. Simply put,
each symptom should be fully explored and an effort made to unify them
into one disease process, or more than one, if it exists. Patient age, patient occupation, side of dominance, and specific job requirements as well as educa-
tional level are important aspects in diagnosis and treatment. Even with a
well-documented diagnosis and excellent treatment, the patient often requires vocational retraining.

Evaluation of Shoulder Girdle Function

Each patient must have 1) a thorough history and physical examination including a peripheral nerve evaluation, 2) strength testing of the muscles of
the upper extremity and the back as they affect the shoulder girdle, and 3)
motion testing of all three joint of the shoulder girdle (glenohumeral, acromioclavicular, and sternoclavicular) and the scapulothoracic articulation
as well as active motion testing of the distal joints (41). A comparison of the

201

involved and uninvolved sides should be made. The surgeon must know if a muscle is partially or completely paralyzed, the time of onset of paralysis, and to what degree spontaneous recovery is still possible, taking into account the muscle atrophy and nerve regeneration if the nerve is damaged (43). For example, is the loss of abduction caused merely by paralysis of the anterior and middle deltoid, of the serratus anterior, or by a combination of both? The clinical examination should attempt to pinpoint the precise level of nerve involvement. The surgeon must know if the loss of muscle groups was so great that there is no possibility of restoring active overhead motion by muscle transfer. Muscle paralysis often enhances the possibility of subluxation of the humeral head from the glenoid. This must be effectively controlled if a disability is to be relieved. Increased paralysis of shoulder muscles places a greater burden on the scapulothoracic muscles, so the surgeon should recognize how a contemplated substitution of one muscle may affect the integrated action of the other muscle groups. The end result should be predictable, to a reasonable degree, before an operation is performed.

In general, the examination starts with an inspection of the thorax, the spine, and the shoulder girdle. The general appearance of the skin, general nourishment, posture, and attitude of the extremity should be noted. The size and shape of scars and stretch marks, for example, along with any skin discoloration or other evidence of skin injury should be recorded. Changes in the contour of the shoulder girdle and muscle development or atrophy of the surrounding tissues should be recorded. For example, atrophy of the muscles around the shoulder in a boy may suggest muscle disease such as muscular dystrophy.

The surgeon should note whether there is normal rounding of the shoulders or abnormal depressions in the skin or in the areas above and below the clavicle. Results of an examination for swelling or a depression around the acromioclavicular or sternoclavicular joints should be recorded, especially when there has been a history of trauma. Obesity may obscure the underlying anatomy. If symmetry is lost, it should be determined if it is due to atrophy, a disruption of the anatomy of the underlying parts, or a combination of both. For example, is there a chronic dislocation leading to a loss of the normal contour, rather than deltoid atrophy? The shoulder girdle should be viewed from behind as well as from the front and sides. The position of the scapulae and the presence or absence of a kyphosis or scoliosis can be observed. The presence of scoliosis may give the false impression of winging of the scapulae. Normally, the scapulae rest in a position between the second and seventh ribs, with the scapula-vertebral borders located 5 cm from the spinous processes. Any deviation from this normal position is considered abnormal. Finally, a comparison of findings for both sides of the body is important when recording the general body contour.

Palpation of the muscles may disclose tenderness. This part of the examination should be gentle. The muscles should be palpated bilaterally, and tone, consistency, size, and shape should be determined. The patient should be asked to contract specific muscles. Defects or abnormal masses may be felt either by inspection or palpation alone or in combination. Muscle atony secondary to acute denervation recognized by flabbiness and a rubbery or woody sensation on palpation suggests muscular dystrophy or polymyositis. Tenderness to palpation can provide useful information in making a diagnosis. For example, tenderness elicited by deep palpation of the suprascapular notch may suggest entrapment of the suprascapular nerve when the history points to this condition.

During testing of the various articulations of the shoulder girdle, the palpation of any subluxations and any grating and grinding sensations should be noted. Loose joints associated with relaxed capsules may be easily overlooked. The palpation of peripheral pulses in the upper extremity may provide information relating to a diagnosis of thoracic outlet syndrome.

Serial examinations of the muscles are important to determine any progression of disease states. Nowhere in the body is the action of multiple muscle groups affected by gravity more than in the shoulder. During the testing of shoulder muscle strength, the examiner should observe and palpate the muscle and its tendon so as to eliminate the action of neighboring muscles. It is important to observe whether the scapula is anchored in position before testing shoulder muscle strengths. For example, the examiner may mistake serratus anterior or trapezius weakness for a loss in deltoid strength. Alternatively, in the presence of a weak deltoid, the scapula can actively rotate, giving the impression that abduction power of the arm is strong. Joint contractures must be overcome before muscle transfer is performed. A transplanted muscle not only loses significant strength but cannot move a joint that is stiff or whose articular surfaces are severely damaged. The muscle must also be large and strong enough to accomplish its intended purposes (57). The surgeon must formulate a workable treatment plan to achieve the best result (52).

Winging of the Scapula

The combined actions of the trapezius and serratus anterior muscles are necessary to keep the scapula in a normal position. Paralysis of either muscle leads to winging of the scapula. The scapula is displaced inward and upward when winging results from serratus anterior weakness. In this case, the inferior angle of the scapula approaches the spine. In the alternative, trapezius paralysis leading to winging of the shoulder blade causes the scapula to be displaced downward and outward (lateral displacement).

There are various degrees of muscle weakness that result in a corresponding winging of the scapula. In less pronounced cases of serratus anterior weakness, winging of the scapula is noted when the patient attempts to raise the arm in forward flexion. Scapular winging is more obvious as the arm is raised against resistance. With complete paralysis of the serratus anterior, the scapula cannot be fixed to the thorax, making it difficult for the patient to elevate the arm. This is made worse when there is weakness of both the serratus anterior and trapezius muscles. Thus, winging is greatly exaggerated if more than one of the major muscles is affected (3). The greater the degree of winging, secondary to increasing paralysis of muscle groups that stabilize the scapula, the greater the disability of the shoulder (20, 21). In this situation, elevation and lifting power is diminished in a corresponding manner with increasing scapula winging.

Serratus Anterior Paralysis

Paralysis of the serratus anterior due to long thoracic nerve injury disturbs shoulder function and can disable normal shoulder function. Most cases of serratus anterior paresis due to a single traumatic episode usually subside spontaneously within 6 to 9 months (14, 16) and certainly within 12 months. Occasionally, the winging does not subside and may become chronic (13, 14, 22, 24, 39, 59). The nerve and its blood supply may be vulnerable to compression and stretching anterior to the lower part of the scapula (25). In some cases in which serratus anterior paralysis is associated with a brachial neuritis or herpes zoster infection, resolution may not occur until 18 to 24 months. Personal experience has shown that when an isolated trauma to the long thoracic nerve of Bell occurs, it is highly unlikely that subsidence of the winging will result after 12 months, especially when there has been no clinical evidence of improvement regardless of the changes in serial EMG studies. In addition, when winging of the scapula persists, it often does not pose a serious problem, especially in individuals who perform sedentary activities and do not stress their shoulders. Thus, the prognosis is good with conservative treatment in most cases. Fery (12, 13) reported a 26% failure rate with conservative treatment, whereas the overall surgical failure rate was only 9%. The condition is often missed or treated as a rotator cuff injury when the shoulder becomes increasingly painful. If painful scapula winging can be controlled, the symptoms of shoulder joint instability may decrease or subside. When symptomatic scapular instability persists without evidence of a timely resolution, surgical stabilization of the scapula may become indicated in selected cases. Each patient must be carefully evaluated, because a substantial number of patients often complain of shoulder joint instability itself. Muscle paralysis often enhances the possibility of subluxation of the humeral head from the glenoid (35).

HISTORICAL REVIEW

In 1723, Winslow (61) first reported on winging of the scapula. In 1837, Velpeau (60) described the condition in association with acromioclavicular dislocation. However, the condition came to the attention of surgeons in 1904 when Tubby (59) described the operation of transferring the sternal portion of the pectoralis major directly into digitations of the paralyzed serratus anterior muscle. This operation did not fully correct the winging, because the transfer was not truly dynamic. The transferred tendon tended to stretch.

Other kinds of operations were designed to dynamically correct the serratus anterior paralysis (18, 33). For example, Chaves (5) transferred the pectoralis minor to the midaxillary border of the scapula, and Rapp (47) used the same muscle-tendon and transferred it to the inferior angle of the scapula. Each operation required fascia lata grafts. The results of each operation were not durable and did not give satisfactory results. Other operations have been tried (55). Herzmark (19) tried to improve residual rhomboid muscle function by reattaching the rhomboid insertion to the posterior surface of the scapula and overlapping the trapezius. Although this procedure helped to stabilize the vertebral border of the scapula, it did not improve elevation of the arm. Steindler (56, 58, 59) tried transferring the levator scapulae to the acromion to substitute for a paralyzed upper trapezius, and transferred the pectoralis major and/or the minor to the inferior scapular angel to effect rotational control of the scapula in the anteroposterior axis if necessary. Dickson (10) used fascia lata grafts sutured into the pectoralis major muscle and the other end of the graft placed through a hole in the scapula. Whitman (62) used strips of fascia lata grafts placed through holes at the vertebral border of the scapula and then attached directly to the spinous process of the four opposing vertebral bodies. In general, all these operations failed and the results were not long-lasting. Also, the grafts tend to stretch. Ketenjian (26) stabilized the scapula to the rib cage in facioscapulohumeral muscular dystrophy using fascia lata strips attached to the vertebral border and then around individual ribs. In the author's experience, when this operation was tried in a small series of patients with isolated serratus anterior paralysis, the operation again failed because the grafts stretched.

Durman (11) used rolled tubular fascia lata strips looped in a hole at the inferior scapular tip after the graft was rolled around the pectoralis major tendon. Iceton and Harris (22) reported 14 cases of winging of the scapula using tubular fascia lata grafts between the pectoralis major tendon and the scapula; there were 4 failures. The grafts apparently stretched in each of these failures. The operation tends to fail when fascia lata grafts are used to correct more than one muscle deficiency but works better with isolated serratus anterior muscle paralysis when no other muscles are affected. Gozna and Harris (15) reported rolling a fascia lata into a tube and holding it with a running heavy nonabsorbable suture. The cut end of the pectoralis major tendon was placed within the tubular graft, and the graft was then passed through a hole in the lower pole of the scapula. Post (44) reported eight cases of severe chronic scapular winging relating to serratus anterior paralysis using fascia lata grafts, with long-lasting and excellent results in all cases. In this latter operation, the fascia lata graft was rolled into a tight spiral and held with a heavy nonabsorbable locking suture. One cut end of the locked spiral graft was woven through the myotendinous junction of the pectoralis major tendon and sutured in place to the pectoralis major tendon and then back upon itself, while the other end of the graft was placed through a hole at the inferior angle of the scapula and sutured to itself. Treated in this manner, the graft does not appear to stretch, in contradistinction to other operations in which the graft does stretch or tear. Recently, Yamaguchi et al. (64) reported that graft stretching can be minimized if the cut end of the sternal head is brought through the hole in the scapula. The fascia lata graft is used to augment the tendon only after it has passed through the hole in the scapula.

EVALUATION

The diagnosis of winging of the scapula due to serratus anterior weakness or paralysis is based on the results of the clinical examination. Patients often complain of a painful popping and clicking sensation that increases with stressful activities. Only when pain subsides is winging of the scapula first observed in most cases and after a prolonged period. The condition most often relates to trauma and may be either direct or by traction injury. For example, prolonged direct compression against the side of the thorax may cause an injury to the long thoracic nerve. Other causes for paralysis of the serratus anterior muscles may relate to brachial neuritis and Parsonage Turner syndrome (40). Herpes zoster (rarely) or electroshock (34, 44) are among other causes that may lead to winging of the scapula.

Serratus anterior weakness or paralysis of the scapula causes inward and upward displacement. The greater the loss of muscle strength, the greater the displacement (winging). The entire back must be examined to be certain that scoliosis is not present, which may create a false impression of winged scapula. In any event, with increasing scapular winging, the winging usually becomes more conspicuous as the arm is raised against resistance. If serratus

Figure 6.1. Winging of scapula in a patient with right serratus anterior palsy demonstrated by pushing against the wall.

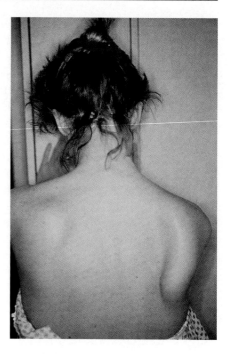

anterior muscle paralysis is severe, the scapula cannot be fixed against the thorax, making it impossible for the patient to raise the arm at all in some cases. When performing a physical examination, the patient is asked to thrust the outstretched arm against the wall or against resistance by the examiner (Fig. 6.1). This causes the winging. Abduction of the arm may cause little winging and is an important clinical difference from the effect of trapezius paralysis. EMG plays an essential role in making the diagnosis. In unusual circumstances when the scapula is exceptionally hypermobile, it may not be possible to obtain EMG confirmatory evidence of muscle paralysis. In other cases associated with multidirectional instability (MDI) of the glenohumeral joint, scapular winging may show mild to severe degrees of winging without actual muscle paralysis. In this latter situation, the symptoms of MDI may be exacerbated.

Imaging studies are not helpful in establishing the diagnosis, except to exclude other pathology such as fracture of the scapula or osteochondroma.

Management of Serratus Anterior Paralysis and Winging of the Scapula

CLOSED TREATMENT

Because most cases of winging of the scapula related to isolated serratus anterior paralysis subside spontaneously within 6 to 9 months (14), these patients should be treated conservatively when the diagnosis is first made. The treatment should consist of rest and avoiding strenuous lifting. Early management of a paralyzed muscle should include immobilization in a functional position, stimulation of the muscle in an attempt to reduce atrophic changes, and reasonable exercises to rebuild viable weakened muscles several times each day (17, 63). An orthosis often helps relieve the pain and control the stability of the shoulder girdle, as described by Johnson and Kendall (24). Serial EMG studies every 3 to 4 months will show whether the nerve is recovering and provide some information as to whether there may be any clinical recovery. The EMG studies cannot be used to evaluate an early recovery, nor is there a firm correlation between improvement in EMG studies and the degree of winging of the scapula. Moreover, in other cases such as the Parsonage-Turner Syndrome or paralytic brachial neuritis with associated winging, a longer period is required for the nerve to recover. Operative treatment should not be considered before conservative treatment has been continued for 18 to 24 months and there is no hope of spontaneous recovery.

OPEN TREATMENT

The purpose of operative treatment is to achieve a stable pain-free scapula, especially during the active use of the upper extremity. An operation should not be performed before 12 months has elapsed and/or there is no hope of spontaneous recovery. In cases of brachial neuritis and other similar neurologic disorders, 18 to 24 months should elapse before surgery is performed.

Pectoralis major transfer with fascia lata grafting is a superior procedure in restoring stability of the scapula relating to serratus anterior paralysis. It is the author's procedure of choice because is has been shown to be very effective (12, 13, 44).

ANATOMY

The serratus anterior is innervated by the long thoracic nerve of Bell (C5-7). Normally it draws the scapula forward, keeping it closely applied to the thorax. When the shoulder girdle is fixed, the muscle acts as an accessory muscle of respiration. The serratus anterior lies on the side of the chest on the medial wall of the axilla and originates from eight digitations from the upper eight ribs and the fascia that cover the intercostal muscles. The first digitation inserts into the deep surface of the superior angle of the scapula. The second to the fourth digitations insert into a strip on the deeper aspect of the medial margin of the scapula. The fifth through the eighth digitations converge on the deep surface of the inferior angle. The muscle aids in fixing the scapula while the trapezius rotates the scapula to direct the arm upward.

OPERATION

The purpose of the pectoralis major transfer is to substitute for the loss of function of the serratus anterior. The sternal portion of the pectoralis major muscle substitutes well for the lost serratus while preserving normal breast contour.

After the administration of general anesthesia, the patient is placed in the modified beach-chair position, taking care to pad all bony prominences. The arm, shoulder, chest, and back to the midline are prepared and draped, as is the ipsilateral thigh. A 10- to 15-cm incision is made in the axillary skin crease. The pectoralis major tendon is identified in its entirety along its humeral insertion. The interval between the sternal and clavicular portions of the muscle is identified with the arm in an abducted, externally rotated position (Fig. 6.2). The tendon of the sternal head is then removed directly

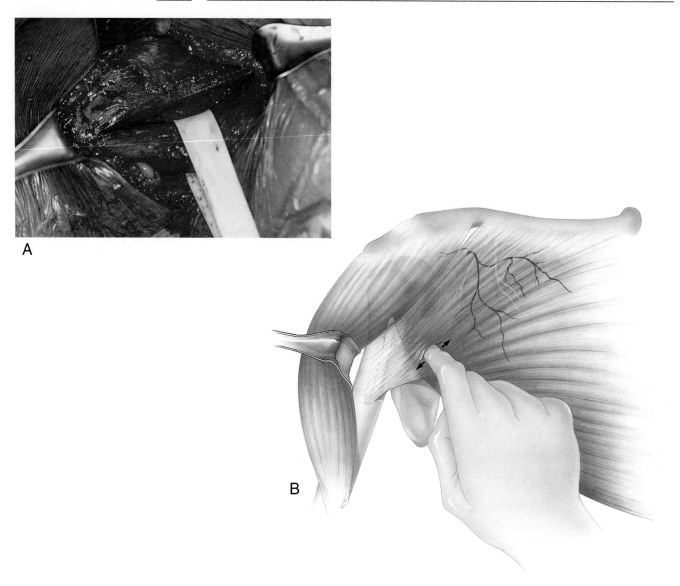

Figure 6.2. **(A)** The interval between the sternal and clavicular heads of the pectoralis major muscle is identified with the arm abducted and externally rotated. **(B)** Schematic drawing of Figure 6.2A.

from its humeral insertion, taking care to avoid injury to the biceps tendon (Fig. 6.3A). Tag sutures are placed in the tendon for retraction. This portion of the pectoralis major is then meticulously released of all fascial restrictions medially to allow mobilization.

Attention is then turned to the lateral thigh. Either one long skin incision over the whole length of the middle aspect of the lateral thigh or two small 3- or 4-cm incisions over the proximal and distal parts of the thigh can be used (Fig. 6.4). With the two-incision technique, a Cobb elevator is used to expose the underlying fascia between the two incisions, and a tendon stripper harvests a long, broad segment of fascia lata approximately 6 × 12 to 15 cm. This fascia is then folded back on itself several times, wrapped tightly, and reinforced with a running zero nonabsorbable suture. The fascia lata graft is then looped through a stab incision at the myotendinous junction of the sternal head of the pectoralis and secured back to itself with two or three non-absorbable sutures (Fig. 6.5). The wound is closed by suturing only the subcutaneous layer and closing the skin with staples. A closed suction drainage system is used for 24 hours.

Using a towel clip, the inferior angle of the scapula is grasped through the thin membranous scapular bone plate, taking care to avoid injury to the thick cortical bone at the axillary edge of the scapular border. The scapula is pulled laterally into the wound. The latissimus dorsi and teres major muscles are retracted downward, facilitating exposure of the inferior angle of the scapula. Using needle-tip electrocoagulation at the edge of the inferior angle of the scapula, the serratus anterior and subscapularis and lower portion of

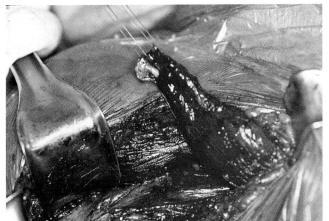

A

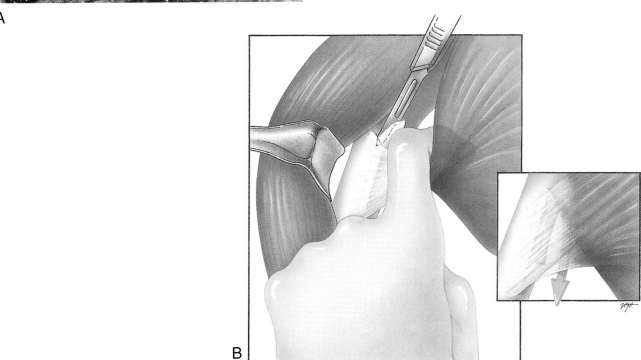

B

Figure 6.3. **(A)** The sternal head tendon of the pectoralis major is removed directly from its humeral insertion. Care should be taken to avoid injury to the underlying biceps tendon and clavicular head insertion. **(B)** Schematic drawing of Figure 6.3A.

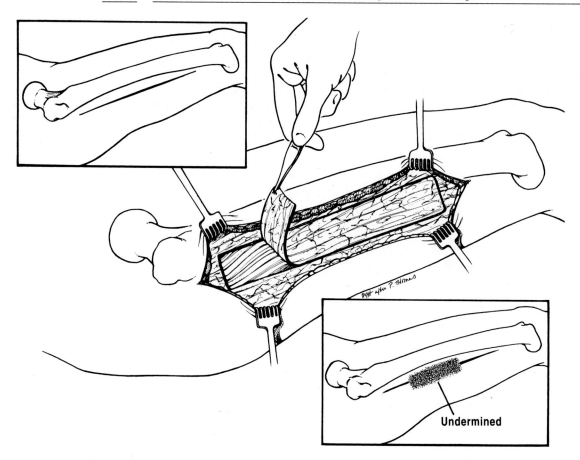

Undermined

Figure 6.4. Fascia lata graft is harvested through either one long or two small incisions.

the rhomboid major and infraspinatus are elevated from the edge of the cortical bone and membranous bone plate of the scapula. After these muscles are elevated and retracted, a 6- to 8-mm hole is drilled through the membranous bone plate 2.5 cm proximal to the lowest point of the apex of the inferior angle. The graft is carefully threaded through the hole, not simply pulled in a forceful manner, to avoid possible fracture of the fragile scapula. The fascia lata graft is then passed through the hole in the inferior angle of the scapula until the tendon of the sternal head of the pectoralis is in direct contact with the scapula itself (Fig. 6.6). This is an important technical aspect of the procedure, because it is believed that if the fascia lata is used as an interposition between the pectoralis tendon and the scapula, it may stretch over time, leading to recurrence of winging. The fascia lata is then folded back on itself and the tendon of the sternal head, thereby acting only as reinforcement of the attachment. After meticulous hemostasis, a layered closure is performed over a suction drain.

The patient is maintained in a custom scapulothoracic orthosis for 6 weeks (Fig. 6.7). This brace is made of a lightweight pad that presses the scapula firmly against the chest wall and away from the midline to prevent winging, both at rest and during elevation. Gentle glenohumeral range of motion exercises and isometric muscle strengthening exercises are performed with the brace during this 6-week period. Thereafter, the brace may be discontinued and progressive strengthening exercises initiated. No heavy lifting or a return to a fully active manual labor occupation is allowed for 6 months.

RESULTS

The results of pectoralis major transfer with fascia lata grafting in the manner described has given consistently excellent, durable results (44, 64). Recently, Yamaguchi et al. (64) reported the results of 11 consecutive patients who had sternal head transfer for symptomatic scapular winging. At an average follow-up of 41 months, 10 of 11 patients (91%) had satisfactory results with significant improvements in pain, function, and scapular tracking (Fig. 6.8). Patients have been quite pleased with the cosmesis of the scar

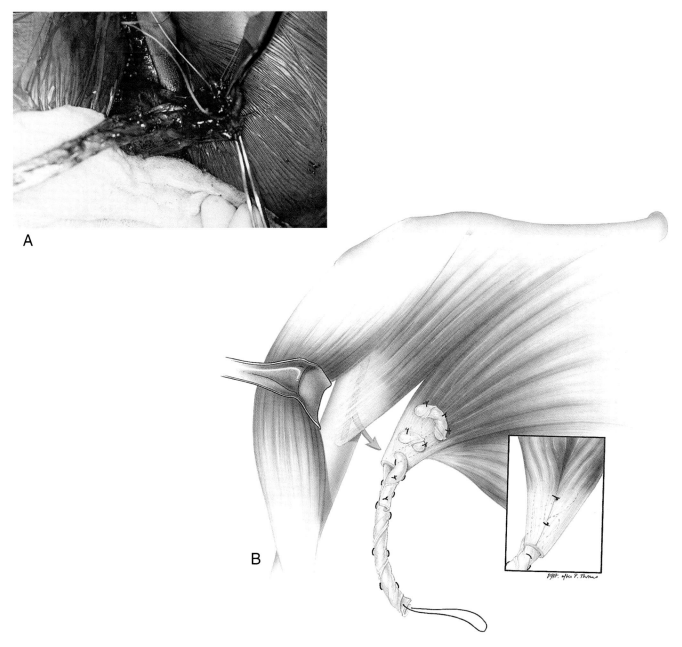

Figure 6.5. **(A)** The fascia lata graft is looped through a stab incision at the myotendinous junction of the pectoralis major and secured back to itself with two or three nonabsorbable sutures. **(B)** Schematic drawing of Figure 6.5A.

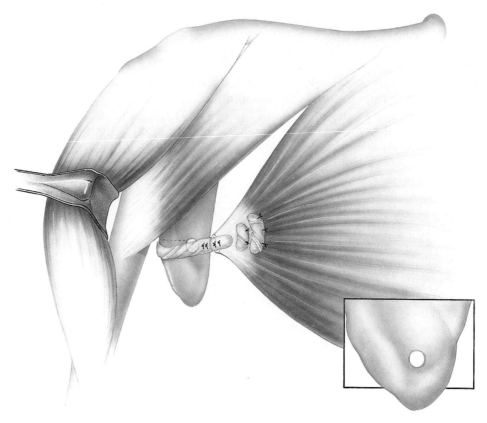

Figure 6.6. The fascia lata graft is passed through the hole in the inferior angle of the scapula until the tendon of the sternal head of the pectoralis is in direct contact with the scapula itself.

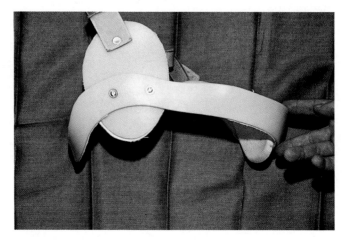

Figure 6.7. A custom scapulothoracic orthosis may be used for 6 weeks.

(Fig. 6.9). The one unsatisfactory result was secondary to noncompliance with the postoperative physical therapy regimen.

Not enough information has been obtained to determine the limits of lifting heavy objects with this operation or whether the treated scapula will withstand high-performance athletic activities such as high-velocity throwing in the overhand position or the lifting of heavier weights against gravity. It has been observed that most patients with severe, painful multidirectional instability (MDI) experience pain relief after the winged scapula is stabilized (44). Experience has shown that a capsular shift operation is not often needed after a sternal head pectoralis major transfer.

COMPLICATIONS

In the author's experience, there has been only one complication of a postoperative hematoma in the axilla that subsided spontaneously (44). No other complications have occurred. Pectoralis major transfer in the manner described has given consistently superior results for isolated serratus anterior paralysis. It should not be used when multiple muscle paralysis is present. The sternal portion of the pectoralis major muscle has the same EMG

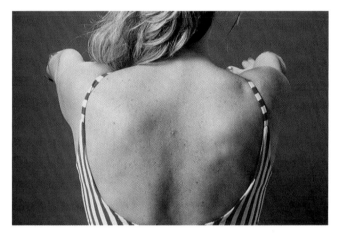

Figure 6.8. Postoperative photograph of patient from Figure 6.1 with elimination of scapular winging.

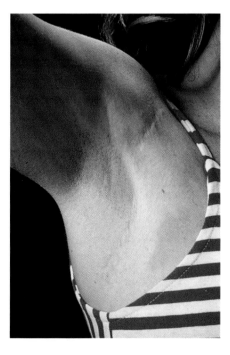

Figure 6.9. Well-concealed scar in the axilla of a postoperative patient.

activity and power as the paralyzed serratus anterior muscle and the fiber orientation of the transferred muscle is the same, which may account for the good results described (12, 13).

Winging of the Scapula Due to Trapezius Paralysis

Injury to the motor spinal accessory (11th cranial) nerve causes paralysis of the trapezius that is often painful, disabling, and deforming. Synchronous scapulothoracic rhythm is lost. The shoulder droops, and the resulting pain can be severe due to muscle spasm, radiculitis from traction on the brachial plexus, frozen shoulder, or subacromial impingement. When paralysis of the trapezius causes severe pain and disability that is not relieved with conservative treatment, as in strengthening of the adjacent muscle groups or nerve grafting through the spinal accessory nerve, muscle transfers to stabilize the scapula may become indicated as a salvage procedure in some select cases.

HISTORICAL REVIEW

Codman (7) recognized the importance of the delicate muscle balance of the shoulder girdle, whereas Inman et al. (23) showed the contribution of the trapezius to the balance of the scapular rotary-force couples.

In an effort to stabilize the winged scapula resulting from a paralyzed trapezius, Dickson (10) tried stabilizing the scapula using fascia lata tubes and anchoring the scapula to the cervical muscles and the spinous process of the first thoracic vertebra. Dewar and Harris (9) tried fixing the scapula with a fascia lata sling and transfer of the levator scapulae. In the author's experience, these operations have not worked well or have failed primarily because the graft stretched or failed and did not provide dynamic balance to the scapula. With exceptionally severe winging of the scapula relating not only to trapezius paralysis but in association with combined serratus anterior paralysis, fusion of the scapula to the rib cage has been tried but seriously limits shoulder motion. On the other hand, dynamic muscle transfer of the levator scapulae and rhomboids, as described by Lange (30, 31), has given uniformly good results in stabilizing the scapula and relieving pain. Several other series have also reported favorable results with this technique (32, 37). In particular, Bigliani (1) reported early favorable results with this technique. More recently, he reported long-term results in a series of 21 patients (2). Furthermore, the surgical technique was modified so that the rhomboid minor was transferred above the scapula. On the other hand, neurolysis and nerve grafting of the spinal accessory nerve have given variable and inconsistent results (1). However, better results have been reported if nerve procedures are done within 1 year of injury.

CLINICAL EVALUATION

Most patients state they can accommodate to the disability caused by winging of the scapula relating to trapezius paralysis, especially if they are elderly or lead a sedentary life. However, more active patients with trapezius paralysis and associated winging may complain of disabling pain that is secondary to muscle spasm, usually involving the levator scapulae and the rhomboid major and minor muscles. Patients may have recurring episodes of radiating pain secondary to radiculitis because of traction on the brachial plexus, especially when the involved extremity has been unsupported as a part of early treatment. Pain may be present that relates to subacromial impingement and/or frozen shoulder. The condition may be misdiagnosed or even mistreated when the surgeon believes that the primary cause of shoulder pain is an impingement syndrome rather than winging of the scapula.

Patients with trapezius paralysis and associated winging can range in age from the teens to the very elderly. The cause may be due to blunt trauma, as in a motor vehicle accident, or may be iatrogenic, such as when the spinal accessory nerve is damaged surgically during the excision of a cervical lymph node or benign tumor from the neck or during a radical neck dissection (1, 37, 41). The author has seen at least one case of a patient who had a herpes zoster infection but who recovered in 20 months with conservative management.

Physical examination may disclose varying degrees of drooping of the involved shoulder, atrophy of the superior trapezius in chronic cases, and winging of the scapula (especially against trapezius muscle resistance). The scapula is displaced downward and outward. There is a loss in contour of the involved side superiorly due to muscle atrophy and a drooping shoulder. The trapezius muscle is weak and demonstrates poor endurance against adduction resistance of the extremity.

Other diagnoses—including stroke, dislocating shoulder, herniated cervical disk, scoliosis, or a progressive neuromuscular disorder—should be ruled out (1, 41).

Although EMG may be useful in confirming an injury to the spinal accessory nerve, negative or inconclusive EMG results do not exclude the diagnosis. This is because severe winging and instability of the scapula may not permit an adequate examination. In addition, imaging studies may be useful in excluding bone trauma.

ANATOMIC AND FUNCTIONAL CONSIDERATIONS

The spinal accessory nerve is the sole motor innervation to the trapezius (1, 41, 53). Although innervation of the third and fourth cervical nerves has been described (18), these branches are usually proprioceptive and not motor. During its course to the trapezius muscle, the spinal accessory nerve is superficial on the floor of the posterior cervical triangle. It lies in subcutaneous tissue and is susceptible to injury. The injury may be penetrating, such as from a stab or gunshot wound, or it may be due to blunt trauma, as in a motor vehicle accident.

The scapula is extremely mobile and is suspended on the chest wall by its musculature. Any imbalance in the muscles results in instability during certain activities and positions. The trapezius is divided into three distinct anatomic components: upper, middle, and lower. The upper portion rotates and elevates the scapula, the middle portion stabilizes and adducts it, and the lower portion rotates the scapula downward and depresses it. The three components of the trapezius muscle work synchronously (Fig. 6.10). One of the most important functions of the trapezius is to elevate the lateral tip of the scapula and, with it, the entire upper extremity. It is the only muscle that can perform this function because it is the only one that passes downward from the neck to insert on the lateral tip of the scapula. Paralysis causes

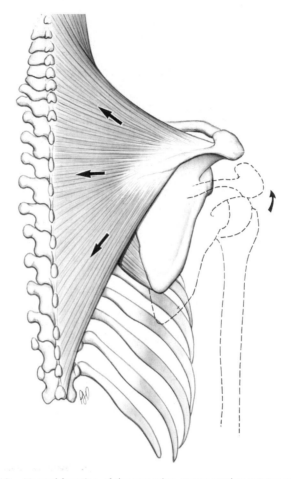

Figure 6.10. Normal function of the trapezius: upper portion rotates and elevates
the scapula, the middle portion stabilizes and adducts it, and the lower
portion rotates the scapula downward and depresses it.

drooping of the entire extremity. In addition, the trapezius is also important
for abduction of the arm and for overhead activities.

To adequately substitute for the complex function of the trapezius muscle, the functions of its three components must be anatomically replaced. Transfer of the levator scapulae and the rhomboid major and minor, the Eden-Lange (30–32) procedure, achieves this goal. All three of these muscles insert on the medial border of the scapula and normally contract as the trapezius acts during rotation, elevation, depression, and medial stabilization of the scapula. When the trapezius is paralyzed, these muscles are unable to prevent winging, lateral displacement, and drooping because their medial insertion places them at a biomechanical disadvantage (Fig. 6.11). Thus, lateral transfer of these muscles to the spine and body of the scapula changes the direction of their pull, allowing them to approximate the function of the trapezius muscle and support the scapula (Fig. 6.12). The levator scapulae substitutes for the upper portion of the trapezius. The rhomboid minor replaces the middle portion of the trapezius, while the rhomboid major replaces the middle and lower portions of the trapezius. When all three muscles act together as a unit, the dynamic equilibrium of the muscle forces that was lost with paralysis of the trapezius is restored.

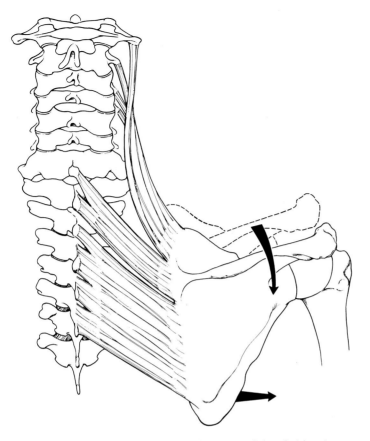

Figure 6.11. The levator scapula, rhomboid minor, and rhomboid major are unable to prevent winging, lateral displacement, and drooping because their medial insertion places them at a biomechanical disadvantage.

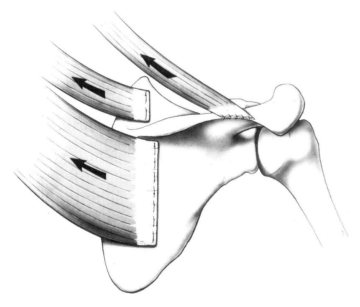

Figure 6.12. Lateral transfer of the the levator and rhomboids changes the direction of their pull, allowing them to approximate the function of the trapezius muscle and support the scapula.

Management of Trapezius Paralysis and Winging of the Scapula

CLOSED TREATMENT

Many patients recover with conservative treatment if the spinal accessory nerve is intact and not severely stretched. If the nerve has been cut, there can be no recovery. Conservative treatment of the trapezius will usually fail in active patients. Narcotic medication may be required in the acute phase to relieve pain; in some cases, narcotic medication may be required for prolonged periods if the pain is severe. Other forms of treatment (including ultrasound, galvanic stimulation, hot packs, and acupuncture) ordinarily provide only temporary pain relief. The arm should be supported in a sling or other device to minimize drooping of the shoulder and traction on the brachial plexus. Overhead activities should be limited.

When there has been no recovery within 15 months, it is unlikely that adequate recovery will result if trauma caused the paralysis. However, when the nerve is injured by infection, such herpes zoster, it is possible for recovery in 18 to 24 months. Accordingly, surgery should be deferred for at least 12 months in most cases relating to trauma and for up to 18 to 24 months in cases involving neuritic infection. The indication for muscle transfers (Eden-Lange [32]) is a failure of conservative treatment after 1 year or after a nerve operation (such as a nerve exploration, lysis, or repair of the spinal accessory nerve or a combination of these measures). In addition, muscle transfers are not ordinarily necessary in older persons who lead a sedentary life, especially if the nondominant extremity is involved.

OPEN TREATMENT

The main indication for operative treatment of trapezius winging of the scapula is shoulder girdle pain (1). The pain usually results from muscle spasm involving the levator scapulae and the rhomboid major and minor. At times, the pectoralis major may be involved. The patient may complain of a dull ache and heavy feeling around the shoulder (1).

SURGICAL TECHNIQUE (EDEN-LANGE [1, 30–32])

The patient is placed on a bean bag in a lateral slightly tilted position, with the arm draped free. The head of the table is elevated 15%. An incision is made midway between the spinous processes and the medial scapular border, starting just above the superior angle and finishing at the base of the scapula (Fig. 6.13). The atrophied trapezius is identified and is transected close to the scapula border. A more medial transection may risk injury to the underlying rhomboid muscles. The levator scapulae, rhomboid minor, and rhomboid major are then identified and are carefully separated from one another (Fig. 6.14). It is important to differentiate the interval between the inferior border of the levator scapulae and the superior border of the rhomboid minor. The arm is supported throughout the procedure, and the scapula is rotated when necessary to achieve adequate exposure. The attachments of the three muscles to be transferred are detached with a narrow osteotome from the medial border of the scapula along with a thin portion of insertional bone (Fig. 6.15). The three individual muscles are then separated and are dissected proximally and medially with great care so that the dorsal scapular nerve

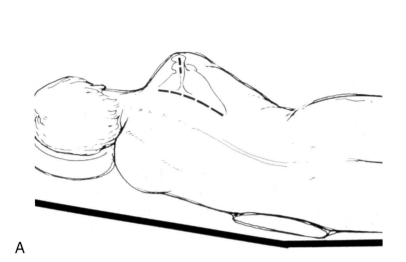

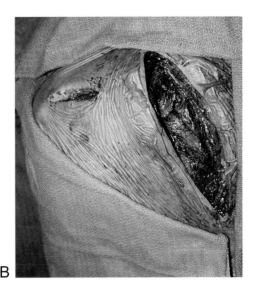

A   B

Figure 6.13. **(A, B)** The first incision is made midway between the spinous processes and the medial scapular border, starting just above the superior angle and finishing at the base of the scapula. The second incision is made starting 3 cm medial to the posterior tip of the acromion and extending approximately 4 cm medially.

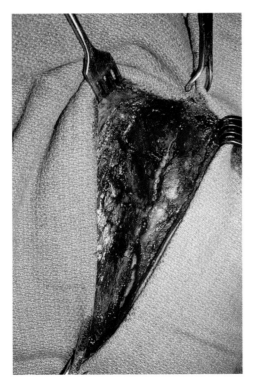

Figure 6.14. The levator scapulae, rhomboid minor, and rhomboid major are identified and separated from one another.

and transverse cervical artery are not injured. It is essential to dissect the levator scapulae far enough proximally and superiorly so that it will reach its new insertion. Sutures are used to tag the ends of each muscle.

The supraspinatus is elevated from the superior fossa of the scapula. Two drill holes are made in the bony plate of the lateral third of fossa 1.5 cm apart. Heavy nonabsorbable sutures are placed through the cut end of the rhomboid minor and then through the holes in the bone plate of the superior fossa. The supraspinatus is imbricated over the repair.

Figure 6.15. The three muscles are detached with a thin portion of bone from their medial insertion with a narrow osteotome.

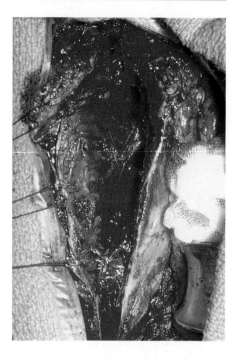

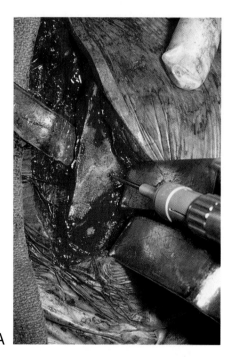

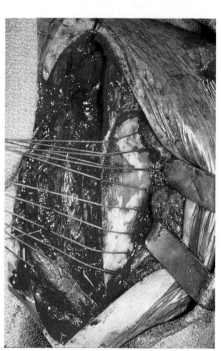

A

B

Figure 6.16. **(A)** Drill holes are placed in the scapula 1.5 to 2.0 cm apart for fixation of the transferred rhomboid minor and major. **(B)** Sutures are placed through the drill holes in the scapula to secure the transferred rhomboid minor and major.

The infraspinatus is then elevated from the inferior fossa of the scapula. Four drill holes are placed in the scapula 1.5 to 2.0 cm apart (Fig. 6.16). The first hole is started approximately 4 to 5 cm lateral to the medial border of the scapula and 1 cm below the spine. Heavy nonabsorbable sutures are passed through the holes with a large needle, taking care to stay close to the scapula and not penetrate the chest wall. Three sutures are used for the rhomboid major. The sutures are tied with the scapula in the reduced position, and the arm is abducted approximately 90° (Fig. 6.17). The infraspinatus is then imbricated over the repair.

Next, the spine of the scapula is palpated, and a 4-cm incision is made starting 3 cm medial to the posterior tip of the acromion and extending medially. The atrophied trapezius, deltoid, and supraspinatus are carefully dissected so that three drill holes can be made through the spine of the scapula. The suprascapular nerve lies beneath this area, and injury to this nerve must be avoided. A tunnel is made through the atrophied trapezius muscle connecting the medial and lateral wounds. The tunnel should be in the line of the upper fibers of the trapezius. The levator scapulae is then passed through the tunnel and secured to the spine of the scapula (Fig. 6.18). The optimum position is 5 to 7 cm from the posterior lateral corner of the scapular spine. Additional sutures can be used to attach the levator tendon to the deltoid and surrounding soft tissues. The incisions are sutured in layers. A foam wedge is used, maintaining the extremity in approximately 60 to 70° of abduction for 4 weeks.

Early passive range of motion above the level of the wedge is begun immediately. Passive elevation in the scapula plane to 130% and external rotation to 30 to 40% are allowed to prevent stiffness that can result from 4 to 6 weeks of immobilization. After 4 weeks, the wedge is removed and gentle strengthening exercises are added. A progressive strengthening program has been devised using rubber tubing, free weights, and medicine ball throws to achieve dynamic scapular stability. These exercises strengthen the transferred levator scapula and rhomboid muscles. Bigliani et al. (2) found that of 22 patients who underwent follow-up for more than 2 years, 13 had excellent results, 6 had satisfactory results, and 3 had unsatisfactory results. All patients in their series had improved function and correction of the deformity, and 19 patients had good pain relief.

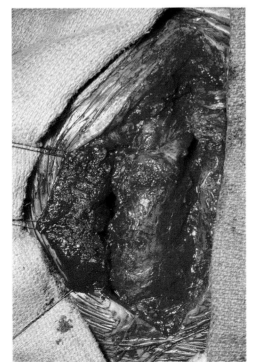

Figure 6.17. Completed transfer of the rhomboid minor and major.

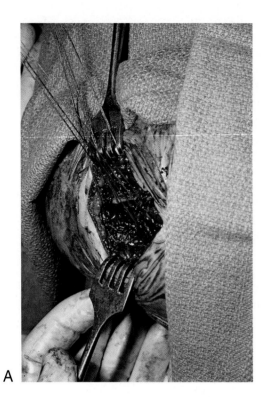
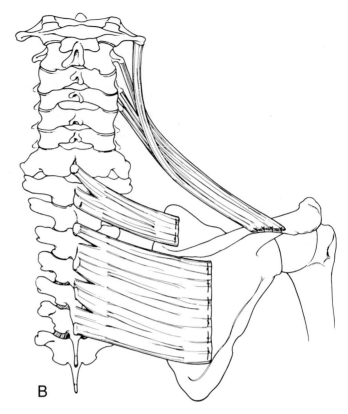

Figure 6.18. **(A)** The levator scapulae is passed through a tunnel and secured to the spine of the scapula. **(B)** Schematic drawing of the completed transfer of all three muscles.

Entrapment Syndromes of the Shoulder Girdle

Many of the conditions causing shoulder pain are easily diagnosed, whereas others are missed or misdiagnosed because of the complex anatomy and physiology of the shoulder girdle. Thus, the surgeon should be precise in establishing the true diagnosis so that correct treatment and relief of pain can be achieved. The exact location of the pathology must be determined early to minimize muscle atrophy, restricted motion, and pain. There are a number of nerve entrapments around the shoulder that may mimic various other diseases. If an incorrect diagnosis is made, a needless operation may be performed that fails to relieve pain and contributes to continuing shoulder disability. Some of the entities causing painful shoulder entrapments include entrapment of the suprascapular nerve and quadrilateral space syndrome.

Suprascapular Nerve Entrapment

HISTORICAL REVIEW

When Kopell and Thompson (28) first described suprascapular nerve entrapment in 1963, they believed that repetitive motion was a mechanism for inducing nerve irritation. Following their report, various causes of suprascapular nerve entrapment were discovered including compression by bone tumors such as an osteochondroma, ganglion cysts, traction injuries, direct trauma including fracture of the scapula, and overuse and repetitive activity of the upper extremity. In some cases, a definite reason cannot be found for the condition; therefore, a significant number of cases are insidious (45). Rengachary et al. (49, 50) described the relatively fixed nature of the suprascapular nerve as it passed through the notch beneath the suprascapular ligament. They showed that repetitive shoulder and scapular motion could cause friction and induce these inflammatory changes and potential constriction of the nerve. In addition, traction forces can also be centered at the notch which may stretch the nerve and cause inflammation and pain as shown by Mayfield and True (36), Seddon (53), and Solheim and Roass (54). Injury to the nerve in its notch by fibrosis and scarring and eventual compression may result after direct trauma as produced by a fall or a blow to the shoulder or perhaps even a scapular fracture. It was not until 1974 that Khalili (27) showed that an increased latency time of the suprascapular nerve at its notch to the supraspinatus and infraspinatus muscles indicated an impaired conductivity and was confirmatory evidence of an entrapment of the suprascapular nerve. Post and Mayer (46) showed the value of early diagnosis of suprascapular nerve entrapment and early decompression in relieving the symptoms and minimizing the chronic effects of atrophy of the external rotator muscles. Early surgical treatment was shown to minimize the chronic effects of atrophy of the external rotators in a long-term, large study performed by Post (45).

CLINICAL EVALUATION

Most cases of entrapment of the suprascapular nerve result from acute trauma (6, 41), encroachment of the suprascapular notch due to a benign or malignant tumor (46), or are idiopathic (65). Unusual cases of selective entrapment of the motor branches to the infraspinatus may be caused by a ganglion cyst. Kopell and Thompson (28) and Post (45) believed that certain extremes of scapular motion or extremes of combined motion of the shoulder joint and scapula render the nerve taut, kinking it over the edge of the foramen. In this manner, abnormal scapular movement may cause a suprascapular neuropathy. Clein (6) stated that although transmitted forces, direct injuries, and traction are important causes, traction injury is the most significant (6, 45, 46).

Diagnosis of suprascapular nerve entrapment is based on patient history, physical examination results, and abnormalities seen on EMG studies. Patients with suprascapular nerve entrapment complain of deep and diffuse pain at the top or back of the shoulder. In many cases, the pain may be referred downward into the arm, to the neck, or to the upper anterior chest wall. The pain may be burning, aching, or crushing. Patients may experience varying combinations of pain complaints together or at different times.

Serial physical examinations may demonstrate early weakness and subtle atrophy of the external rotators and provide a clue as to the diagnosis. In severe cases of neuropathy, atrophy and weakness of the supraspinatus and infraspinatus may exist. Infraspinatus atrophy may be present to a greater degree than in the supraspinatus, when for example, entrapment occurs at the spinoglenoid notch due to compression by a ganglion cyst. The longer the condition exists, the more easily the diagnosis can be made because of the increasing pronounced findings that may appear relating to muscle atrophy.

Thus, it is essential to test muscle power carefully during each examination to detect any weakness or decreased muscle endurance.

Specific scapular motions may be painful, and the patient may restrict shoulder motion, thereby simulating adhesive capsulitis. However, if full external rotation is present with the arm held close at the side, adhesive capsulitis is an unlikely diagnosis. Adduction of the extended arm across the body tenses the nerve and may increase pain. Thumb pressure over the suprascapular notch causes severe tenderness in the majority of patients (42). However, suprascapular notch tenderness is not pathognomonic for suprascapular nerve entrapment alone and should not be relied on as a definitive test.

Rose and Kelly (51) used a small-gauge spinal needle and 1% local anesthetic injected into the suprascapular notch to effect pain relief. However, a negative test does not exclude a diagnosis of entrapment, because the surgeon cannot be certain the nerve was paralyzed. This test should not be relied on to establish the diagnosis.

Confirmation of the diagnosis does depend on the EMG results (23). Nerve conduction time during the performance of the EMG study may show that the conduction time is delayed. If needed, a comparison with the opposite side is made. Kraft (29) showed that the usual mean normal latency is 2.7 ± 0.5 msec (average, 1.7 to 3.7 msec) to the supraspinatus and 3.3 ± 0.5 msec (average, 2.4 to 4.2 msec) to the infraspinatus. Significant neuropathic changes may be associated with a reduction in the interference pattern to a severe degree of denervation in the supraspinatus and infraspinatus muscles.

Magnetic resonance imaging studies may help to rule out a ganglion cyst, which may be the cause of a suprascapular nerve entrapment. Plain radiographs may demonstrate a fracture, callus formation at the notch causing the entrapment, or other pathology that will aid in planning operative treatment and management of entrapment of the suprascapular nerve.

CLOSED TREATMENT

In the author's experience, pain may subside in a very small number of patients over a prolonged period. However, these patients ordinarily go on to have increasing and severe muscle atrophy and a corresponding loss of shoulder function (45, 46). Once the diagnosis is established, it is best to treat the patient operatively as the best means of relieving pain and restoring function. The earlier a patient is operated on before atrophy occurs, the greater the chance that function will be restored.

OPEN TREATMENT

Anatomy

The suprascapular nerve originates from the upper trunk of the brachial plexus formed by the roots of C5 and C6 at Erb's point. The nerve courses downward, usually behind the brachial plexus and parallel to the omohyoid muscle beneath the trapezius to the superior edge of the scapula and then through the scapular notch. The roof of the notch is formed by the transverse scapular ligament. The ligament is taut but usually feels slightly ballottable when it is palpated. For this reason, it is not possible to palpate the notch until the ligament is transected. In unusual and uncommon circumstances, the ligament may be ossified, making easy identification of the suprascapular ligament difficult.

The notch may assume various shapes such as a letter U or V and may be deep and narrow or shallow and wide (49). The floor of the notch may be relatively sharp (49, 50). The suprascapular artery and vein pan above the transverse scapular ligament while the nerve passes below and through the notch and supplies the supraspinatus and infraspinatus muscles. Also, the nerve provides articular branches to both the glenohumeral and acromioclavicular joints (28). Sensory and sympathetic fibers of the nerve innervate two-thirds of the shoulder capsule (51). The nerve then turns around the lateral edge of the scapular spine to innervate the infraspinatus. The suprascapular nerve has no sensory endings to the skin.

The chief indication for surgery is to relieve pain, and this goal is achieved in most patients. Conservative treatment generally is not indicated with entrapment of the suprascapular nerve. Rengachary et al. (49, 50) performed anatomic dissections on cadavers to study the configuration of the suprascapular notch and measurements. They believed that certain notch configurations predispose individuals to suprascapular nerve entrapment. They stated that the inciting irritative motion beneath the suprascapular ligament was not translatory but rather angulatory, as different movements of the shoulder caused a bending of the nerve under the suprascapular ligament, creating a type of sling effect. After release of the suprascapular ligament, notch resection is unnecessary in most patients except when it is being compressed by a callus from a previous fracture or tumor. Similarly, neurolysis is unnecessary in the routine case.

SURGICAL TECHNIQUE

In contrast to other surgical approaches (38), the author recommends a posterior surgical approach because it is safe, easy, and unlikely to cause nerve and muscle damage (45, 46).

The patient is placed either in a semiprone position on a bean bag or in a sitting beach-chair position with the arm draped free. If the patient is positioned in the semiprone position, an axillary roll is placed beneath the contralateral shoulder. The patient is tilted forward 20% with the involved shoulder pointed upward. A soft pillow or blankets are placed between the knees and ankles to avoid contact of the bony parts. The skin incision is made parallel and slightly above the spine of the scapula and is approximately 10 to 12 cm long (Fig. 6.19). It is important to sharply elevate the whole trapezius from the scapular spine to avoid injury to the spinal accessory nerve when the muscle is retracted. The trapezius muscle should not be split in a longitudinal manner. Electrocoagulation is used for hemostasis. As the fibers of the trapezius and the periosteum are elevated, a thin, fatty layer is observed between the undersurface of the trapezius and the underlying supraspinatus muscle. The supraspinatus should not be elevated from its fossa. The trapezius muscle is retracted cephalad with a wide blunt retractor. With blunt dissection, the suprascapular ligament overlying its notch is palpated. Only minimal distal retraction of the supraspinatus muscle is required.

With a blunt elevator and moist cottonoid, the suprascapular ligament can be cleaned to show its glistening white structure. If the ligament is ossified, the suprascapular notch can be identified by gently inserting a 1-mm diameter, blunt-tipped malleable probe into the suprascapular foramen. The suprascapular artery and vein immediately superficial to the suprascapular

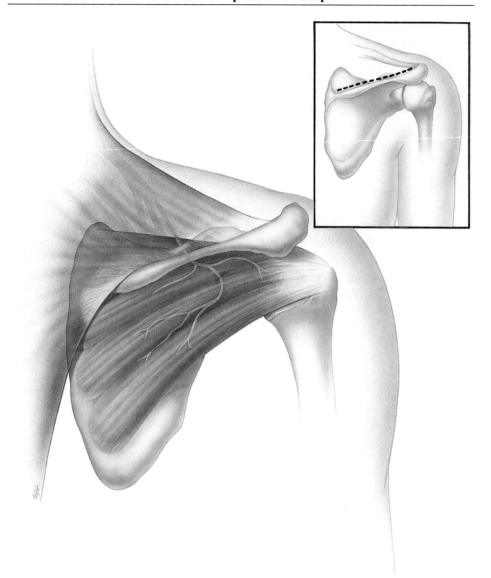

Figure 6.19. The skin incision is made parallel and slightly above the spine of the scapula and is approximately 10 to 12 cm long.

ligament should be teased to one side using a moist cottonoid (Fig. 6.20). If the vessels bleed, hemostasis can be obtained with one or two small vascular clips. The ligament is then sharply released while protecting the suprascapular nerve beneath (Fig. 6.21). Direct suction of blood or irrigation of fluid around the nerve should be avoided.

In the uncommon case of an ossified suprascapular ligament, it is carefully resected using a small-tipped, angled Kerrison rongeur while the nerve is protected with a malleable probe in the foramen. Once the nerve is freed, further exploration of the nerve or neurolysis is unnecessary unless a tumor, osteophyte, or exostosis causes compression. In this event, the lesion should be resected. The surrounding region should be inspected and gently palpated to rule out any abnormal masses. If a ganglion is known to be the cause of the entrapment, it should be fully excised using a nerve stimulator to identify nerve tissue and avoid accidental injury.

The trapezius muscle is then reattached to the spine of the scapula using no. 2 nonabsorbable sutures placed through several drill holes in the bone. The wound is then closed in layers. The arm is placed in a sling and immobilized postoperatively. Gentle active assistive and passive motion exercises may be started in the first week postoperatively. Active motions are permitted

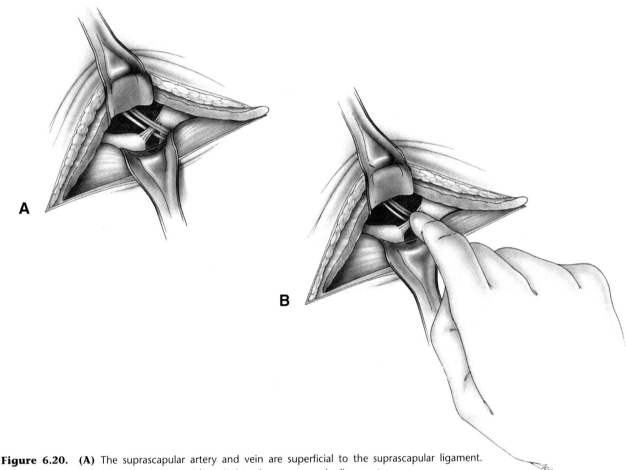

Figure 6.20. **(A)** The suprascapular artery and vein are superficial to the suprascapular ligament. **(B)** The vessels should be teased to one side to isolate the suprascapular ligament.

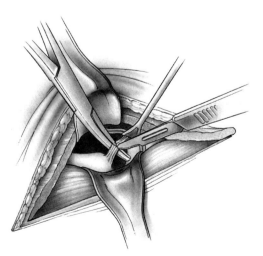

Figure 6.21. The ligament is sharply released while protecting the suprascapular nerve beneath.

within 10 to 14 days. Using the posterior approach, the author has not observed any complications.

Quadrilateral Space Syndrome

Quadrilateral space syndrome is a rare condition caused by the compression of the posterior humeral circumflex artery and the axillary nerve or one or more of its major branches in the quadrilateral space. Patients are usually between the ages of 22 and 35 years and may exhibit psychophysiologic overlay. Quadrilateral space syndrome often interferes with the patient's occupation and daily activities (4, 8). It is usually observed in the dominant upper extremity with no significant history of shoulder trauma, although Reeder et al. (48) have reported the condition in the throwing athlete. Regardless of a history of shoulder injury of even minimal degree, the onset is usually insidious. The patient may complain of tingling in the upper extremity. Motion such as forward flexion, abduction, and external rotation of the arm increases the pain, which may awaken the patient at night. The pain is diffuse and is manifested by an atypical distribution of pain and paresthesias, thereby making the diagnosis difficult. The patient may undergo a variety of treatments that usually do not relieve their symptoms.

Point tenderness may be found posteriorly over the quadrilateral space. Abduction and external rotation of the arm for 1 to 2 minutes will often cause symptoms. An inequality of the peripheral radial pulses may cause the examining physician to make a diagnosis of thoracic outlet syndrome. Results of a neurologic examination are usually normal, as are the EMG results.

A diagnosis is very difficult to make. Patients who have a history and physical findings suggesting quadrilateral space syndrome should have a subclavian arteriogram performed according to the Seldinger technique (4). In this imaging study, radiopaque dye is injected with the arm in abduction and external rotation. The dye is followed distally to the extent that the posterior humeral circumflex artery is observed.

With a positive arteriogram, the posterior humeral circumflex artery may be patent with the humerus at the side but will occlude when the arm is abducted to 60° or more. In other cases, additional passive elevation and external rotation may be needed to achieve positive results. If the dye is not followed peripherally, the diagnosis of compression of the posterior humeral circumflex artery may be missed.

ANATOMY

The anatomic structures constituting the boundaries of the quadrilateral space from the posterior view are the teres minor superiorly, the glenohumeral capsule and humerus laterally, the long head of the triceps medially, and fascia and adipose tissue along with the teres major inferiorly.

CLOSED TREATMENT

Most patients have had oral antiinflammatory medications, steroid injections, exercise programs, and physical therapy, all of which tend to fail to relieve the painful symptoms of this condition.

OPERATIVE TREATMENT

If adequate conservative treatment has failed, the patient has had intractable pain for a long period, and other causes of the pain have been excluded, a diagnosis of quadrilateral space entrapment can be made after confirmation by a positive arteriogram. The patient may benefit from surgical decompression of the quadrilateral space; however, decompression does not guarantee that pain will be relieved.

The patient is placed on a bean bag in the lateral decubitus position and tilted toward the prone position 30%. The prone position may also be used. In either case, the upper extremity is draped into the field. A pad is placed beneath the axilla, and a pillow is placed between the knees and ankles. A skin incision is made parallel and just below the entire length of the scapular spine and then curved downward at the lateral border of the incision over the humerus (Fig. 6.22). The inferior skin flap must include the subcutaneous

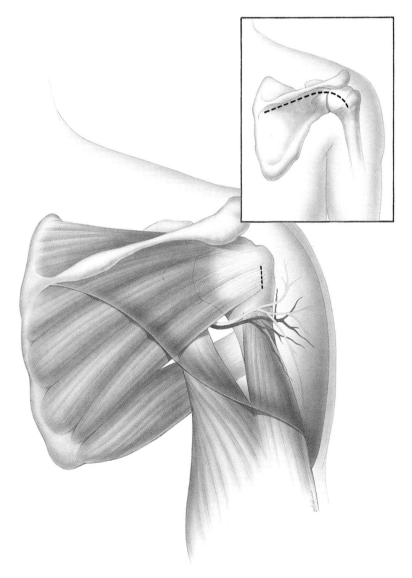

Figure 6.22. A skin incision is made parallel and just below the entire length of the scapular spine and then curved downward at the lateral border of the incision over the humerus.

layer. Hemostasis is obtained with electrocautery. The deltoid is identified, and the fascia overlying it is opened at the inferolateral border and directed superomedially. In a large individual, a portion of the deltoid may be elevated from the scapular spine if greater exposure of the quadrilateral space is needed. The entire deltoid muscle flap is retracted superiorly with its neurovascular bundle intact. The teres minor is detached at its insertion into the rotator cuff and reflected medially, allowing demonstration of the small portion of the posterior glenohumeral joint capsule (Fig. 6.23).

The quadrilateral space is then decompressed by blunt and sharp dissection. Fibrous bands that are encountered traversing the space are removed. Neurovascular structures are protected. Cormier et al. (8) and Cahill and Palmer (4) recommend elevation of the arm while palpating the posterior humeral circumflex artery to test the pulse to determine whether adequate decompression has been accomplished. Thereafter, the teres minor is allowed to remain retracted and is not reattached over the quadrilateral space. This does not weaken the external rotators in any significant way. If a small rent ap-

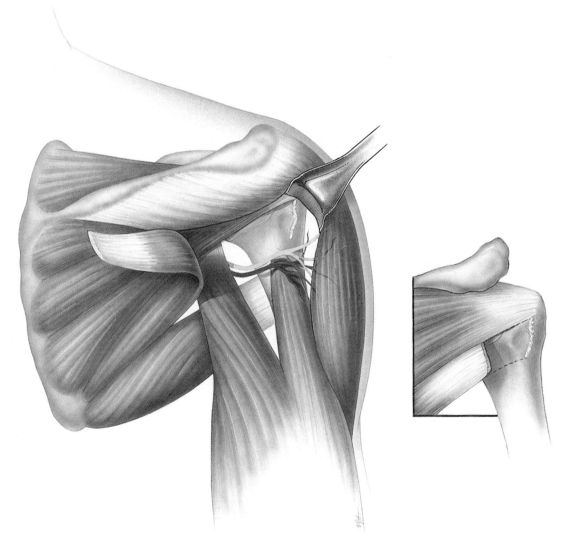

Figure 6.23.   The teres minor is detached at its insertion into the rotator cuff and reflected medially, allowing demonstration of the small portion of the posterior glenohumeral joint capsule.

pears in the posterior capsule after the teres minor is retracted, it is not closed. The deltoid is reapproximated to the spine with no. 2 nonabsorbable sutures placed through four or five drill holes in the spine, if it has been elevated. The arm is placed in a sling for 2 to 10 days. Gentle pendulum exercises are started when pain subsides for several days. Gentle passive and active assistive exercises are begun thereafter. After 6 weeks, gentle progressive muscle resistance exercises are performed as tolerated.

REFERENCES

1. Bigliani LU, Perez-Sanz JR, Wolfe IN. Treatment of trapezius paralysis. J Bone Joint Surg 1985;67A:871–877.
2. Bigliani LU, Compito CA, Duralde XA, et al. Levator scapulae and rhomboid transer for trapezius paralysis. J Bone Joint Surg 1996;78A(10):1534–1540.
3. Brunnstrom S. Muscle testing around the shoulder girdle: a study of the function of shoulder blade fixators in seventeen cases of shoulder paralysis. J Bone Joint Surg 1941;23:253–272.
4. Cahill BR. Palmer RE. Quadrilateral space syndrome. J Hand Surg 1983;8:65–69.
5. Chaves JP. Pectoralis minor transplant for paralysis of the serratus anterior. J Bone Joint Surg 1951;33B:228–230.
6. Clein LJ. Suprascapular entrapment neuropathy. J Neurosurg 1975;43(3): 337–342.
7. Codman EA. The shoulder. Rupture of the supraspinatus tendon and other lesions in or about the subacromial bursa. Boston: Thomas Todd, 1934.
8. Cormier PJ, Matalon TA, Wolin PM. Quadrilateral space syndrome: a rare cause of shoulder pain. Radiology 1988;167:797–798.
9. Dewar FP, Harris RI. Restoration of function of the shoulder following paralysis of the trapezius by fascial sling fixation and transplantation of the levator scapulae. Ann Surg 1950;132:1111–1115.
10. Dickson FD. Fascial transplants in paralytic and other conditions. J Bone Joint Surg 1937;19:405–412.
11. Durman DC. An operation for paralysis of the serratus anterior. J Bone Joint Surg 1945;27:380–382.
12. Fery A. Results of treatment of anterior serratus paralysis. In: Post M, Morrey BF, Hawkins TR, eds. Surgery of the shoulder. St. Louis: Mosby-Yearbook, 1990: 325–329.
13. Fery A, Sommelet M. Serratus anterior paralysis—results of treatment of twelve cases and review of the literature. French J Orthop Surg 1987;1:168–179.
14. Foo CL, Swann M. Isolated paralysis of the serratus anterior: a report of 20 cases. J Bone Joint Surg 1983;65B:552–556.
15. Gozna ER, Harris WR. Traumatic winging of the scapula. J Bone Joint Surg 1979; 61A:1230–1233.
16. Gregg JR, Labosky D, Harty M, et al. Serratus anterior paralysis in the young athlete. J Bone Joint Surg 1979;61A:825–832.
17. Hansson KG. Serratus magnus-paralysis. Arch Phys Med 1948;29:156–161.
18. Hass J. Muskelplastik bei serratuslahmung. Orthop Chir 1931;55:617–622.
19. Herzmark MD. Traumatic paralysis of the serratus anterior relieved by transplantation of the rhomboidei. J Bone Joint Surg 1951;33A:235–238.
20. Horwitz MT, Tocantins LM. An anatomical study of the role of the long thoracic nerve and the related scapular bursae in the pathogenesis of local paralysis of the serratus anterior muscle. Anat Rec 1938;71:375–385.
21. Horwitz MT, Tocantins LM. Isolated paralysis of the serratus anterior (magnus) muscle. J Bone Joint Surg 1938;20:720–725.
22. Iceton J, Harris WR. Results of pectoralis major transfer for winged scapula. J Bone Joint Surg 1985;67B:327.

23. Inman VT, Saunders JB, Dec M, et al. Observations on the function of the shoulder joint. J Bone Joint Surg 1944;26:1–30.

24. Johnson JT, Kendall HO. Isolated paralysis of the serratus anterior muscle. J Bone Joint Surg 1955;37A:567–574.

25. Kauppila LI. The long thoracic nerve: possible mechanisms of injury based on autopsy study. J Shoulder Elbow Surg 1993;2:244–248.

26. Ketenjian AY. Scapulocostal stabilization for scapular winging in fascioscapulohumeral muscular dystrophy. J Bone Joint Surg 1978;60A:691–695.

27. Khalili AA. Neuromuscular electrodiagnostic studies in entrapment neuropathy of the suprascapular nerve. Orthop Rev 1974;3:27.

28. Kopell HP, Thompson WAL. Peripheral entrapment neuropathies. Baltimore: Williams & Wilkins, 1963:131.

29. Kraft G. Axillary, musculocutaneous and suprascapular nerve latency studies. Arch Phys Med Rehabil 1972;53:383–387.

30. Lange M. Die behandlung der irreparablem trapeziuslahmung. Langenbecks Arch Klin Chir 1951;270:437–439.

31. Lange M. Die operative behandlung der irreparablem trapeziuslahmung. TIP Fakult Mecmuasi 1959;22:137–141.

32. Langenskiold A, Ryoppy S. Treatment of paralysis of the trapezius muscle by the Eden-Lange operation. Acta Orthop Scand 1973;44:383–388.

33. Lowman CL. The relationship of the abdominal muscles to paralytic scoliosis. J Bone Joint Surg 1932;14:763–772.

34. Marmor L, Bechtol CO. Paralysis of the serratus anterior due to electric shock relieved by transplantation of the pectoralis major muscle: a case report. J Bone Joint Surg 1963;45A:156–160.

35. Mayer L. Operative reconstruction of the paralyzed upper extremity. J Bone Joint Surg 1939;21:377–383.

36. Mayfield FH, True CW. Chronic injuries to peripheral nerves by entrapment. In: Youmans J, ed. Neurological surgery. Philadelphia: WB Saunders, 1973:1158–1159.

37. Mayr H. Trapeziuslahmung nach operativer behandlung tuberkuloser halslymphdrusen. Munchneer Med Wochenschr 1953;95:170–172.

38. Murray JW. A surgical approach for entrapment neuropathy of the suprascapular nerve. Orthop Rev 1975;3:33.

39. Osterhaus K. Obstetrical paralysis: a preliminary report of 2 cases. N Y Med J 1908;88:887–891.

40. Parsonage MJ, Turner JW. Neuralgic amyotrophy. the shoulder girdle syndrome. Lancet 1948;:973–978.

41. Post M. Physical examination of the shoulder girdle. In: Post M, ed. Physical examination of the musculoskeletal system. Philadelphia: Lea & Febiger, 1987: 13–55.

42. Post M. Miscellaneous painful conditions of the shoulder. In: Post M, ed. The shoulder—surgical and nonsurgical treatment. Philadelphia: Lea & Febiger, 1988: 345–347.

43. Post M. Orthopaedic management of neuromuscular disorders. In: Post M, ed. The shoulder—surgical and nonsurgical treatment. Philadelphia: Lea & Febiger, 1988:187.

44. Post M. Pectoralis major transfer. J Shoulder Elbow Surg 1995;4:1–9.

45. Post M, Grinblat E. Suprascapular nerve entrapment: diagnosis and results of treatment. J Shoulder Elbow Surg 1993;2:190–197.

46. Post M, Mayer J. Suprascapular nerve entrapment: diagnosis and treatment. Clin Orthop 1987;223:126–136.

47. Rapp IH. Serratus anterior paralysis treated by transplantation of the pectoralis minor. J Bone Joint Surg 1954;36A:852–854.

48. Reeder MR, Ruland LJ, McCue FC. Quadrilateral space syndrome in a throwing athlete. Am J Sports Med 1986;14:511–513.

49. Rengachary SS, Burr D, Lucas S, et al. Suprascapular entrapment neuropathy: a clinical, anatomical and comparative study. part 2: anatomical study. Neurosurgery 1979;5(4):447–451.

50. Rengachary SS, Neff MP, Singer PA, et al. Suprascapular entrapment neuropathy: a clinical, anatomical, and comparative study. part 1: clinical study. Neurosurgery 1979;5(4):441–446.

51. Rose DL, Kelly CR. Shoulder pain: suprascapular nerve block in shoulder pain. J Kansas Med Soc 1969;70:135.

52. Schottstaedt ER, Larsen LJ, Bost FC. The surgical reconstruction of the upper extremity paralyzed by poliomyelitis. J Bone Joint Surg 1958;40A:633–643.

53. Seddon JH. Symposium on reconstructive surgery of the paralysed upper limb. Proc R Soc Med 1949;42:831–838.

54. Solheim LF, Roaas A. Compression of the suprascapular nerve after fracture of the scapular notch. Acta Orthop Scand 1978;49:338–340.

55. Spira E. The treatment of dropped shoulder: a new operative technique. J Bone Joint Surg 1948;30A:229–233.

56. Steindler A. Tendon transplantation in the upper extremity. Am J Surg 1939;44:26–27.

57. Steindler A. Orthopedic operations. Springfield, IL: Charles C. Thomas, 1940.

58. Steindler A. The traumatic deformities and disabilities of the upper extremity. Springfield, IL: Charles C. Thomas, 1946.

59. Tubby AH. A case illustrating the operative treatment of paralysis of the serratus magnus muscle by muscle grafting. Br Med J 1904;2:1159–1160.

60. Velpeau AM. Luxations de l epaule. Arch Gen Med 1837;14:269–305.

61. Winslow M. Sur quelques mouvements extraordinaires des omoplates et des bras, et sur une nouvelle espece de muscles. Mem Acad Royale Sci 1723:98–112.

62. Whitman A. Congenital elevation of the scapula and paralysis of serratus magnus muscle. JAMA 1932;99:1332–1334.

63. Wolf J. The conservative treatment of serratus palsy. J Bone Joint Surg 1941;23:959–961.

64. Yamaguchi K, Connor PM, Manifold SG, et al. Split pectoralis major transfer for serratus anterior palsy. Presented at the American Shoulder and Elbow Surgeon's Annual Open Conference, Atlanta, Georgia, February 26, 1996.

65. Zoltan JD. Injury to the suprascapular nerve associated with anterior dislocation of the shoulder: case report and review of the literature. J Trauma 1979;19:203–206.

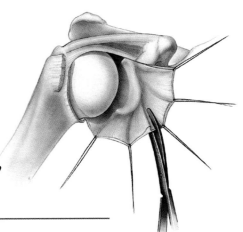

Acromioclavicular Joint, Clavicle, and Sternoclavicular Joint

R O G E R   G .   P O L L O C K

Introduction

Most shoulder problems involve either the glenohumeral joint or the subacromial articulation. Thus, many of the procedures described in this chapter are addressed at reconstruction or repair of the structures comprising these articulations. However, the shoulder complex is additionally composed of the acromioclavicular, sternoclavicular, and scapulothoracic articulations. Although disorders at these articulations do not commonly require surgical intervention, problems do occur and interfere with the smooth functioning of the shoulder complex. This chapter describes the surgical management of disorders involving the acromioclavicular joint, the clavicle, and the sternoclavicular joint.

Acromioclavicular Joint

The acromioclavicular (AC) joint is a diarthrodial joint, the articular surfaces of which are covered by fibrocartilage. As DePalma (31) has pointed out, this joint has variable inclination, ranging from near vertical to angled downward medially up to 50°. A fibrocartilaginous disc is contained in the joint, which undergoes degeneration with advancing age and the function of which is not well understood. Of major structural significance are the ligaments stabilizing the AC joint: the AC ligaments and the coracoclavicular ligaments. The AC ligaments are credited chiefly with stabilizing the joint against posterior displacement of the clavicle, whereas the coracoclavicular ligaments are the primary stabilizers against superior translations and axial compression (40). Finally, the fibers of the deltoid and trapezius muscles blend with the AC ligaments to add further stability to the joint.

Disorders of the AC joint requiring surgical treatment can be divided into two types: those in which the joint is stable (i.e., degenerative disorders) and those in which joint stability has been compromised (usually traumatic disorders). When a stable AC joint has become painful due to arthritis or to osteolysis of the distal clavicle (Fig. 7.1) and nonoperative treatment has been unsuccessful, then excision of the distal clavicle is the surgical treatment of

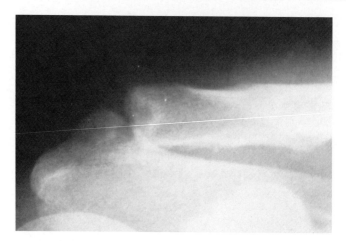

Figure 7.1. Anteroposterior radiograph demonstrates cystic changes of the distal clavicle consistent with osteolysis in a young male weight-lifter.

choice. As will be described, this can be performed using open, modified open, or arthroscopic means. On the other hand, when the stability of the joint has been compromised by ligamentous injury, then the operative treatment of the painful AC joint will involve reconstruction rather than excision alone.

EXCISION OF THE DISTAL CLAVICLE

In 1941, Gurd (47) and Mumford (60) independently described their results with excision of the distal clavicle for treating symptomatic AC injuries. Whereas Gurd originally recommended this procedure for treating a symptomatic complete AC separation, Rockwood (78) has pointed out that excision alone in the setting of ligamentous disruption can allow for posterior abutment of the remaining posterior clavicular stump against the base of the acromion. Thus, excision of the distal clavicle is reserved for disorders in which the AC joint is painful and stable. The most common diagnoses amenable to treatment by distal clavicle excision are degenerative arthritis, posttraumatic arthritis after intraarticular clavicle fractures, and osteolysis of the distal clavicle after the failure of nonoperative treatments (e.g., nonsteroidal antiinflammatory medications and intraarticular cortisone injections).

   Diagnosis of these disorders requires careful clinical and radiographic assessment. Pain is usually well-localized to the superior aspect of the shoulder (over the AC joint) but may radiate to the trapezial region. Symptoms are often increased with activities that result in compression of the AC joint, such as weight-lifting or lying on the affected shoulder. On examination, there is tenderness with palpation directly over the AC joint. Symptoms are usually reproduced with adduction (especially with the arm flexed to 90°) and with internal rotation of the shoulder (with the hand reaching posteriorly up the back). In addition to standard shoulder radiographs, specific assessment is made with anteroposterior radiographs of the AC joint with and without a 10° cephalic tilt using reduced penetration (so-called "soft tissue" technique). This technique provides the best visualization of the distal clavicle and demonstrates subtle changes, such as small cysts in the distal clavicle. The radiographs allow for more precise diagnosis of the specific disorder (osteoarthritis versus osteolysis). However, the radiographic findings may be normal even though the joint is quite symptomatic. An intraarticular injection of local anesthetic (2 to 3 mL 1% lidocaine) allows for confirmation that the AC joint is the source of the patient's symptoms. Complete elimination of symptoms within several minutes of injection provides strong evidence that the pathology is localized to the AC joint.

Traditionally, distal clavicle excision had been performed by open means. Satisfactory results have been reported with this procedure for patients with degenerative arthritis and osteolysis of the AC joint in a number of series (22, 24, 46, 61, 70, 75, 100). More recently, arthroscopic approaches to the AC joint have been introduced to perform excision of the distal clavicle (15, 37, 38, 42, 43, 50, 51, 85). The arthroscopic procedure may be performed using a bursal approach, in which the distal clavicle is viewed from the subacromial bursa (15, 42, 43, 50, 51, 85). This is the author's favored approach when the distal clavicle is excised in conjunction with the performance of an anterior acromioplasty, such as in patients with both subacromial impingement and AC symptoms. Alternatively, when pathology is isolated to the AC joint, the author prefers to perform the arthroscopic excision through direct anterior and posterior superior portals, which allow direct visualization of the joint surfaces without violation of uninvolved structures (15, 37, 38, 50). Both open and arthroscopic procedures for resecting the distal clavicle have had high degrees of success when performed in the context of a stable AC joint.

As suggested above, distal clavicle excision may also be performed as part of another procedure, such as in rotator cuff surgery. As Neer (64, 66) pointed out, inferior osteophytes on the clavicle may encroach on the subacromial space and contribute to impingement symptoms. In this situation, these undersurface osteophytes are removed as part of the decompression procedure in conjunction with an anterior acromioplasty, performed by either arthroscopic or open technique. However, when the AC joint is tender preoperatively and demonstrates degenerative changes radiographically, a formal distal clavicle excision is also performed. This can be accomplished either as part of an open acromioplasty procedure or as described above, using a subacromial bursal arthroscopic approach. More recently, in cases of larger rotator cuff tears in which open surgery is performed, the author has preferred to excise the distal clavicle using a power burr from beneath the joint, a technique adapted from arthroscopic experience. In this way, using the modified open technique, the distal clavicle can be resected while leaving the posterior and superior AC capsule intact. Thus, although formal distal clavicle excision is necessary in only 10 to 15% of patients undergoing surgery for rotator cuff problems who have symptoms referable to the AC joint and not merely radiographic changes, in these patients there are several options for performing this excision, depending on the surgical approach chosen for dealing with the subacromial pathology.

Open Technique

A 6- to 7-cm incision is made in the skin lines over the AC joint (Fig. 7.2A). Using electrocautery, the subcutaneous tissue is widely undermined to expose the AC joint and distal clavicle. The joint capsule and deltotrapezial fascia are incised longitudinally (parallel to the axis of the clavicle) to expose the distal clavicle (Fig. 7.2B). The electrocautery and a sharp elevator are used to carefully dissect the soft tissues off the distal clavicle both anteriorly and posteriorly. Blunt (Darrach) elevators are used to protect the deltoid flap anteriorly and the trapezial flap posteriorly, and an osteotome or microsagittal saw is used to resect 1 to 2 cm of the distal clavicle (Fig. 7.2C). Care is taken to create a smooth edge, and slightly more bone is resected superiorly and posteriorly to prevent later abutment. The coraco-clavicular ligaments are left intact, as the resection is carried out lateral to their insertion on the undersurface of the clavicle. The deltoid and trapezial flaps are then reapproximated using interrupted, nonabsorbable sutures, thus closing the dead space created by the bony resection (Fig. 7.2D). The skin is closed using a continuous subcuticular suture. Postoperatively, a sling is used for 4 to 6 weeks to allow for healing of the deltoid. Passive motion is begun on the first postoperative day.

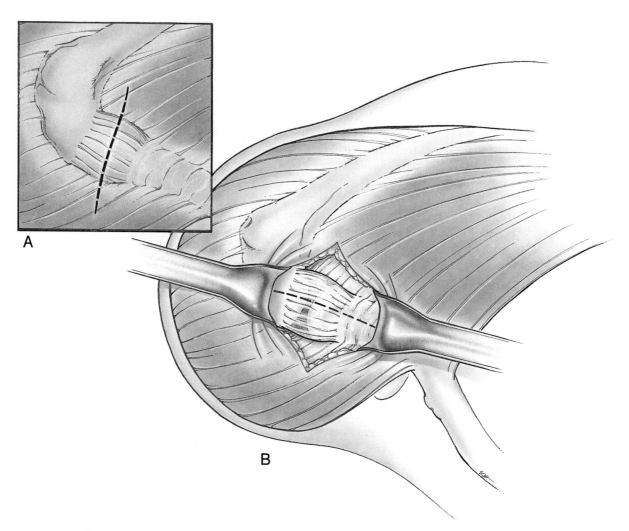

Figure 7.2. Open distal clavicle excision. **(A)** The skin incision is made in the skin lines over the AC joint and measures approximately 5 cm. **(B)** After widely undermining the subcutaneous flaps, the deltopectoral fascia is split along the long axis of the clavicle. The split starts at the AC joint and extends for 3 to 4 cm.

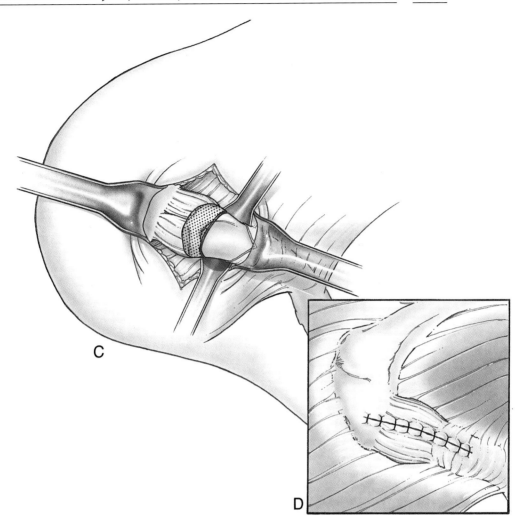

Figure 7.2. **(C)** After carefully dissecting the distal clavicle in subperiosteal fashion, a microsagittal saw is used to excise approximately 2 cm of the distal clavicle. **(D)** The deltotrapezial fascial flaps are carefully closed using zero nonabsorbable sutures.

Arthroscopic Techniques

Direct Superior Approach

In the direct superior approach, the arthroscope and instruments are placed into the AC joint through anterosuperior and posterosuperior portals (Fig. 7.3). The patient is in the beach-chair position, and the procedure is performed under regional anesthesia (interscalene block). The bony anatomic landmarks, namely the distal clavicle and acromion, are outlined on the skin with a marking pen. It is crucial to make a precise determination of the joint location before creating the portals. To assist in joint localization, three 22-gauge needles are useful: one placed anteriorly into the joint at the site of the proposed anterosuperior portal, one placed posteriorly into the joint at the site of the posterosuperior portal, and the final one directly in the center of the joint. In this manner, the joint location and its inclination can be better appreciated. The joint is insufflated with normal saline, and the proposed

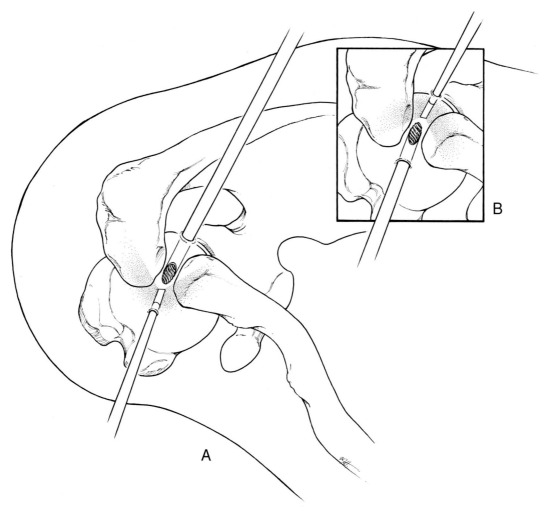

Figure 7.3. **(A,B)** Direct superior approach. For cases involving distal clavicle excision alone, direct anterosuperior and posterosuperior portals can be used to perform the arthroscopic excision. This eliminates the need to violate the subacromial bursa.

portal sites are injected using 1% lidocaine with epinephrine to minimize skin bleeding.

The anterosuperior portal is created in line with the AC joint and 0.75 cm anterior to it, using an 11-blade scalpel to incise the skin and pierce the joint capsule. Similarly, the posterosuperior portal is made in line with the joint and 0.75 cm posterior to it. Initially, if the AC joint is quite narrow, the 2.7-mm (wrist) arthroscope is used to start the procedure, placing it into the AC joint through the anterosuperior portal. A small motorized resector (2 or 3.5 mm) placed into the posterosuperior portal can begin the resection of the meniscal remnant and joint debris, thus better exposing the articular surfaces. Normal saline with epinephrine (1:300,000 units concentration) is used for irrigation during the procedure. A small burr (2 or 3.5 mm) is then used to start the bony resection of the distal clavicle, widening the joint space sufficiently to allow the insertion of the standard 4-mm arthroscope.

The 4-mm arthroscope affords a panoramic view of the entire distal clavicle. Electrocautery is helpful both in maintaining hemostasis and also in subperiosteally releasing the ligamentous envelope from the distal clavicle.

Starting at the 12 o'clock position and proceeding in circular fashion, the electrocautery shells out the distal clavicle while preserving the roof and the floor provided by the AC ligaments. This allows excellent visualization of the distal clavicle and allows for a precise, even resection of bone. A larger burr is then used to complete the resection of the distal clavicle. The arthroscope is switched to the posterosuperior portal and the burr to the anterosuperior portal to allow for access to the most anterior corner of the clavicle and to prevent leaving any ridges of bone. A probe may be placed into the joint and used to palpate the periphery of the resected clavicle under direct visualization to assure that there are no retained bony ridges. Because the arthroscopic procedure maintains the integrity of the surrounding ligamentous envelope, the author has found that it is only necessary to remove 5 to 7 mm of the distal clavicle as long as the resection is performed evenly (Fig. 7.4). Final beveling of the bone surface can be performed with a manual arthroscopic rasp. A meniscal resector is used to remove any remaining bony or soft tissue debris. The arthroscopic portals are closed in subcuticular fashion with absorbable sutures.

Postoperatively, the patient wears a sling for comfort for 1 or 2 days. Because the deltoid origin has not been detached, active use may be started as soon as comfort allows. Early emphasis is on regaining full range of motion, followed by strengthening and a return to heavy activities. Flatow et al. (38) have reported satisfactory results using this technique in patients with isolated osteoarthritis or osteolysis of the distal clavicle, situations in which the AC joint is stable. However, the author has seen less satisfactory results in patients with low-grade clavicular instability, such as after a Type II AC separation, or in patients with hypermobility of the AC joint in association with generalized ligamentous laxity. In these situations, an open excision with stabilization of the distal clavicle using a transfer of the coracoacromial ligament may be more appropriate to prevent pain due to residual instability.

Bursal Approach

This procedure for distal clavicle excision is preferred when the clavicular resection is being performed in conjunction with a subacromial procedure,

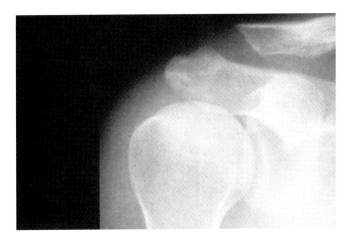

Figure 7.4. Postoperative radiograph after arthroscopic distal clavicle excision. Note that only 5 to 7 mm of bone are resected as the ligamentous envelope is preserved around the AC joint.

such as an arthroscopic anterior acromioplasty. The arthroscopic acromioplasty is carried out through anterolateral and posterolateral subacromial portals, as previously described in Chapter 4. Resection of the undersurface of the medial or clavicular facet of the acromion will afford better visualization of and access to the distal clavicle. The electrocautery and meniscal resector are used to remove the fat pad at the undersurface of the AC joint. Because this tissue can be rather vascular, the electrocautery is particularly helpful in maintaining hemostasis. The joint capsule inferiorly is also resected to expose the distal clavicle for resection. Working with the arthroplasty burr in the anterolateral subacromial portal, the distal clavicle resection is begun (Fig. 7.5A). An assistant pushes downward over the distal clavicle, thus bringing more of the clavicle into the field of view. Although the entire procedure

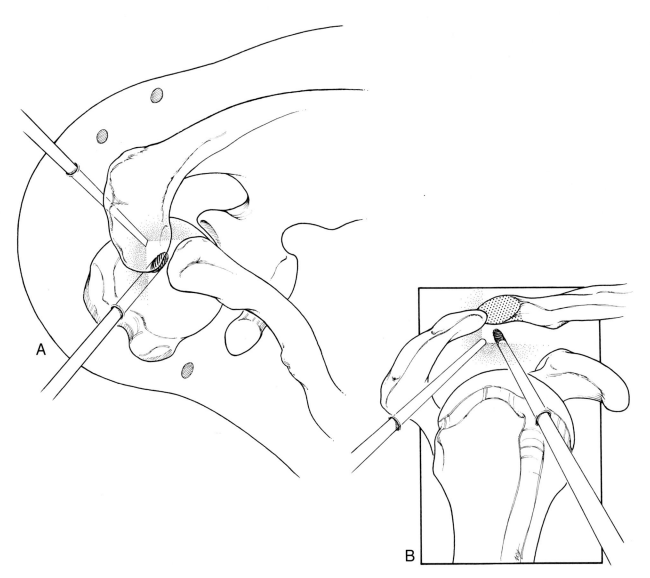

Figure 7.5. **(A,B)** Bursal approach. The distal clavicle can be arthroscopically resected using the anterolateral and posterolateral subacromial portals. This is usually the method chosen for distal clavicle excision in cases in which an arthroscopic anterior acromioplasty is also performed. A direct anterosuperior portal can be added to complete the distal clavicle excision and to view the resection directly from inside the AC joint.

can be performed through the subacromial portals, the author usually prefers to create one direct superior portal to complete the resection (Fig. 7.5B). The arthroplasty burr is placed into this superior portal, and visualization continues through the subacromial portal. This allows for easier access to the superior portion of the distal clavicle and particularly to the posterosuperior region, where ridges may be left due to inadequate visualization from below. As described above, the electrocautery is used to peel the capsule subperiosteally off the distal clavicle to facilitate the bony excision. The arthroscope can then be placed directly into the AC joint through the superior portal to assess the adequacy of the resection from another perspective. As described in the previous section on excision from a direct superior approach, a manual arthroplasty rasp is used through the superior portal to perform the final bony contouring. Remaining bony and soft tissue debris are removed with the resector, and the portals are closed in subcuticular fashion with absorbable sutures.

Postoperatively, the patient wears a sling for 1 or 2 days for comfort. Range of motion exercises are begun on the first postoperative day to prevent stiffness, and light active use of the arm is permitted, as previously described for the rehabilitation after arthroscopic acromioplasty.

Modified Open Technique

In patients undergoing open rotator cuff surgery, if the AC joint is also symptomatic preoperatively due to degenerative arthritis, then a concomitant distal clavicle excision will also be performed at the time of anterior acromioplasty and rotator cuff repair. Recently, the author has preferred to perform this resection using a modified open approach, in which a burr is placed into the joint from below and used to excise 5 to 10 mm of the distal clavicle. This technique allows for preservation of the superior and posterior joint capsule, theoretically causing less disruption of AC stability. It is thus an application of an arthroscopic technique to open rotator cuff surgery.

In this technique, after the anterior acromioplasty has been performed, attention is directed toward the AC joint. A small curette is placed into the joint from below to define the location and inclination of the joint as well as to remove soft tissue and any remaining cartilage on the distal clavicle. If there is any doubt about the location of the joint, the AC joint capsule can be incised anteriorly, but the integrity of the superior and posterior ligaments is maintained. After the joint orientation has been assessed and the remaining soft tissues have been removed, an oval arthroplasty burr is placed into the AC joint from below and used to perform the bony resection (Fig. 7.6). To assess the adequacy of the resection, the surgeon's index finger can be placed into the AC joint from below, and the arm can be adducted. Resection of 5 to 10 mm of bone is usually all that is required to prevent impingement of the surgeon's finger when the arm is adducted. Thus, this technique allows for preservation of much of the ligamentous architecture and also avoids the cosmetic deformity that was once associated with excision of greater than 2 cm of the distal clavicle.

ACROMIOCLAVICULAR SEPARATION

The usual mechanism of AC separation is a fall onto the point of the shoulder with the arm in an adducted position. The clavicle is maintained in its

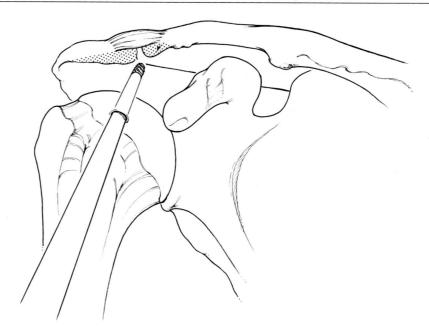

Figure 7.6.   Distal clavicle excision, modified open technique. A burr is used to resect the distal clavicle from below, leaving the superior AC ligaments intact.

anatomic position by the sternoclavicular ligaments and the action of the trapezius muscle, while the scapula is driven inferiorly, damaging the ligamentous structures that stabilize the AC joint and causing the scapula to droop. Traditionally, these injuries had been classified into three groups (Types I, II, and III) (3, 90). However, Rockwood has further subdivided the complete injuries (Type III) into three further groups (Type III, IV, and V) and has added a final, rare group (Type VI) to the classification system (77). These injuries are classified according to the relative displacement of the distal clavicle and the amount of damage to the AC capsular ligaments, the coracoclavicular ligaments, and the fascia of the deltoid and trapezius muscles. A Type I injury represents a sprain of the AC ligaments, and radiographic findings are normal. A Type II injury represents a tear of the AC ligament and a sprain of the coracoclavicular ligaments. Radiographs demonstrate widening of the AC joint but no significant increase in the coracoclavicular distance. In a Type III injury, both the AC and coracoclavicular ligaments are torn, with resulting dislocation of the joint. In addition, there is damage to the fascia of the deltoid and trapezius overlying the distal clavicle. Radiographically, the coracoclavicular distance is 25 to 100% greater than on the uninjured side (Fig. 7.7). A Type IV injury is similar to a Type III injury, but there is more significant posterior displacement of the distal clavicle through the trapezius, and the skin may even be tented (Fig. 7.8). A Type V injury includes the damage described in a Type III injury, but there is a greater degree of displacement of the clavicle toward the base of the neck. The coracoclavicular distance is 100 to 300% greater than on the uninjured side. Finally, the Type VI injury is a subcoracoid or subacromial dislocation of the distal clavicle and is exceedingly rare (44, 74).

The treatment of acute Type I and II AC injuries is nonoperative. Ice, analgesics, and immobilization in a sling for a short period are generally recommended, followed by gradual resumption of use as pain diminishes. The

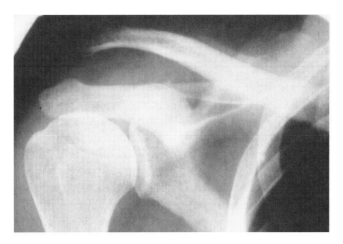

Figure 7.7. Anteroposterior radiograph demonstrates a Type III or complete AC separation. Both the AC and coracoclavicular ligaments are torn in this injury.

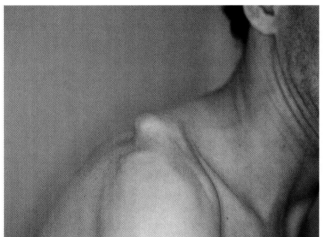

A

Figure 7.8. **(A,B)** Type IV AC separation with tenting of the skin posteriorly from displacement of the clavicle through the trapezial fascia.

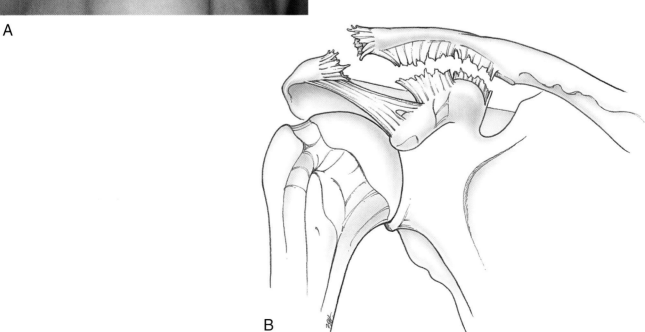

B

treatment of acute Type III separations, however, remains controversial, and there are proponents for both operative and nonoperative treatment. Many authors have reported satisfactory results with nonoperative treatment (4, 5, 26, 33, 88, 89, 92, 99), and a number of series comparing operative and nonoperative treatment have failed to demonstrate superior results after surgery (11, 41, 49, 56, 57, 81, 87, 93). Currently, the trend is toward nonoperative treatment of many of these injuries. Such treatment consists of accepting the deformity, using a sling for comfort in the early post-injury period, and then rehabilitating the shoulder with range of motion and strengthening exercises. The use of straps or splints to attempt to maintain a reduction is generally contraindicated, as they are usually ineffective and may cause breakdown of the skin overlying the clavicle.

However, some patients with Type III injuries will continue to have pain and loss of function after conservative treatment (29, 54, 99). In particular, young athletic patients and patients who perform heavy labor or overhead work are considered to be at a higher risk for failure of nonoperative treatment; the author will generally recommend operative stabilization for patients in these groups with Type III AC separations. In addition, operative stabilization is routinely recommended acutely for patients with more severe AC injuries (Types IV, V, and VI). In these cases, there is even more damage to the deltotrapezial aponeurosis, leading to greater deformity and instability.

Cooper (25) first reported on internal fixation of an AC dislocation in 1861. Since then, many methods of internal fixation have been used to treat these injuries. These have included transarticular pins or screws (9, 10, 16, 20, 57, 72, 76, 86, 87), coracoclavicular screws (11, 17, 41, 54, 81, 87, 91, 97), coracoclavicular wire or suture fixation (2, 6, 7, 12, 13, 17, 19, 34, 48, 66, 72, 76, 86, 91, 95, 97), coracoclavicular fixation with synthetic grafts (39, 45, 52, 73, 80), and transfer of the coracoid muscles to the clavicle (8, 14, 32, 35, 98). The author prefers using coracoclavicular fixation with heavy sutures (no. 5 Tevdek or Ethibond) because this avoids the use of metallic fixation, which can loosen, migrate, or break. Moreover, no additional surgical procedures are needed to retrieve hardware. Although late bone erosion has been reported with the use of synthetic grafts (such as Dacron arterial grafts) (39, 45), the author has not seen this with no. 5 sutures. Additionally, the author performs a transfer of the coracoacromial ligament to the distal clavicle (21, 53, 68, 96) (a modified Weaver-Dunn technique) in chronic cases (longer than 3 or 4 weeks from the time of injury), as well as an excision of 5 to 7 mm of the distal clavicle.

OPERATIVE TECHNIQUE FOR ACROMIOCLAVICULAR RECONSTRUCTION

The procedure (66, 96) is performed with the patient in the beach-chair position, and regional anesthesia (interscalene block) is usually used. A skin incision is made over the superior aspect of the shoulder from just posterior to the AC joint to the coracoid in the direction of the skin lines (Fig. 7.9A). The subcutaneous tissue is undermined, exposing the deltotrapezial fascia. The deltotrapezial fascia is then incised, starting at the AC joint and proceeding medially for approximately 5 cm. Because the clavicle has been displaced posteriorly relative to its normal position, this fascial incision will not lie over the middle of the clavicle (as this would incise the trapezial muscle belly), but somewhat anterior to this point (Fig. 7.9B). Using an electrocautery and a sharp elevator, the soft tissue flaps are carefully subperiosteally elevated off the distal clavicle both anteriorly and posteriorly. The AC meniscus is usually detached or torn and is excised. In chronic cases and often in acute cases in which there is osteochondral damage to the distal clavicle, a minimal distal clavicle resection (4 to 5 mm of bone) is performed using a microsagittal saw to prevent the later development of degenerative arthritis.

Starting at the AC joint, the anterior deltoid may be split in the direction of its fibers for a distance of 2 to 3 cm. This will afford access to the coracoacromial ligament, which is harvested at its insertion along the anterior aspect and undersurface of the anterior acromion. This ligament is tagged and later transferred to the distal clavicle in chronic cases of AC separation (longer than 3 or 4 weeks after injury) (Fig. 7.9C). The anteromedial flap of deltoid can then be gently retracted to gain access to the coracoid process.

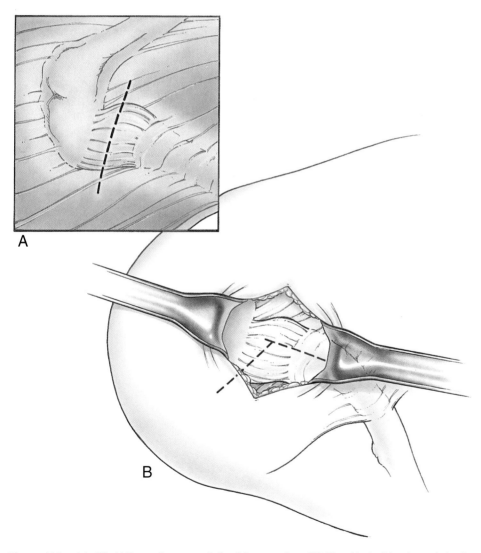

Figure 7.9.   Modified Weaver-Dunn repair for AC separation. **(A)** The skin incision is made in the skin lines over the superior aspect of the shoulder and measures approximately 7 cm. **(B)** The delto-trapezial fascia is split along the long axis of the clavicle, starting over the AC joint and proceeding medially for 4 for 5 cm. An L-shaped extension is used distally to split the deltoid to allow access to the coracoacromial ligament and the coracoid.   *(continued)*

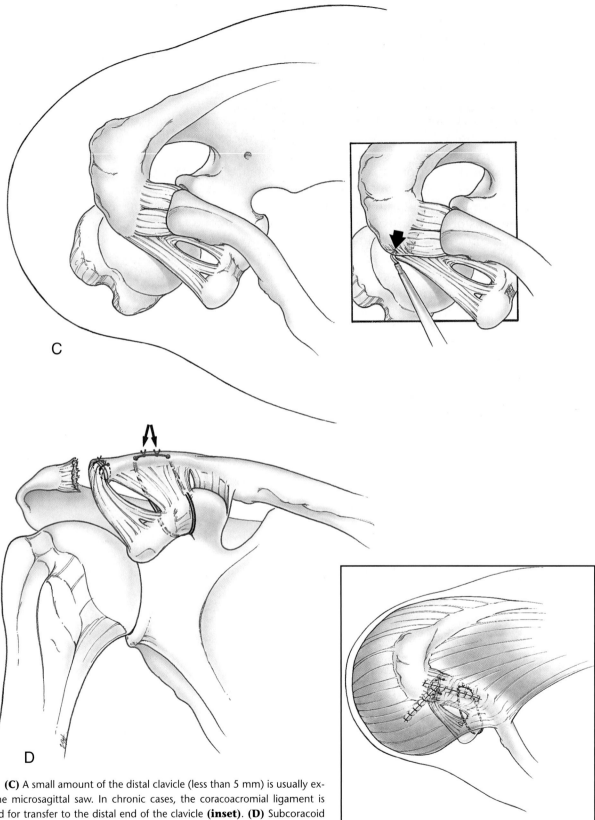

Figure 7.9. **(C)** A small amount of the distal clavicle (less than 5 mm) is usually excised using the microsagittal saw. In chronic cases, the coracoacromial ligament is then harvested for transfer to the distal end of the clavicle **(inset)**. **(D)** Subcoracoid fixation using several no. 5 braided nonabsorbable sutures (e.g., Tevdek) is used. The coracoacromial ligament is then transferred to the distal clavicle and repaired through drill holes in the clavicle using no. 2 nonabsorbable braided sutures. The deltoid split and deltotrapezial fascia are repaired with no. 1 braided nonabsorbable sutures **(inset).**

A large curved clamp (e.g., the type used in gallbladder surgery) is then passed around the coracoid process, starting medially, proceeding along the inferior surface of the coracoid, and exiting on the lateral aspect of the coracoid process. Two or three no. 5 nonabsorbable sutures are then passed around the coracoid using this clamp to accomplish subcoracoid fixation of the clavicle. Two small drill holes, spaced 1 cm apart, are placed in the middle of the clavicle at a point directly over the coracoid process. The ends of each of the sutures are then passed through these holes. Next, the distal clavicle is slightly overreduced by pushing directly down on it and also by pushing upward on the elbow while the sutures are snugly tied. Passing sutures through the clavicle in this manner, rather than simply passing them around the clavicle, prevents excessive anterior translation of the distal clavicle and eliminates concerns about transection of the clavicle from bone erosion by the sutures. The coracoacromial ligament, which has been harvested earlier (maintaining as much length as possible), is then transferred to the distal clavicle and secured using no. 2 nonabsorbable sutures passed through drill holes in the superior aspect of the distal clavicle (Fig. 7.9D). The deltotrapezial flaps are then carefully imbricated to add further stability, and the skin is closed with a continuous subcuticular suture.

Postoperatively, the shoulder is immobilized in a sling for 6 weeks, after which time range of motion exercises are begun. Resistive exercises are added 8 weeks after surgery. Patients are advised to avoid high-demand or contact activities for at least 6 to 9 months after surgery.

Most severe AC injuries that will require operative treatment can be satisfactorily reconstructed using this approach. In rare cases, in which the AC joint is dislocated and the coracoid is fractured, then obviously subcoracoid fixation cannot be achieved. In these unusual cases, reduction and transacromial pinning of the AC joint with heavy threaded Steinmann pins to prevent migration or breakage or, alternatively, open reduction and internal fixation of the coracoid fracture with screws, can be used.

Clavicle

The clavicle serves as an osseous strut between the scapula and the chest midline, maintaining the width of the shoulder. Biomechanically, it functions as a yoke system when the arm is carrying a weight, giving the muscles that elevate the clavicle and the scapula a fulcrum around the sternoclavicular joint to suspend the load at a distance from the midline (1, 36). Moreover, by spacing the shoulder complex, the clavicle acts as a lateral fulcrum for the muscles extending from the chest wall to the humerus, such as the pectoralis major (36). When the clavicle is fractured, these mechanisms are disrupted and the shoulder droops downward and forward.

FRACTURES OF THE CLAVICLE

Clavicle fractures are generally classified into three groups according to their location along the length of this bone. Fractures of the middle third of the clavicle are, by far, the most common, accounting for up to 80% of all clavicle fractures (Fig. 7.10) (65). These can be caused by either an indirect shearing force or a direct blow to the clavicle. Fractures of the lateral third of the

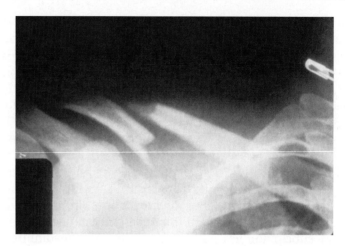

Figure 7.10. Anteroposterior radiograph of a fracture of the middle third of the clavicle. Most of these fractures are treated nonoperatively with a sling and heal uneventfully.

clavicle comprise approximately 15% of these injuries. They are usually the result of a direct blow to the point of the shoulder, similar to the mechanism for an AC separation. Neer (62, 63, 65) has further subdivided distal clavicle fractures into three types. Type I is a minimally displaced fracture. Type II is a displaced fracture in which the proximal fragment is detached from the coracoclavicular ligaments, which remain with the distal fragment. Type III is an intraarticular distal clavicle fracture. Medial third fractures are quite uncommon, accounting for only 5% of clavicle fractures and usually occur as a result of direct trauma.

Most clavicle fractures can be treated nonoperatively using some form of immobilization for the shoulder—a clavicular cast, figure-of-eight harness, or in most instances a simple sling. The indications for operative treatment of an acute clavicle fracture include the following: 1) neurovascular injury, 2) open fractures, 3) severe displacement with potential skin compromise (skin tenting), 4) a clavicle fracture in the context of multiple trauma, 5) segmental fractures with a rotated intermediate fragment, 6) severe deformity that is not cosmetically acceptable to the patient, and 7) many Type II distal fractures.

OPERATIVE TREATMENT OF MIDDLE THIRD CLAVICLE FRACTURES

The two major options for operative treatment of fractures of the middle third of the clavicle are intramedullary fixation with a Knowles or Steinmann pin (27, 69, 82) and fixation with a plate and screws (59). In the author's experience, the most common acute fracture pattern requiring operative treatment involves a segmental fragment with a small intermediate fragment, which is rotated 90° to the long axis of the clavicle (Fig. 7.11). Thus, the author prefers the use of fixation with a plate and screws and additional interfragmentary screw(s) as required to gain stable fixation. The use of weak semitubular plates has been avoided because of their higher rate of breakage. Instead, the author usually uses either a 3.5-mm reconstruction plate or a dynamic compression plate (Fig. 7.12). The reconstruction plate offers the advantage of being more malleable, making it easier to contour to the clavicle and allowing it to be less prominent on this subcutaneous bone than a dynamic compression plate. Bone grafting is usually reserved for the operative treatment of nonunions of the clavicle in conjunction with plate fixation.

With the patient in the beach-chair position and under general anesthesia, a vertical, lazy S-shaped incision is made in the skin lines, centered over the fracture site. This incision yields a more cosmetically acceptable scar than one directed transversely over the clavicle. Subcutaneous branches of the supraclavicular nerves are carefully dissected out and gently retracted out of harm's way. The deep fascia and muscle overlying the clavicle is split in a direction parallel to the long axis of the clavicle, using electrocautery to minimize bleeding. Meticulous subperiosteal dissection is undertaken with an elevator to expose the proximal and distal fragments (Fig. 7.13A). If there is a rotated intermediate segment, it is carefully retrieved, recognizing that this fragment may be pointed directly at the underlying neurovascular structures. The risk to the subclavian vessels increases with more medial fractures.

When the fracture fragments have been exposed and mobilized, they are manually reduced anatomically, and the reduction is maintained using at least two A-O bone clamps. One or two 3.5-mm interfragmentary cortical screws may be placed in lag fashion in an anteroposterior direction to provide initial fixation, if the fracture lines are directed obliquely. A reconstruction plate is contoured to the clavicle and is then affixed using 3.5-mm

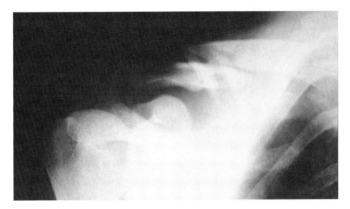

Figure 7.11. Segmental middle third fracture of the clavicle with a rotated intercalated fragment.

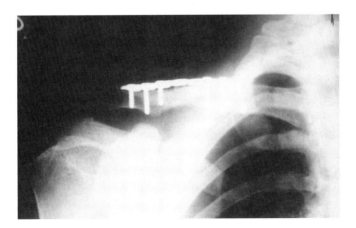

Figure 7.12. Postoperative radiograph of the segmental clavicle fracture pictured in Figure 7.11. Fixation was achieved using a 3.5-mm reconstruction plate and an additional interfragmentary screw.

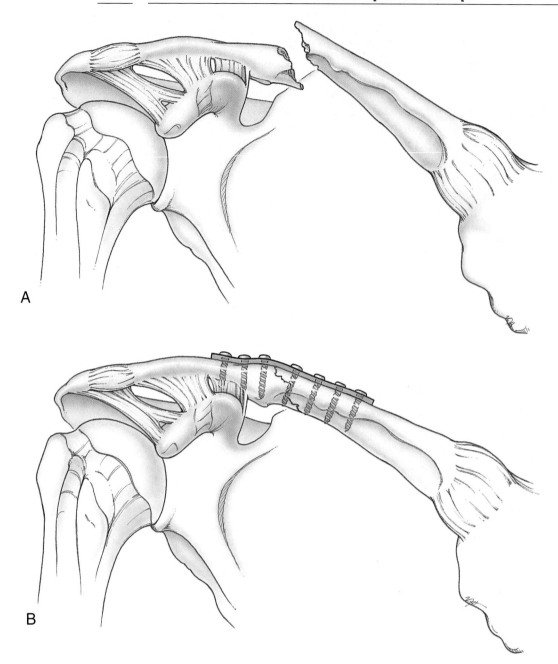

Figure 7.13. Technique of plate fixation for middle third clavicle fractures. **(A)** Meticulous subperiosteal dissection is used to expose the proximal and distal fragments. **(B)** Fixation is achieved with an A-O or reconstruction plate so that there are at least six cortices of fixation both proximal and distal to the fracture site. Bone grafting is used in cases of nonunion of middle third clavicle fractures.

bicortical screws. The length of the plate is chosen so that there will be at least six cortices of fixation both proximal and distal to the fracture (Fig. 7.13B). Small Bennett retractors are helpful in protecting inferiorly during drilling and screw placement. Quite stable fixation can be achieved in this manner. The deep tissues are reapproximated over the plate, and the skin is closed with a continuous subcuticular suture.

Postoperatively, the shoulder is immobilized in a sling until there are signs of clinical and radiographic healing, which usually occurs by 6 to 8 weeks. Range of motion exercises and light active use of the shoulder may be started after healing occurs. If the hardware is symptomatic or prominent, consideration may be given to plate removal 1 year after fracture healing. However, plate and screw removal will temporarily weaken the clavicle, and activity must be restricted afterward to reduce the risk of refracture.

OPERATIVE TREATMENT OF TYPE II DISTAL CLAVICLE FRACTURES

The author's operative technique for repairing Type II distal clavicle fractures is quite similar to the technique described for the reconstruction of AC separations. Functionally, the two injuries are somewhat analogous, in that the proximal segment in both injuries has been separated from the suspensory coracoclavicular ligaments, allowing the scapula to droop (Fig. 7.14). Subcoracoid fixation with heavy (no. 5) nonabsorbable sutures has proven quite effective in restoring the proximal clavicle fragment to its anatomic position, where it is held so that bony healing to the distal fragment (with the attached coracoclavicular ligaments) can occur (65, 66). The distal fragment is often not very large and may even be comminuted, thus making attempts at fixation with screws or plates and screws problematic. Moreover, the use of transacromial pins necessitates violation of the AC joint and can result in the development of later degenerative arthritis. The technique of subcoracoid fixation avoids these pitfalls and provides effective fixation for Type II distal clavicle fractures.

The procedure is performed with the patient in the beach-chair position. An incision is made in the skin lines over the superior aspect of the shoulder, starting over the fracture site and proceeding anteriorly to the coracoid (Fig. 7.15A). The deltotrapezial fascia is incised, starting over the fracture site and proceeding laterally a short distance, but especially medially for several centimeters to expose the displaced proximal fragment of the clavicle (Fig. 7.15B). The distal fragment will be located in its normal position with respect to the AC joint, and the coracoclavicular ligaments will be attached to its undersurface. Unless this distal fragment is very small with comminution extending into the articular surface (in which case excision may be considered), it is left undisturbed and the proximal fragment is brought down to it. Often, the fracture pattern in these distal fractures will be somewhat oblique, so that the proximal fragment can be brought down into a cancellous bed formed by the distal fragment. To hold the proximal fragment reduced, subcoracoid fixation is performed. The anterior soft tissue sleeve is elevated off the clavicle, so that access to the coracoid can be obtained. As in reconstructions of the AC separations, a large curved (gallbladder-type) clamp is then passed around the coracoid from its medial to lateral side. This clamp is used for passage of several no. 5 nonabsorbable sutures around the coracoid. Two drill holes are then placed in the clavicle, and one end of each suture is passed through each of these holes. The proximal fragment is then manually reduced, and the sutures are tied snugly, thus anchoring this fragment (Fig. 7.15C). Several nonabsorbable sutures (no. 5 or 2) can also be used to secure the proximal and distal fragments to each other. Occasionally, the distal fragment will be large enough to allow for an interfragmentary screw to be placed from the distal to the proximal fragment (Fig. 7.16). The deltotrapezial fascia is then repaired, and skin closure is carried out with a continuous subcuticular suture.

Postoperatively, the shoulder is immobilized for approximately 6 weeks to allow bony healing. The sling is then removed, and range of motion and later strengthening exercises are progressively implemented.

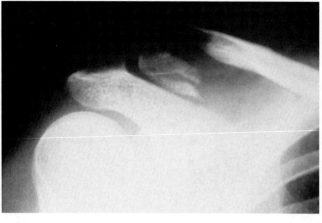

A

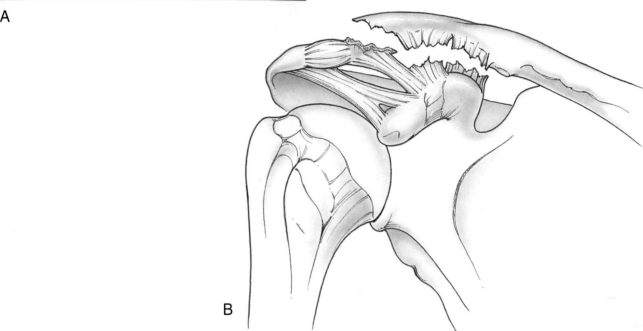

B

Figure 7.14. **(A)** Anteroposterior radiograph of a typical Type II distal clavicle fracture. The cora-coclavicular ligaments remain with the distal fragment (which is split into at least two pieces). The proximal fragment no longer has any attachment to the coracoclavicular ligaments. **(B)** Schematic of Type II distal clavicle fracture. When there is large displacement between the fragments, there is a significant risk of nonunion of this fracture, and operative treatment is usually considered.

Sternoclavicular Joint

The sternoclavicular (SC) joint is the only true joint that connects the upper extremity to the body. It is a diarthrodial joint with both articular surfaces covered by fibrocartilage. Half the medial end of the clavicle articulates with the sternum, and the other half forms a portion of the sternal notch. The SC joint is characterized by relative bony incongruity, relying on a number of surrounding ligaments for its stability (the intraarticular disc ligament, the costoclavicular ligament, the interclavicular ligament, and the anterior and posterior capsular ligaments) (36, 79). Due largely to this strong set of ligamentous stabilizers, the SC joint is rarely dislocated. In fact, symptomatic pathologic conditions involving the SC joint are much less common than

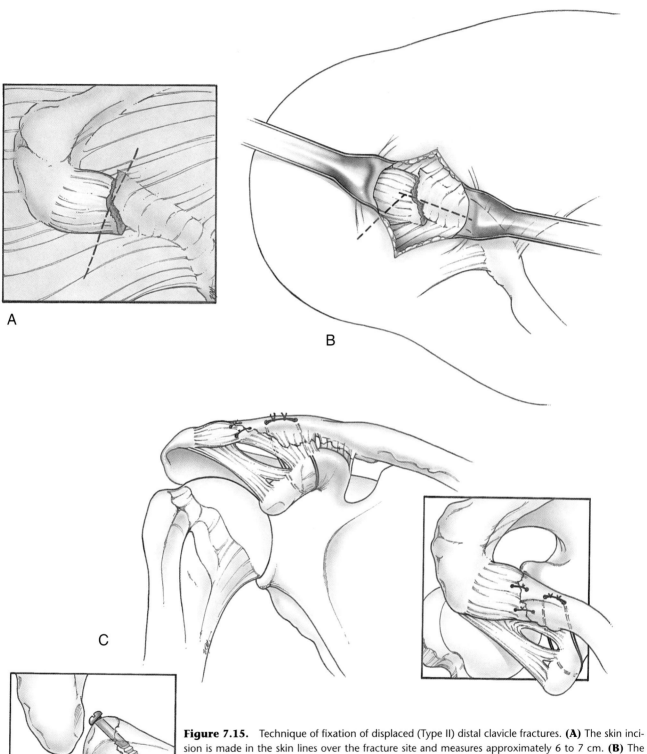

Figure 7.15. Technique of fixation of displaced (Type II) distal clavicle fractures. **(A)** The skin incision is made in the skin lines over the fracture site and measures approximately 6 to 7 cm. **(B)** The deltotrapezial fascia is split in its raphe along the long axis of the clavicle over the proximal fragment. An L-shaped fascial split into the deltoid is chosen to allow better access to the coracoid. Care is taken not to disrupt the ligamentous attachment to the distal fragment. **(C)** Subcoracoid fixation with several no. 5 nonabsorbable braided sutures passed through drill holes in the proximal fragment is achieved as this fragment is reduced down into the cancellous bed formed by the distal fragment. Additional sutures are passed from the distal to the proximal fragment, incorporating the coracoclavicular ligaments in the repair. **(D)** An interfragmentary screw can be used to augment the fixation when the distal fragment is large and not comminuted.

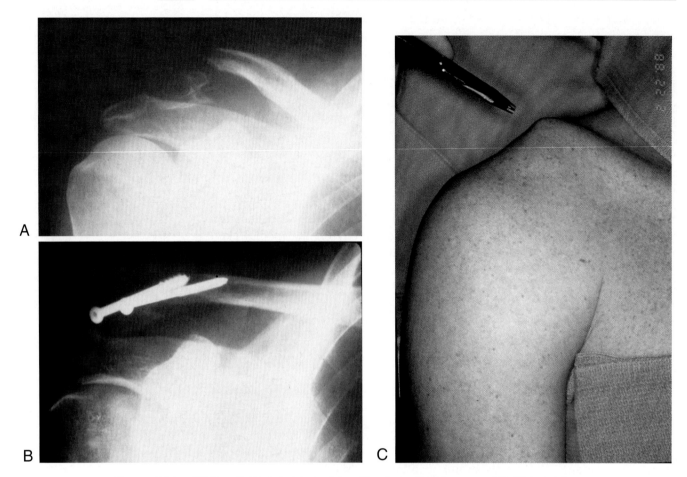

Figure 7.16. **(A)** Type II distal clavicle fracture with a large distal fragment. **(B)** Clinical deformity seen with these fractures resembles that seen with a complete AC separation. **(C)** Because the deltoid fragment is of good size and quality (i.e., not comminuted), screw fixation was used in this case.

those involving the other components of the shoulder complex. Similar to the AC joint, indications for operative treatment may include traumatic instability and degenerative arthritis, although these problems are seen much less frequently at the SC joint than the AC joint.

STERNOCLAVICULAR INSTABILITY

Sternoclavicular dislocations are uncommon but may occur with violent trauma, such as in motor vehicle accidents and contact sports (71, 79, 83, 94). They may occur in either an anterior or posterior direction, and anterior dislocations occur far more frequently. The mechanism for these injuries may be either a direct blow to the medial aspect of the clavicle or an indirect force to the lateral aspect of the shoulder. In the literature, greater attention has been paid to posterior dislocations because they may cause life-threatening injury to the trachea, lungs, and great vessels.

Clinically, a patient with a posterior SC dislocation may present with hoarseness, dysphagia, dyspnea, or venous congestion of the neck and upper extremity. On physical examination, the diagnosis of a posterior dislocation of the SC joint can be difficult to make. Anterior dislocations are more easily diagnosed on examination by the prominence of the medial end of the clavicle. The circulation and neurologic status of the extremity should always be assessed in a patient with a suspected SC dislocation. Anteroposterior radiographs can be difficult to interpret, and a 40° cephalic tilt view (79) and tomograms can be helpful. Computed tomography is also quite useful in assessing SC injuries, clarifying the bony abnormalities and the relationship of the trachea, esophagus, and subclavian vessels to the bony structures (Fig. 7.17). Computed tomography can also differentiate between a true SC dislocation and a displaced physeal fracture of the medial end of the clavicle (a pseudodislocation), which is seen in adolescents after trauma to the SC joint (Fig. 7.18) (18, 30).

Anterior SC dislocations are generally treated nonoperatively. An attempt at closed reduction may be made in an acute anterior SC dislocation by placing traction on the arm while pushing directly on the medial clavicle. However, it is difficult to maintain the reduction, and if redislocation occurs, the deformity is usually accepted and the shoulder is treated symptomatically. Operative attempts at stabilization of anterior SC dislocations have been marked by high complication rates, with serious morbidity resulting from mediastinal or even intracardiac migration of fixation pins (23, 28, 58, 67, 84).

Posterior SC dislocations may imperil the mediastinal structures, and closed reduction is indicated. The patient is placed supine with a bolster between the scapulae, and lateral traction is exerted on the abducted and extended arm. Further mechanical advantage may be gained by grasping the clavicle with a sterile towel clip and pulling anteriorly. A closed reduction that is stable can usually be obtained using these maneuvers. However, if the attempt at closed reduction is unsuccessful, then open reduction is undertaken. The patient is left in the supine position with the bolster between the scapulae posteriorly, and general anesthesia is administered. A 6-cm incision is made over the SC joint, parallel to the clavicle. Dissection is carried through the cervical fascia down to but not through the anterior joint capsule, which is preserved to provide stability once the reduction has been achieved. Again, a towel clip is placed directly on the clavicle, to reduce it by pulling anteriorly, as an assistant places traction on the extremity. Once the reduction has been achieved, it will usually be stable with the shoulders held back. If the anterior capsule is damaged or there is concern about the stability of the reduction, the clavicle can be secured to the sternum using no. 5

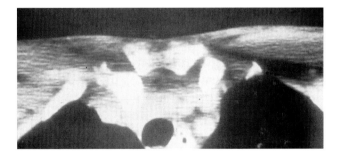

Figure 7.17. Computed tomography scan demonstrates a posterior SC dislocation. These can be life-threatening injuries because they may result in injury to or compression of the great vessels, trachea, and esophagus. A closed reduction should be attempted. If unsuccessful, open reduction should usually be used.

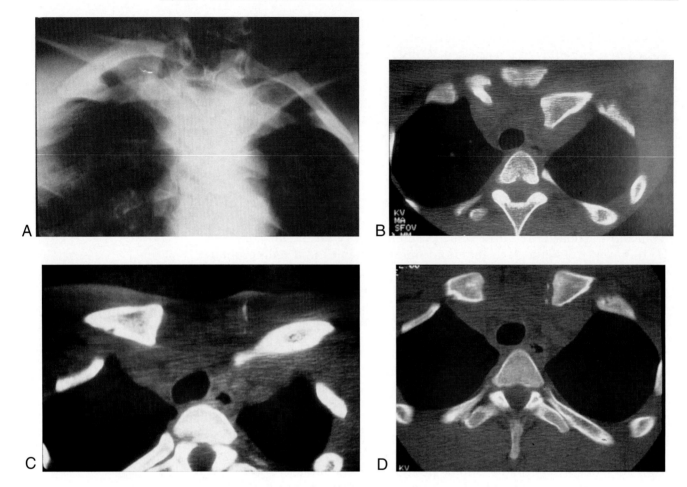

Figure 7.18.   Pseudodislocation of the SC joint. **(A)** Plain radiograph is suggestive of a SC dislocation in this adolescent patient. **(B)** Computed tomography scan indicates that this injury represents a posterior SC dislocation. **(C)** Another computed tomography scan slice, however, demonstrates that there is a small epiphyseal fragment, which is separated from the remainder of the clavicle. Thus, this represents a displaced physeal fracture of the medial end of the clavicle. **(D)** Computed tomography appearance of the SC joint after reduction of the displaced physeal fracture using a towel clip to grasp the distal fragment.

nonabsorbable sutures passed through drill holes (66). Postoperatively, the shoulders should be held back through the use of a figure-of-eight harness or shoulder spica cast for 6 weeks.

STERNOCLAVICULAR ARTHRITIS

Degenerative arthritis of the SC joint is radiographically not uncommon but is usually asymptomatic (55). Mild symptoms can usually be managed with nonsteroidal antiinflammatory medications and heat, and only rarely will surgery become necessary. When the symptoms do not respond to these measures and if the pain is eliminated with an intraarticular lidocaine injection, then surgery may be considered. This consists of excision of 1 cm of the medial clavicle (66).

For this procedure, the patient is placed in the beach-chair position, and a general anesthetic is administered. A 5-cm skin incision is made horizontally in line with the long axis of the clavicle and proceeding from the SC joint laterally (Fig. 7.19A). The skin is undermined, thus exposing the

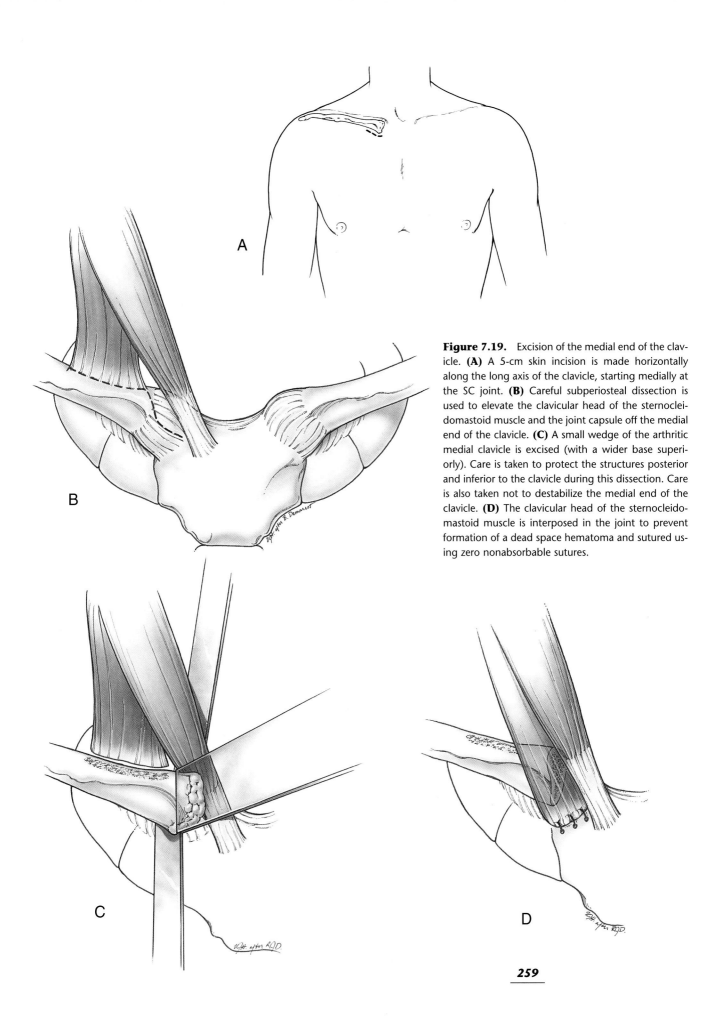

Figure 7.19. Excision of the medial end of the clavicle. **(A)** A 5-cm skin incision is made horizontally along the long axis of the clavicle, starting medially at the SC joint. **(B)** Careful subperiosteal dissection is used to elevate the clavicular head of the sternocleidomastoid muscle and the joint capsule off the medial end of the clavicle. **(C)** A small wedge of the arthritic medial clavicle is excised (with a wider base superiorly). Care is taken to protect the structures posterior and inferior to the clavicle during this dissection. Care is also taken not to destabilize the medial end of the clavicle. **(D)** The clavicular head of the sternocleidomastoid muscle is interposed in the joint to prevent formation of a dead space hematoma and sutured using zero nonabsorbable sutures.

underlying joint capsule. Subperiosteal dissection using electrocautery and a small elevator is undertaken to elevate the clavicular head of the sternocleidomastoid muscle and the capsule off the medial clavicle (Fig. 7.19B). After the clavicle is exposed superiorly, similar subperiosteal dissection is undertaken along the inferior aspect of the medial clavicle, but care is taken not to damage the costoclavicular ligament (this would destabilize the medial clavicle). A wedge of 0.5 to 1 cm of the medial clavicle with a wider base superiorly is then excised, carefully protecting the structures posterior and inferior to the clavicle with small Bennett retractors (Fig. 7.19C). The edge of the remaining medial clavicle is then made smooth, removing any sharp bony edges. The clavicular head of the sternocleidomastoid muscle is interposed into the joint and sutured with zero nonabsorbable sutures (Fig. 7.19D). The superficial layers are reapproximated with absorbable sutures, and the skin is closed with a continuous subcuticular suture.

Postoperatively, the arm is placed in a sling for several days for comfort. Use of the arm is gradually increased.

REFERENCES

1. Abbott LC, Lucas DB. The function of the clavicle: its surgical significance. Ann Surg 1954;140:583–597.
2. Alldredge RH. Surgical treatment of acromioclavicular dislocations. J Bone Joint Surg 1965;47A:1278.
3. Allman FL Jr. Fractures and ligamentous injuries of the clavicle and its articulation. J Bone Joint Surg 1967;49A:774–784.
4. Anderson R, Burgess E. Acromioclavicular dislocation: a conservative method of treatment. Northwest Ed 1939;38:40–46.
5. Anzel SH, Streitz WL. Acute acromioclavicular injuries: a report of nineteen cases treated nonoperatively employing dynamic splint immobilization. Clin Orthop 1974;103:143–149.
6. Arner O, Sandahl U, Ohrling H. Dislocation of the acromioclavicular joint: review of the literature and a report on 56 cases. Acta Chir Scand 1957;113:140–152.
7. Aufranc OE, Jones WN, Harris WH. Complete acromioclavicular dislocation. JAMA 1962;180:113–114.
8. Bailey RW. A dynamic repair for complete acromioclavicular joint dislocation. J Bone Joint Surg 1965;47A:858.
9. Bakalim G, Wilppula E. Surgical or conservative treatment of total dislocation of the acromioclavicular joint. Acta Chir Scand 1975;141:43–47.
10. Baker DM, Stryker WS. Acute complete acromioclavicular separation: report of 51 cases. JAMA 1965;192:105–108.
11. Bannister GC, Wallace WA, Stableforth PG, et al. The management of acute acromioclavicular dislocations. J Bone Joint Surg 1989;71B:848–850.
12. Bargren JH, Erlanger S, Dick HM. Biomechanics and comparison of two operative methods of treatment of complete acromioclavicular separation. Clin Orthop 1978;130:267–272.
13. Bearden JM, Hughston JC, Whatley GS. Acromioclavicular dislocation: method of treatment. Am J Sports Med 1973;1:5–17.
14. Berson BL, Gilbert MS, Green S. Acromioclavicular dislocations: treatment by transfer of the conjoined tendon and distal end of the coracoid process to the clavicle. Clin Orthop 1978;135:157–164.
15. Bigliani LU, Nicholson GP, Flatow EL. Arthroscopic resection of the distal clavicle. Orthop Clin North Am 1993;24:133–141.

16. Bloom FA. Wire fixation in acromioclavicular dislocation. J Bone Joint Surg 1945;27:273–276.
17. Bosworth BM. Acromioclavicular separation: new method of repair. Surg Gynecol Obstet 1941;73:866–871.
18. Brooks AL, Henning GD. Injury to the proximal clavicular epiphysis. J Bone Joint Surg 1972;54A:1347–1348.
19. Browne JE, Stanley RF, Tullos HS. Acromioclavicular joint dislocations: comparative results following operative treatment with and without primary distal clavisectomy. Am J Sports Med 1977;5:258–263.
20. Bundens WD Jr, Cook JI. Repair of acromioclavicular separations by deltoid-trapezius imbrication. Clin Orthop 1961;20:109–115.
21. Cadenat FM. The treatment of dislocations and fractures of the outer end of the clavicle. Int Clin 1917;1:145–169.
22. Cahill BR. Osteolysis of the distal part of the clavicle in male athletes. J Bone Joint Surg 1982;64A:1053–1058.
23. Clark RL, Milgram JW, Yawn DH. Fatal aortic perforation and cardiac tamponade due to a Kirshner wire migrating from the right sternoclavicular joint. South Med J 1974;67:316–318.
24. Cook FF, Tibone JE. The Mumford procedure in athletes: an objective analysis of function. Am J Sports Med 1988;16:97–100.
25. Cooper ES. New method of treating long-standing dislocations of the scapuloclavicular articulation. Am J Med Sci 1861;41:389–392.
26. Copher GH. Upward dislocation of the acromial end of the clavicle. Am J Surg 1933;22:507–508.
27. Craig EV. Fractures of the clavicle. In: Rockwood CA Jr, Matsen FA III, eds. The shoulder. Philadelphia: WB Saunders, 1990.
28. Daus GP, Drez D Jr, Newton BB Jr, et al. Migration of a Kirshner wire from the sternum to the right ventricle: a case report. Am J Sports Med 1993;21:321–322.
29. Dawe CJ. Acromioclavicular joint injuries. J Bone Joint Surg 1980;62B:269.
30. Denham RH Jr, Dingley AF Jr. Epiphyseal separation of the medial end of the clavicle. J Bone Joint Surg 1967;49A:1179–1183.
31. DePalma AF. Surgical anatomy of the acromioclavicular and sternoclavicular joints. Surg Clin North Am 1963;43:1541–1550.
32. Dewar FP, Barrington TW. The treatment of chronic acromioclavicular dislocation. J Bone Joint Surg 1965;47B:32–35.
33. Dias JJ, Steingold RF, Richardson RA, et al. The conservative treatment of acromioclavicular dislocation: review after five years. J Bone Joint Surg 1987;69B:719–722.
34. Ejeskär A. Coracoclavicular wiring for acromioclavicular joint dislocation: a ten year follow-up study. Acta Orthop Scand 1974;45:652–661.
35. Ferris BD, Bhamra M, Paton DF. Coracoid process transfer for acromioclavicular dislocations: a report of 20 cases. Clin Orthop 1989;242:184–187.
36. Flatow EL. The biomechanics of the acromioclavicular, sternoclavicular, and scapulothoracic joints. American Academy of Orthopaedic Surgeons Instructional Course Lectures 1993;42:237–245.
37. Flatow EL, Bigliani LU. Arthroscopic acromioclavicular joint debridement and distal clavicle resection. Operative Tech Orthop 1991;1:240–247.
38. Flatow EL, Duralde XA, Nicholson GP, et al. Arthroscopic resection of the distal clavicle with a superior approach. J Shoulder Elbow Surg 1995;4:41–50.
39. Fleming RE Jr, Tornberg DN, Kiernan HA. An operative repair of acromioclavicular separation. J Trauma 1978;18:709–712.
40. Fukuda K, Craig EV, An K-N, et al. Biomechanical study of the ligamentous system of the acromioclavicular joint. J Bone Joint Surg 1946;28:813–837.

41. Galpin RD, Hawkins RJ, Grainger RW. A comparative analysis of operative versus nonoperative treatment of grade III acromioclavicular separations. Clin Orthop 1985;193:150–155.

42. Gartsman GM. Arthroscopic resection of the acromioclavicular joint. Am J Sports Med 1993;21:71–77.

43. Gartsman GM, Combs AH, Davis PF, et al. Arthroscopic acromioclavicular joint resection: an anatomical study. Am J Sports Med 1991;19:2–5.

44. Gerber C, Rockwood CA Jr. Subcoracoid dislocation of the lateral end of the clavicle: a report of three cases. J Bone Joint Surg 1987;69A:924–927.

45. Goldberg JA, Viglione W, Cumming WJ, et al. Review of coracoclavicular ligament reconstruction using Dacron graft material. Aust N Z J Surg 1987;57:441–445.

46. Grimes DW, Garner RW. The degeneration of the acromioclavicular joint: treatment by resection of the distal clavicle. Orthop Rev 1980;9:41–44.

47. Gurd FB. The treatment of complete dislocation of the outer end of the clavicle: a hitherto undescribed operation. Ann Surg 1941;63:1094–1098.

48. Horn JS. The traumatic anatomy and treatment of acute acromioclavicular dislocation. J Bone Joint Surg 1954;36B:194–201.

49. Jacobs B, Wade PA. Acromioclavicular joint injury: an end-result study. J Bone Joint Surg 1966;48A:475–486.

50. Johnson LL. Diagnostic and surgical arthroscopy. St. Louis: CV Mosby, 1981.

51. Kay SP, Ellman H, Harris E. Arthroscopic distal clavicle excision: technique and early results. Clin Orthop 1994;301:181–184.

52. Kappakas GS, McMaster JH. Repair of acromioclavicular separation using a Dacron prosthesis graft. Clin Orthop 1978;131:247–251.

53. Kawabe N, Watanabe R, Sato M. Treatment of complete acromioclavicular separation by coracoacromial ligament transfer. Clin Orthop 1984;185:222–227.

54. Kennedy JC. Complete dislocation of the acromioclavicular joint: 14 years later. J Trauma 1968;8:311–318.

55. Kier R, Wain S, Apple J, et al. Osteoarthritis of the sternoclavicular joint: radiographic features and pathologic correlation. Invest Radiol 1986;21:227–233.

56. Lancaster S, Horowitz M, Alonso J. Complete acromioclavicular separations: a comparison of operative methods. Clin Orthop 1987;216:80–88.

57. Larsen E, Bjerg-Nielsen A, Christensen P. Conservative or surgical treatment of acromioclavicular dislocation: a prospective, controlled, randomized study. J Bone Joint Surg 1986;68A:552–555.

58. Leonard JW, Gifford RW. Migration of a Kirshner wire from the clavicle into the pulmonary artery. Am J Cardiol 1965;16:598–600.

59. Mueller ME, Allgower N, Willenegger H. Manual of internal fixation. New York: Springer-Verlag, 1970.

60. Mumford EB. Acromioclavicular dislocation: a new operative treatment. J Bone Joint Surg 1941;23:799–802.

61. Murphy OB, Bellamy R, Wheeler W, et al. Post-traumatic osteolysis of the distal clavicle. Clin Orthop 1975;109:108–114.

62. Neer CS II. Fracture of the distal clavicle with detachment of coracoclavicular ligaments in adults. J Trauma 1963;3:99–110.

63. Neer CS II. Fractures of the distal third of the clavicle. Clin Orthop 1968;58:43–50.

64. Neer CS II. Impingement lesions. Clin Orthop 1983;73:70–77.

65. Neer CS II. Fractures of the clavicle. In: Rockwood CA Jr, Green DP, eds. Fractures in adults. Philadelphia: JB Lippincott, 1984.

66. Neer CS II. Shoulder reconstruction. Philadelphia: WB Saunders, 1990.

67. Nettles JL, Linscheid R. Sternoclavicular dislocations. J Trauma 1968;8:158–164.

68. Neviaser JS. Acromioclavicular dislocation treated by transference of the coracoacromial ligament. Arch Surg 1952;64:292–297.

69. Neviaser RJ, Neviaser JS, Neviaser T, et al. A simple technique for internal fixation of the clavicle. Clin Orthop 1975;109:103–107.

70. Novak PJ, Bach BR Jr, Romeo AA, et al. Surgical resection of the distal clavicle. J Shoulder Elbow Surg 1995;4:35–40.
71. Omer GE. Osteotomy of the clavicle in surgical reduction of anterior sternoclavicular dislocation. J Trauma 1967;7:584–590.
72. Paavolainen P, Björkenheim JM, Paukku P, et al. Surgical treatment of acromioclavicular dislocation: a review of 39 patients. Injury 1983;14:415–420.
73. Park JP, Arnold JA, Coker TP, et al. Treatment of acromioclavicular separations: a retrospective study. Am J Sports Med 1980;8:251–256.
74. Patterson WR. Inferior dislocation of the distal end of the clavicle. J Bone Joint Surg 1967;49A:1184–1186.
75. Petersson CJ. Resection of the lateral end of the clavicle: a 3 to 30 year follow-up. Acta Orthop Scand 1983;54:434–438.
76. Phemister DB. The treatment of dislocation of the acromioclavicualr joint by open reduction and threaded wire fixation. J Bone Joint Surg 1942;24:166–168.
77. Rockwood CA Jr. Injuries to the acromioclavicular joint. In: Rockwood CA Jr, Green DP, eds. Fractures in adults. 2nd ed. Philadelphia: JB Lippincott, 1984.
78. Rockwood CA Jr. Disorders of the acromioclavicular joint. In: Rockwood CA Jr, Matsen FA III, eds. The shoulder. Philadelphia: WB Saunders, 1985.
79. Rockwood CA Jr. Disorders of the sternoclavicular joint. In: Rockwood CA Jr, Matsen FA III, eds. The shoulder. Philadelphia: WB Saunders, 1990.
80. Roper BA, Levack B. The surgical treatment of acromioclavicular dislocations. J Bone Joint Surg 1982;64B:597–599.
81. Rosenorn M, Pedersen EB. A comparison between conservative and operative treatment of acute acromioclavicular dislocation. Acta Orthop Scand 1974;45:50–59.
82. Rowe CR. An atlas of anatomy and treatment of mid-clavicular fractures. Clin Orthop 1968;58:29–42.
83. Salvatore JE. Sternoclavicular joint dislocation. Clin Orthop 1968;58:51–54.
84. Smolle-Juettner FM, Hofer RH, Pinter H, et al. Intracardiac malpositioning of a sternoclavicular fixation wire. J Orthop Trauma 1992;6:102–105.
85. Snyder SJ. Arthroscopic acromioclavicular joint debridement and distal clavicle resection. Tech Orthop 1988;3:41–45.
86. Stewart R. Acute acromioclavicular joint dislocation: internal fixation of the clavicle and coracoid process of the scapula with a vitallium screw. Minn Med 1946;29:357–360.
87. Taft TN, Wilson FC, Oglesby JW. Dislocation of the acromioclavicular joint: an end-result study. J Bone Joint Surg 1987;69A:1045–1051.
88. Thorndike A Jr, Quigley TB. Injuries to the acromioclavicular joint: a plea for conservative treatment. Am J Surg 1942;55:250–261.
89. Tibone J, Sellers R, Tonino P. Strength-testing after third-degree acromioclavicular dislocations. Am J Sports Med 1992;20:328–331.
90. Tossy JD, Mead NC, Sigmond HM. Acromioclavicular separations: useful and practical classification for treatment. Clin Orthop 1963;28:111–119.
91. Tsou PM. Percutaneous cannulated screw coracoclavicular fixation for acute acromioclavicular dislocations. Clin Orthop 1989;243:112–121.
92. Urist MR. Complete dislocations of the acromioclavicular joint: the nature of the traumatic lesion and effective methods of treatment with an analysis of forty-one cases. J Bone Joint Surg 1946;28:813–837.
93. Walsh WM, Peterson DA, Shelton G, et al. Shoulder strength following acromioclavicular injury. Am J Sports Med 1985;13:153–158.
94. Waskowitz WJ. Disruption of the sternoclavicular joint: an analysis and review. Am J Orthop 1961;3:176–179.
95. Watkins JT. An operation for the relief of acromioclavicular luxations. J Bone Joint Surg 1925;7:790–792.
96. Weinstein DM, McCann PD, McIlveen SJ, et al. Surgical treatment of complete acromioclavicular dislocations. Am J Sports Med 1995;23:324–331.

97. Weitzman G. Treatment of acute acromioclavicular joint dislocation by a modified Bosworth method: report on 24 cases. J Bone Joint Surg 1967;49A:1167–1178.

98. Weaver JK, Dunn HK. Treatment of acromioclavicular injuries, especially complete acromioclavicular separation. J Bone Joint Surg 1972;54A:1187–1194.

99. Wojtys EM, Nelson G. Conservative treatment of grade III acromioclavicular dislocations. Clin Orthop 1991;268:112–119.

100. Worcester JN, Green DP. Osteoarthritis of the acromioclavicular joint. Clin Orthop 1968;58:69–73.

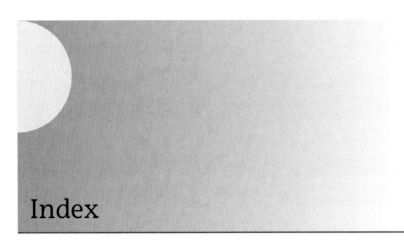

Index

Page numbers in *italics* refer to illustrations; numbers followed by t indicate tables.